Epilepsy and Seizures

Building Care in the Community

Aditi Malhotra

Todd Jailer

hesperian
health guides

Oakland, California USA

hesperian
health guides

Published by:
Hesperian Health Guides
2860 Telegraph Avenue
Oakland, California 94609 USA
www.hesperian.org

ISBN: 978-0-942364-21-7
First ebook edition: April 2026
ISBN: 978-0-942364-26-2

Help us improve this book!

We developed this book in partnership with people with epilepsy and health workers committed to improving care at the community level. Your feedback will help make future editions better.

Contact us at:

epilepsy@hesperian.org to tell us how you are using this book and what you think.

This book was printed in the USA by EPAC.

Credits

Editorial oversight: Amy Hill, Sarah Shannon
Research coordination: Aditi Malhotra
Additional writing: Amy Hill
Medical review: Eddie Chengo, ClinMed/MSc, Epilepsy Practice
Medicines editor: Dani Behonick
Copy editing and proofreading: Cynthia Peters
Index: Todd Jailer
Networking and community review coordination: Amy Hill, Aditi Malhotra
Design and production: Luis Aspeitia, Rosemary Jason, Kathleen Tandy
Cover design: Luis Aspeitia, Rosemary Jason
Art coordination: Amy Hill, Aditi Malhotra

Cover photos: iStock.com

Illustrations: Special thanks to Shu Ping Guan for her skilled and compassionate drawings. Thanks also to the other artists whose illustrations make this book come alive: Namrata Bali, Sara Boore, Heidi Broner, Debasmita Dasgupta, Regina Faul-Doyle, Barbara Carter, Sandy Frank, Susie Gunn, May Haddad, Jesse Hamm, Haris Ichwan, Rosemary Jason, Anna Kallis, Rodney Kawaayi, Mabel Negrete, Gabriela Nuñez, Leana Rosetti, Petra Raul-Rouendaal, Chengyu Song, Lihua Wang, Paula Worby, and Mary Ann Zapalac.

Thanks

Dozens of individuals provided the expertise and support that made this book possible.

Hesperian staff and volunteers

Hesperian's staff, interns, and volunteers worked to bring this book to the world: special thanks to Jessica Barrera, Alicia Flores, Jade Fong, Shivranjani Gandhi, Gretchen Herbkersman, Maile Hernández, Tawnia Litwin, Purnima Mane, Susan McCallister, Kimiye Owens, Shawn Philips, Amol Ray, Linda Spangler, Keziah Sullivan, Vanessa Tran, Dominique Tzou, Sarah Whitney, and Paula Worby

Funders

The development of this book was generously underwritten by a gift from the Gertrude Hochschild Sergievsky Charitable Trust. Timely funding from the Band Foundation allowed us to complete the resource and expand its impact. General support funding (covering a host of necessary activities and bridging gaps) was provided by the Cogan Family Foundation, West Foundation, and Hesperian's individual donors. We are deeply grateful for their support.

Special appreciation

Our heartfelt thanks to the International Bureau for Epilepsy (IBE) for their invaluable partnership. IBE's support in facilitating connections with reviewers was instrumental in bringing this resource to fruition. The enthusiasm, expertise, and dedication of the IBE team expanded our network and strengthened the book's content. Their *Advocate's Toolkit for Reducing Epilepsy Stigma in Africa* provided the definition and classifications for stigma we used as well as inspiration for one of the book's stigma-related illustrations.

Eddie Chengo, Director of the Foundation for People with Epilepsy (FPE) Neurology Centre in Kenya, graciously reviewed the entire manuscript to ensure that complex medical and pharmaceutical information was accurately presented, and perhaps more importantly, to lend us the benefit of his years of committed interactions supporting people with epilepsy.

We deeply admire the work of Espacio Epilepsia, Keilah Foundation, the Nakivale refugee camp "Care for All" project, Kenya Association for the Welfare of People with Epilepsy (KAWE), Neurology on Wheels, Purple Bench Initiative, and Samman Association, whose community-centered care and advocacy programs are featured in this book. We are particularly grateful to those who shared with us their personal journeys to live well with epilepsy: Vinay Jani, Priti Vishwakarma, and Bright Bwalya. We are indebted to Mauricio Olave Aguirre, who prepared Spanish translations of many chapters and coordinated invaluable feedback from Latin America.

Grassroots community groups and organizational collaborators

Medical professionals, epilepsy advocates, people with epilepsy, and epilepsy caregivers from different parts of the world participated as advisors and reviewers, individually and in groups. Their diverse perspectives, critiques, and suggestions have improved the book's accuracy, usability, and cultural relevance.

David Naboare Foundation (Ghana)

Epilepsy Association of Zambia

Epilepsy Foundation of Hong Kong

Epilepsy Foundation of India

Epilepsy South Africa

International Bureau for Epilepsy (IBE)

International Bureau for Epilepsy, Africa Region

International Bureau for Epilepsy, Community Council

International League Against Epilepsy (ILAE)

Kenya Association for the Welfare of People with Epilepsy (KAWE)

Neurological Association of Zambia

Pretola Global Health & Consulting

Purple Bench Initiative (Uganda)

Samman Association (India)

STOP Epilepsy India

Tanzania Epilepsy Organization

Advisers, reviewers, interviewees

Silvia Abente
Vanesa Diaz Acuña
Afzal
Silvia Castellón Agamez
Nikhil Agarwal
Nitin Agarwal
Mauricio Olave Aguirre
Iván Molinares Amaris
Action Amos
Richard Andwilile
Nakato Annet
Naziya Ramzan Ansari
Melody Asukile
Iasmin Omar Ata
Isrey Ayubu Athumani
Mercy Atieno
Jose David Ospino Ayola

Jesca Babonerawo
Julio Eduardo Pestana Balbutin
Cecilia Banda
Naomi Banda
Max Abu Bangura
Loren Elena Gasca Barba
Danna Baldovino Barrios
Harriet Barlow
Jeremiah Bazaale
Omaira Zuleta Beleño
Yusenin Paola Martínez Beltrán
Debashish Bhaindarkar
Prakash Bhaindarkar
Naomi Bowa
Merle Bron
Bright Bwalya
Aloysius Byekwaso

Juan Cabañas
Nancy Cabrera
Sharlene Cassel
Patricia Chaguamate
Bhakti D Chachada
Mandy Chan
Violet Chanda
Anchal Chaudhari
Om Chaudhari
Parth Chauhan
Sunita Deepak Chauhan
Shradha Chaurasia
Shubham Chaurasia
Susan Chawirima
Sudesh Chawla
Eddie Maraga Chengo
Daphne Cheung
Natasha Chewe
Samuel Chiagmba
Evelyn Chikopa
Fellistus Chikwatu
Francis Ananda Chipukunya
Ted Chiu
Julie Cliff
Caroline Cox
Eli Cripps
Peg Cumberland
Bruce Curtis

Sharifa Damba
Milenis Pitre Daza
Chirag Deshmukh
Megha Deshmukh
Sofia Di Noia
Lenie Hoegen Dijkhof
Aimee Dollman
Aneeta Dominic
Nimmy Dominic
Narasimha Reddy Donthi
Carol D'Souza

Ekpanaka Jesynta Ekpeni
Sarelis Escorcia
Promise Eze

Abigail Farfán
Jazmin Ferreira
Rebecca Figueroa
Abraham D Flaxman
Karla Florez
Chia Benard Ful

Kshitija Vijay Gaikwad
Ivana Garcia
Matovu Gerald
Nellie Gogoda
Utpal Gogoi
Alisson Gonzalez
Kristen Graser
Jesus Guido
Radhika Rao Gupta
Isishaj Blondin Rivera Gutierrez
Anays Valiente Guzman

Rowan Haffner
Katie Hamilton
Charles Kumi Hammond
Nafisa Haveliwala
Shenaz Haveliwala
Nancy Henderson
Margaret Holladay
Stephanie Homer

Carlos Mario Villadiego Humanez
Anchor Hung

Noemí Canales Iturriaga

Namita Jacob
Kuldeep Jain
Rachana Jain
Yogesh Jain
Vinay Jani
Marleine Jansen

Hari K
Cynthia Kabamba
Mumba Kachomba
Siddhi Kadam
Mariam Kajiru
Kiran Kanth
Chisomo Kapiseni
Symon Kariuki
Veronica Kasonde
Jyoti Katkar
Charles Kato
Annastacia Kavemba
Nfwama Kawatu
Prince Kazadi
Ansh Keluskar
Avantika Keluskar
Usha Khanapur
Edward Kija
Mary Kipingili
Neha Kirpal
Fred Kiserem
Rachel Katondo
Deborah Koltai
Ajit Kumar
Anand Kumar
Millie Kumwenda
Kwalela Kwalela
Jacob Kwame

Susan Lapowsky
Rafael Lizama
Emma Lovise Larsen
Manuel Tomas Mesa Latorre
Mariola Lesiak-Bzdak
Kelly Less
Mabel Li
Diane Lockhart
Leslie London
Lombabo J. Llyod
Maria Lujan
Ruth Lupando
Miyanda Lupiya

Anita Mago
Nina Mago
Majid Mago-Mulangwa
Marci Manderscheid
Raphael Mandevu
Jayanti Mani
Neo Matjeka
Robert Matovu
Sharon Mbugua
Matisse McCullough
Pam McLaren
Man Mohan Mehndiratta
Dana Marcela Padilla Miller
Maria Eugenia de Morales
Aditya Mehta
Marly Patricia Villareal Mendoza
Akanksha Mirji
Leocardia Miti
Jane Mkandawire
Zarine Mogal
Elvira Vacas Montero
Jaya Motwani
Christina Msokwa
Pamela Mtema
Suzana Mukoyi
Florence Mulenga
Zacharie Mulumba
Rose Munuo
Rachael Mwange
Peggy Mwansa
Rose Mwanza
Naluca Mwendaweli
Grenda Mwiinga

Pooja Nandi
Maria Nabakyejjo
Joan Nabalanzi
Reste Nabasumba
David Naboare
Josephine Nabukenya
Patricia Nakamanya
Aginesi Nakazzi
Rachel Nakirya
Josephine Nakku
Maria Nakyejjo
Mary Naluwaga
Sarah Nambajjwe
Agnes Nampijja
Hellen Namulindwa
Gladys Maria Carrascal Navarro
Betty Ncachilwa
Wendy Nefdt
Balaji Nemala
Brenda Ngulu
Carolina López Nieto
Ariane Dora Niteka
Gladys Joanne Njenga
Mundih Noelar Njohjam
Ukundi Nkya
Sally Noguera

Claire Nolan
Betty Nsachilwa
Priscilla M. Nsama
Bruna Nucera
Sally Nyakanyanga
Halima Nyinandege
Beatrice Nyirenda
Esther Nyirenda
Jessie Nyirenda

Tolu Olaniyan
Nicholas Otieno Okayo

Deepesh Palkar
Karina Pandya
Saniya Patil
Patricia Peñalosa
Gabriela Pesantez
Ann Petru
Daniela Pesse
Amos Phiri
Rhoda Phiri
Narendra Pillai
Pamela Pipan
Suneela Pradhan

Ishan Rahate
Rahul Ranjan
Abigail Rattin
Suresh Rijhwani
Ximena Pesantez Rios
Liezel Pardo Rocha
Claudia Barrios Rodriguez
Rosmery Vizcaino Rodriguez
Yulis Gaviria Rojas
Jerusha Ranshinge Rungta
Tushar Rungta
Dzenana Rustempasic
Andrea Ryan

Ley Sander
Palmira Fortunato dos Santos
Christopher Sakala
Wendy Sanchez
Deanna Saylor
Lacey Schmeidler
Mary Secco
Martin Senyunja
Moses Serumaga
Jina Shah
Urvashi Shah
Mayna Shaikh
Zeba Shaikh
Divyasiny Sharma
Mayank Sharma
Marissa Shaw
Naveen Shukla
Maala Sichintu
Roxanne Simmons
Ananya Singh
Babaljeet Singh
Gagandeep Singh
Madhu Singh
Mamta Bhushan Singh
Surender Singh
Adriana Smith
Sarah Snow
Desiree Lee Son
Siddhita Sonavane
Norman Ssemmambo
Nirmal Suraya

Sophie Taggart
Hermes Tebulo
Michael Terry
Hemant Tiwari
Leslie Toledo
Carolina Traslaviña Torres
Manjari Tripathi
Amarnath Trivedi
Oyungerel Tsedevdamba

Fides Uiso
Paula Ullauri

Mercy Gomez Valdez
Laura Elena Hernández Vanegas
Norma Hernández Vanegas
Jessica Veach
Giselle Mejía Vergara
Srishti Verma
Kollencheri Puthenveettil Vinayan
Sanjana Vishwakarma
Sudhindra Vooturi

Sitawa Wafula
Donna Walsh
Donald Wetlieb
Jo Wilmshurst
Carey Wilson
Nick Woolfield
Leonie Wollscheid

Sandeep Yadav
Jacob Yankah

Rachel Zaslow
Doris Zimba
Narhajid Zuunnast

Contents

Chapter		Page
1	Introduction	2
2	How to help a person having a seizure	14
3	Types of seizures and how to identify them	34
4	Medicines for epilepsy and seizures	82
5	Acting against epilepsy stigma	124
6	Living well with epilepsy	160
7	Pregnancy and birth with epilepsy	202
8	Talking with children about epilepsy and seizures	232
9	Preventing violence can prevent epilepsy and seizures	262
	Where to find more information	276
	Glossary: Words related to epilepsy	284
	Index of seizure types, causes, and treatments	287
	About Hesperian Health Guides	290

Chapter 1

In this chapter

Understanding epilepsy and seizures **4**
What is a seizure? 5
How do we support people with epilepsy? **5**
Seizure first aid 6
Access to treatment and medicines 6
Severe forms of epilepsy 7
Epilepsy stigma 8
Improving care for people with epilepsy **8**
Global campaigns against epilepsy 9
Community action makes change happen **11**
Preventing epilepsy 12
Adapt this information for your community 12

Introduction

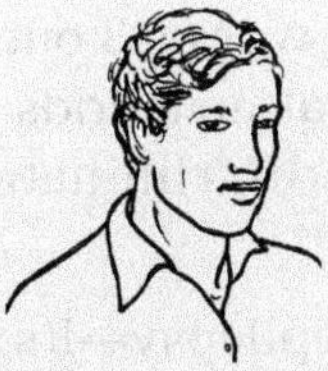

One Sunday, Alfredo was driving his family home from church when their car was hit by a truck. It was a bad accident—his brother was killed and Alfredo spent weeks in the hospital. After his head injuries healed, he went back to work. His company valued him as lead accountant and held his job for him. He could still find and fix errors better than anyone else in the company. But now, Alfredo sometimes gets an odd feeling in his stomach and his coworkers tell him he starts rocking from side to side, no longer paying attention to what they were doing together. After a minute or so, he feels a little tired but returns to normal.

Sultana is a popular young woman, always involving her friends in projects around town. After painting a mural about protecting the environment, she was walking home when suddenly she stopped, fell to the ground, and began shaking. Her friends called her mother, who came and gently comforted her and brought her home. Sultana's mother knew about seizures because her sister used to have them before she started taking medicines to control them.

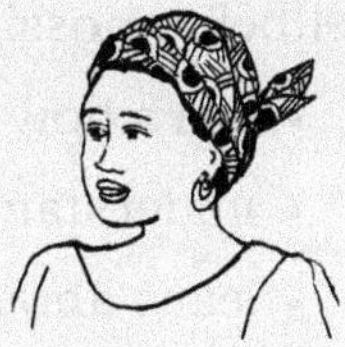

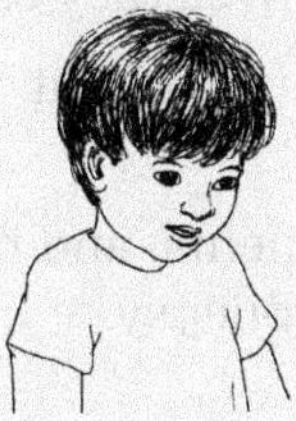

Everyone thought Kinjal was a sweet, spacey child. He enjoyed helping with household chores, but sometimes he just seemed to be off in his own world. It wasn't until he started school that people noticed how often he would drift off. His teacher suggested he visit a clinic at their city hospital. He and his family went and the doctors there explained that they thought epilepsy was causing him to have absence seizures. They gave him a medicine which helped. Now Kinjal's absence seizures happen much less frequently. He has gotten into the habit of checking with his friend Ran to make sure he does not miss homework assignments or anything else important at school due to his seizures.

What Alfredo, Sultana, and Kinjal have in common is epilepsy, which each experiences as a different kind of seizure. One of the most common brain (neurological) conditions in the world, epilepsy affects 50 to 70 million people. Even though epilepsy occurs in every country, among people from every walk of life, and in every age group, religion, ethnic group, and gender, there is a lack of clear, accessible information about epilepsy.

Alfredo, Sultana, and Kinjal were also fortunate that the people around them—in their families, schools, workplaces, and clinics—were aware of epilepsy and seizures and had access to medicines, so their right to health was respected. For more than half of the people with epilepsy in the world, over 25 million people, that is not the case. Despite the need, there is a lack of epilepsy training among health workers and a lack of access to the medicines that treat it, creating a huge "treatment gap" that prevents most people with epilepsy from getting the care they need. Some data shows that people in low-income countries (LICs) are up to 3 times more likely to have epilepsy than those in wealthier countries. And to make matters worse, 3 out of every 4 people with epilepsy in LICs cannot get treatment. Lack of treatment adds to misinformation about epilepsy, fear of people who have epilepsy, and discrimination and stigma against them.

The goal of this book is to share clear, accurate information about epilepsy—its medical and physical effects as well as its social and emotional effects. It is different than other medical books because it focuses on care and treatment for epilepsy and seizures in communities where people may lack adequate access to healthcare, education, safety, decent housing, enough food, and all the other things that make wellbeing possible. We hope you will use this book to:

- learn how to give first aid when someone has a seizure.
- understand different kinds of seizures and what can cause or trigger them.
- learn about medicines that treat seizures.
- stop the spread of epilepsy stigma, misinformation, and discrimination.
- support healthy pregnancies and births for people with epilepsy.
- talk to children about epilepsy.
- support people with epilepsy to live the healthiest, most fulfilling lives they can.
- stop the physical and structural violence that can cause epilepsy and make it worse.
- convince people in your community, in local and national governments, and in the health system to protect the health and rights of people with epilepsy.

Understanding epilepsy and seizures

Epilepsy is a brain condition that causes a person to have seizures repeatedly. It is not an illness that can spread seizures from one person to another. Antiseizure medicines, which are usually taken every day, can stop most types of seizures from happening. To achieve that, a person needs medical support to find out what kind of seizure they have and which medicine will best treat it. When someone's seizures are well-controlled by medicines, the people around them would probably never know they have epilepsy.

What is a seizure?

The brain is the center of electrical activity in our bodies. Every thought, feeling, and body movement we have is a result of the brain's electrical activity. A seizure is a sudden, uncontrolled, and temporary disturbance to the brain's electrical activity.

Seizures can make a person lose control over their muscles and sometimes fall to the ground. Their muscles may stiffen and cause their arms and legs to make jerking movements. With some seizures, a person may stare blankly, become unresponsive for a few seconds, move suddenly, or do things like smack their lips, drool or chew, or pick at their clothing.

How a seizure affects a person's awareness is different for each person. Some people lose consciousness. Others can hear but cannot respond, while some can hear but are confused and take longer to respond. Sometimes people feel a tingling in their arms or legs, hot or cold flashes, or other sensations, including emotions such as fear, anxiety, or unexpected joy.

Most seizures last less than 2 minutes. Some are only a few seconds.

After a seizure, people may feel tired, confused, dizzy, or have a headache. Although they feel poorly, most cannot remember anything about their seizure.

Not all seizures are caused by epilepsy, but a main feature of epilepsy is that seizures happen repeatedly.

How do we support people with epilepsy?

For many years, health and medical systems wrongly regarded epilepsy as a mental illness rather than a brain condition with physical causes. Many cultures believe epilepsy is a spiritual illness, caused by a curse, witchcraft, possession by evil spirits, or sins committed by the person, their relatives, or ancestors. This widespread misinformation combines with a lack of easy-to-understand and accurate information about epilepsy and adds to stigma and the poor treatment of people with epilepsy. This book provides updated information to help people with epilepsy and their families act against stigma and improve their quality of life.

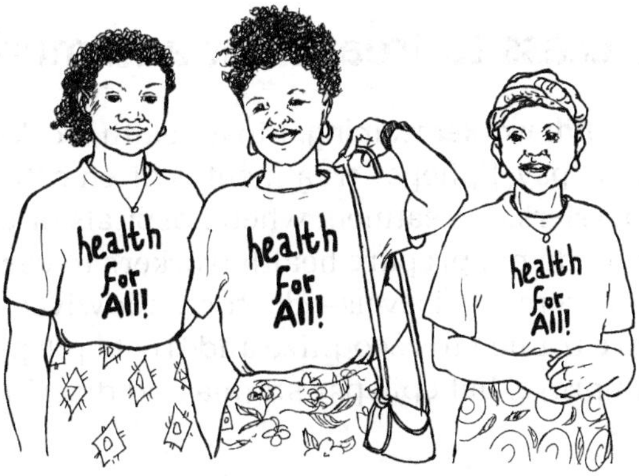

Raising awareness and improving care and support for people with epilepsy should not just be the concern of the person who has it or their family—it is a community responsibility. This book contains practical, actionable information about epilepsy that will be useful for everyone. Understanding epilepsy is important and possible for people with limited formal education or medical training, for community health promoters, frontline health workers, and midwives, for social workers, teachers, religious leaders, and faith healers, and for government, administrative, and law-enforcement personnel—for all community members.

Seizure first aid

A seizure can look alarming or scary to a person seeing one for the first time. People witnessing a seizure often freeze because they do not know how to respond, and sometimes they even run away in fear.

Training people in seizure first aid is simple and can transform negative responses to seizures into helpful ones. By understanding the basics of seizures and how to help a person having a seizure safely recover, many injuries can be prevented (see Chapter 2: How to help a person having a seizure).

Holding seizure first aid trainings also helps to break the silence that surrounds epilepsy. As people learn more about the condition, they may also begin to understand how much of the "problem" of epilepsy lies in their lack of understanding, not in those who have epilepsy.

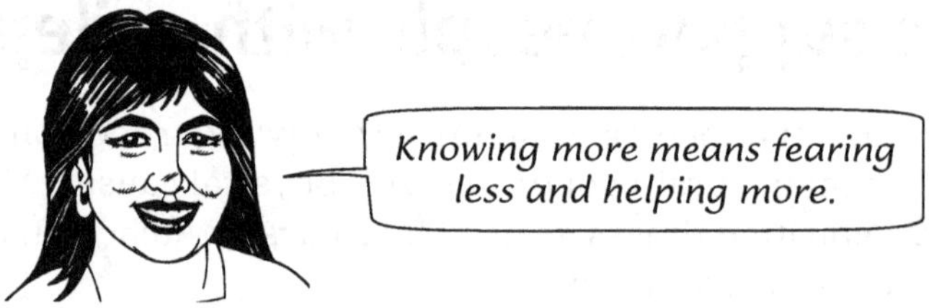

Access to treatment and medicines

Health worker training. Most health workers receive little or no training about epilepsy. Epilepsy treatment is often categorized as a "specialty." This creates barriers to treatment when hospitals or clinics do not hire enough "specialists" and do not prepare health workers to care for people with epilepsy. When health workers at all levels—doctors, midwives, nurses, health promoters, and others—are trained to recognize and treat epilepsy and seizures, not only will healthcare improve, but epilepsy stigma and discrimination will decrease.

Health access. When medical systems, insurance rules, and disability policies do not include epilepsy, antiseizure medicines and services for epilepsy are often difficult to find and afford. Social security and health institutions must recognize people's right to accessible and affordable epilepsy treatment.

Access to medicines. New medicines better target different types of epilepsy and have fewer side effects. Unfortunately, they are often unavailable in low-resource settings or have a higher price. Due to financial pressures as well as inadequate supply chains, pharmacies and clinics often run out of stock of antiseizure medicines, which is a big problem since these medicines must be taken daily. A variety of antiseizure medicines must be included in essential drug lists globally and made available at affordable prices.

Nonmedical treatments. Medicines are not the only treatment for epilepsy, which is good because some seizures are not well-controlled by them. Medicines work best when combined with enough rest, nutritious food, special diets, exercise, and learning how to avoid seizure triggers. Health workers need to learn more about and promote these other treatments.

Social acceptance. Organizations, businesses, and institutions need to change rules that create barriers to full participation by people with epilepsy. Social barriers that limit access to medicines and treatment must be removed as well.

Severe forms of epilepsy

Some forms of epilepsy can be severely disabling. Some rare childhood epilepsy syndromes can delay or impair the development of speech and other brain functions. When medical treatment is delayed, for epilepsy or for the treatment of infections that can result in epilepsy, the frequency of seizures and the damage they cause can increase. Also, when epilepsy occurs with another health condition, for example, with cerebral palsy, treatment can become more complicated. People with epilepsy have the same rights as everyone else to live a full life, on their own terms, and that means they have a right to the treatment and support they need.

Even when a person's seizures are well-controlled, it is possible that their health may change suddenly with no clear reason why. A rare condition called sudden unexpected death in epilepsy (SUDEP) can result in immediate death. This condition is especially shocking for family members who, like most people, are unaware that epilepsy can cause death. Regular access to medicine and ongoing care seems to lower the risk of SUDEP. More research on its prevention is needed.

Epilepsy stigma

The negative feelings, unfair behaviors, discouragement, discrimination, and fear directed at people with epilepsy make living with the condition more difficult. Some people say the stigma directed at them is much harder to deal with than the physical effects of seizures.

Epilepsy stigma can be internalized and make a person feel bad about themselves and their abilities. Interpersonal stigma can cause others to avoid, exclude, or deny the rights of people with epilepsy. And institutional stigma can prevent people with epilepsy from attending school, getting the care they need from the health system, and finding the employment they need to survive.

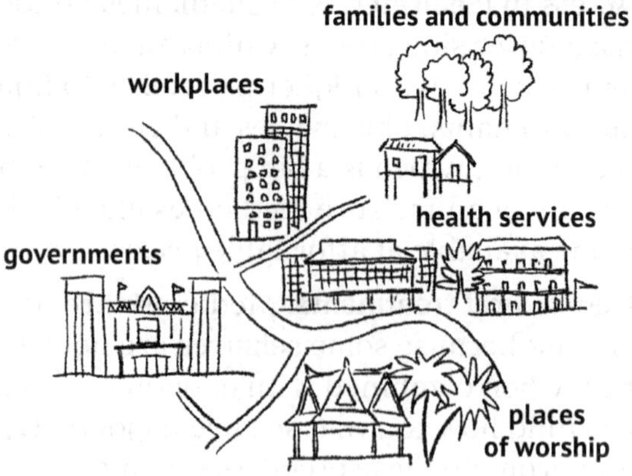

Where can epilepsy stigma be found?

Some of the most powerful forms of epilepsy stigma are directed at people wanting to get pregnant and have children. Some people with epilepsy are told they should never get pregnant, undermining their confidence and denying them the joy of building a family. Women's needs are often ignored by pharmaceutical companies—few medicines are safe to use during pregnancy, and the ones that are can be difficult to access. But with the right medical and social support, people with epilepsy can have healthy pregnancies and safe deliveries, and can breastfeed and raise their children.

People with epilepsy are challenging all forms of stigma. Through support groups and community education, they are helping people understand epilepsy. By lobbying to change policies, practices, and laws that limit what people with epilepsy can achieve, they are changing our societies for the better.

Improving care for people with epilepsy

Epilepsy was first written about almost 4000 years ago, on ancient Mesopotamian tablets found in Iraq. Two centuries later, Ayurvedic healers in India and the Greek doctor Hippocrates recognized that epilepsy seemed to have a physical cause in the body, rather than being the result of a curse or demonic possession.

But given the amount of time that has passed, little progress has been made to help people with epilepsy until more recently. It is worth looking at that progress—and at the challenges that remain—since the World Health Organization (WHO) began suggesting that governments prioritize epilepsy as a global health issue.

Global campaigns against epilepsy

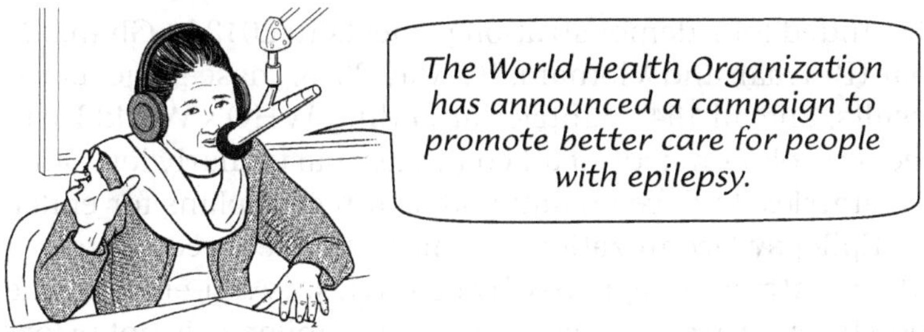
The World Health Organization has announced a campaign to promote better care for people with epilepsy.

In June 1997, WHO launched the campaign "Out of the Shadows" to improve epilepsy awareness and treatment worldwide. The campaign pledged to address "the hidden suffering" of more than 40 million people throughout the world affected by epilepsy forced to "live secret lives because of ill-informed public attitudes." WHO organized this effort with the International League Against Epilepsy (ILAE), an association of doctors and scientists, and the International Bureau for Epilepsy (IBE), a network of national epilepsy organizations. (Hesperian worked closely with both organizations during the development of this book.)

The campaign had two general goals: 1) to raise awareness that epilepsy was a treatable brain condition, and 2) to identify people's needs and encourage governments and health agencies to promote diagnosis, treatment, and care for people with epilepsy.

Little changed for people with epilepsy during the campaign's first phase, so in 2001, WHO launched a second phase to move from awareness to practical action. The campaign began demonstration projects to create real-world models of diagnosis, treatment, care, and prevention, and to encourage government health ministries to develop services and reduce the treatment gap and stigma. This second phase built upon two learnings from the first phase: 1) without access to treatment, working to end stigma cannot succeed, and 2) medical training on epilepsy is poor, and health professionals need better epilepsy education.

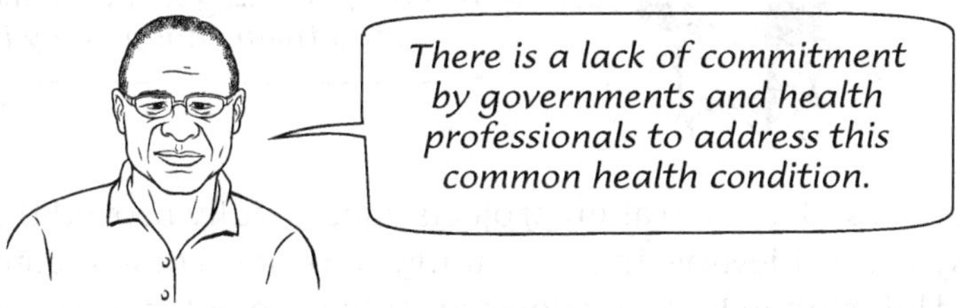
There is a lack of commitment by governments and health professionals to address this common health condition.

continues

Global campaigns against epilepsy *(continued)*

WHO funded four demonstration projects in 2012 in Ghana, Mozambique, Myanmar (Burma), and Vietnam. By May 2015, these projects were showing good results, and all 194 countries attending WHO's World Health Assembly approved a resolution urging all countries, particularly low- and middle-income countries, to develop national health care plans for epilepsy. As the Eswatini Epilepsy Organization summarized a few years later: "There is very little investment in epilepsy by countries... Anti-epilepsy medicines and neurologists are scarce in poor countries... Epilepsy is not prioritized by governments."

In 2019, WHO, ILAE, and IBE published *Epilepsy: A public health imperative,* the first report to summarize conditions facing people with epilepsy worldwide. Using the experiences of the demonstration projects as a guide to what was possible, the report promoted changes that would ensure people with epilepsy receive the care and treatment they deserve and need.

"Stigma is a significant contributor to poor physical and mental health in people with epilepsy."

—World Health Organization, *Epilepsy: A public health imperative*, 2019

In only a few years, the demonstration projects had increased the numbers of people accessing treatment by 23% in Ghana, 45% in Myanmar, and 38% in Vietnam. Thousands of people participated in campaigns to reduce stigma. However, when the demonstration projects and their funding ended in 2017, the numbers of people getting treatment declined significantly.

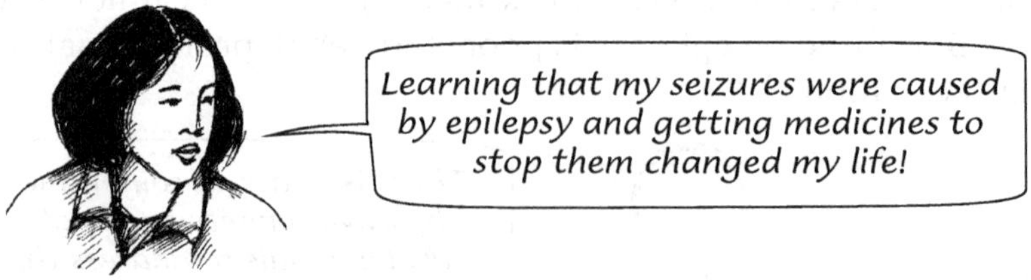

These low-cost demonstration projects successfully proved that treatment for epilepsy was achievable in any country if its government committed to provide it. Unfortunately, many governments have not made epilepsy a priority and treatment remains out of reach for most people with epilepsy.

Community action makes change happen

Although better access to epilepsy treatment has not yet been achieved, it is not the fault of the WHO. As part of the United Nations system, the WHO has no real power to make change in the world. That power lies in our communities and with our governments. By partnering with organizations like ILAE and IBE, the WHO extended its reach into the medical community and among people affected by epilepsy. It is up to all of us to do more.

Few governments acknowledge and ensure people's right to health, including people with epilepsy. That is why working with neighbors, places of worship, community organizations, and local schools and health centers is more likely to bring quicker results, as well as to build the support necessary to achieve larger changes at district, state, and national levels. Community education about epilepsy and seizures, and how to respond with seizure first aid, can help normalize the discussion of epilepsy. By talking with our local health workers, we can challenge our health promoters, nurses, and midwives, as well as our doctors, to learn how to treat people with epilepsy and make epilepsy treatment part of primary health care. We can make sure our local institutions, schools, markets, and services welcome rather than discriminate against people with epilepsy.

As our societies become more accepting and better incorporate people with epilepsy into community life, the number of people concerned about equality for people with epilepsy grows. As we gain more power and influence, we can have a bigger cultural impact, especially in challenging the misinformation and stigma surrounding epilepsy. We can also demand our health systems plan for and make more and better services available for people with epilepsy, including access to affordable medicines.

From raising a child with the skills to reject feelings of self-stigma, to participating in support groups, to campaigning for local and national changes, you will find examples throughout this book (especially in Chapters 6 and 9) of how individuals and groups began working to improve conditions for people with epilepsy both inside and outside of their communities.

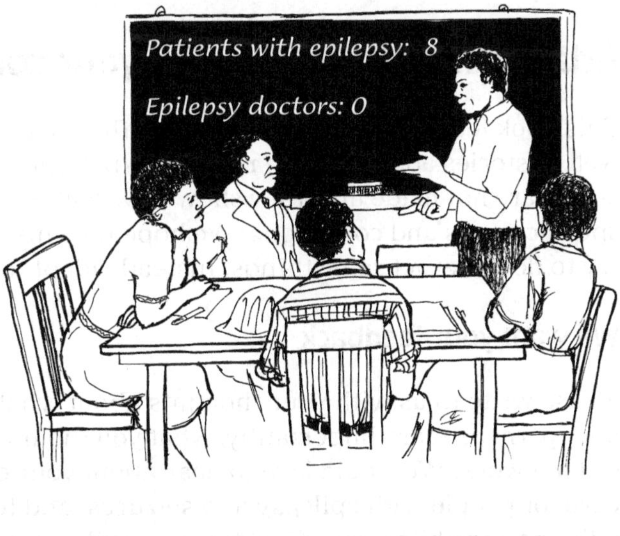

Preventing epilepsy

It can be challenging, and sometimes impossible, to determine the cause of a person's epilepsy. This makes epilepsy prevention difficult. Sometimes epilepsy is "genetic," caused either by genes inherited from a parent or by a mutation (a sudden change) that could be random or caused by something in the environment.

The cause of epilepsy for many other people is more evident: a violent injury to the head. Preventing those injuries, caused by crashes and transit accidents, dangerous workplaces, war and conflicts, domestic violence, contact sports, etc., is one way to prevent epilepsy. Another way to prevent epilepsy is to change the social conditions that make injuries more likely: the harms (structural violence) caused by poverty, gender discrimination, lack of access to food, shelter, and education, and other social causes. Recognizing health care as a human right, so infections do not go untreated and cause epilepsy, is another important way to prevent epilepsy. And guess what? Making changes like these will improve life for everyone, not just people concerned about epilepsy.

Working with others on any of these issues is also an opportunity for them to learn about epilepsy and change attitudes produced by epilepsy stigma. While making the community better for everyone, the community will become more open to people with epilepsy.

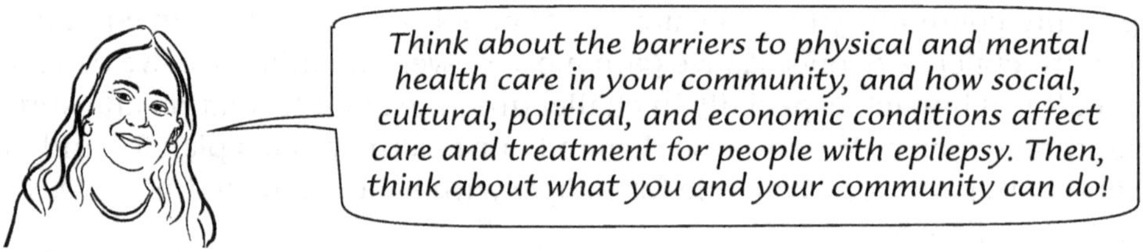

Adapt this information for your community

This book features stories of people with epilepsy shared in their own words, as well as stories adapted from real-life experiences. The examples of community action are not made up—they show how real organizations responded to their specific needs and conditions. We hope they inspire you. Do not just copy them and try to do the exact same things. Instead, adapt them to your situation and strengths.

We want your feedback

Please write to us with your thoughts about what you found useful in this resource and, perhaps more importantly, what you did not agree with or what you tried that did not work. We would love to hear about your experiences organizing for better care for people with epilepsy and seizures, and to share your wisdom in future editions or publications. Contact us at epilepsy@hesperian.org to tell us what you think.

Chapter 2

In this chapter

First aid for seizures **15**
Steps of seizure first aid 16
Tips for giving seizure first aid 17
How to help a person having a seizure in a wheelchair 18
What not to do during a seizure 19
Seizure emergencies **19**
If a person has a seizure that lasts longer than 5 minutes (status epilepticus) 19
If a person has a seizure while swimming 20
If a person has a seizure in the bathroom 20
If a person falls from a height 21
If a person has difficulty breathing or stops breathing after a seizure 21
If a person does not regain consciousness after a seizure 21
If a person chokes on food or drink during a seizure 21
After the seizure **24**
Other problems that can happen with seizures **26**
If a person vomits 26
If a person loses bladder or bowel control 26
If a person wants to sleep right away 27
If a person is injured or bleeding 27
If a person breaks or knocks out a tooth 28
If a person is burned 28
If a person is aggressive or shows unusual behaviors 30
When to see a health worker **30**
Training the community in seizure first aid **30**
Story: Purple Bench's community-driven approach to seizure first aid training 31

How to help a person having a seizure

Seizures can happen anywhere, at any time. Usually, seizures end quickly by themselves and no medical help is needed. Family and community members can learn how to help a person stay safe and prevent injuries during seizures, and to recover comfortably. Because seizures do not spread from one person to another, it is completely safe to help someone having a seizure.

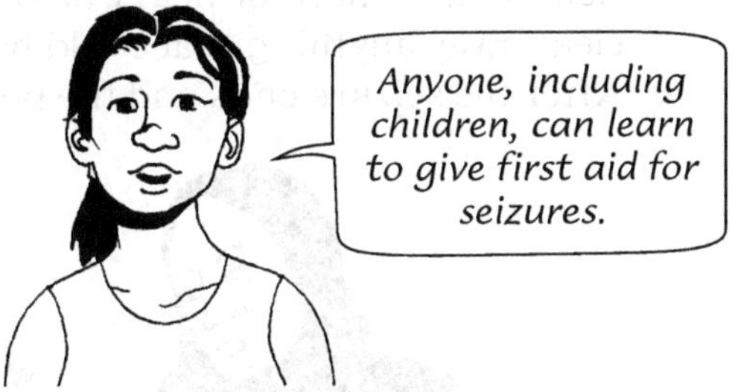
Anyone, including children, can learn to give first aid for seizures.

First aid for seizures

When people are asked what happens to someone during a seizure, they will often describe a person falling down, their body getting stiff and making jerking movements, and the person losing consciousness. This is one of the most commonly recognized type of seizures, called a tonic-clonic seizure.

There are other types of seizures that may cause only some of these effects. In some seizures, the person does not fall down and does not lose consciousness. A person having an absence seizure may stare blankly for a few moments and then recover. A person having a myoclonic seizure may have a quick muscle jerk (like what happens sometimes when you are falling asleep) and recover almost immediately.

The kind of seizure first aid you can offer depends on the effects of the seizure on the person. No matter what type of seizure a person has, they will benefit from first aid that offers them comfort and helps them stay safe and recover. For information about different types of seizures, see Chapter 3.

Because tonic-clonic seizures are common and are most likely to have harmful effects, from falling down or losing consciousness, we focus on them in this chapter. If the person you are helping has a different kind of seizure, please keep reading. You will find descriptions of other aspects of seizures and information that will help you support the safety and recovery of the person having the seizure.

Steps of seizure first aid

To help a person having any type of seizure, remain calm and alert, and follow these steps. Remember that quick, calm, and gentle action is more important than getting every detail right.

1. **Stay calm and stay close.** Speak gently, they may be able to hear you even if they cannot respond. If appropriate, let others around you know the person is having a seizure. Do not leave them alone.
2. **Protect them from injury.** If the person is standing or walking, guide them away from streets, stairs, hot or hard surfaces—anything that might hurt them. Remove any sharp or heavy objects that could cause injury. If they have fallen, clear away anything that could harm them, and ask people to give them space. After the seizure ends and the person is awake, help them move to a safer place.

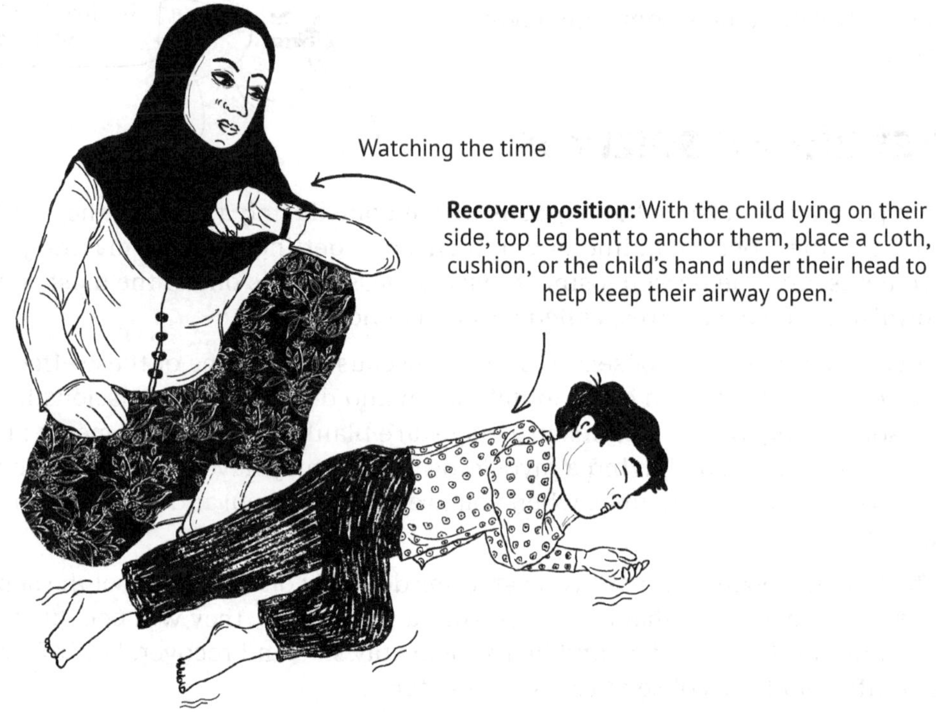

3. **If a person falls during a seizure,** gently roll them into the recovery position with the top leg bent so they do not roll over. Place a cushion or their arm under their head. Tilt the head back slightly and raise their chin gently to help keep their airway open. During a seizure, muscles may relax or may contract, and because the tongue is a large muscle, it can block the airway. This slight tilt and lift with a person lying on their side instead of their back will help saliva, vomit, or other fluids drain from the mouth.

4. **Loosen any tight or buttoned clothing around the neck** to support breathing and prevent choking. If a person wears glasses, remove them carefully.
5. **Do not restrain.** Do not hold a person down or try to stop their movements during a seizure. This can injure both you and the person having the seizure.
6. **Do not put anything in their mouth or between their teeth.** This can cause them to bite their tongue or cheek and bleed in their mouth. If they swallow something, it could block their airway and make breathing difficult. (It is not possible for someone having a seizure to swallow their own tongue.)
7. **Comfort and reassure the person as they recover.** As the person wakes up, gently help them recover. Talk to them about what happened, offer comfort, and make sure they are all right. Eventually, help them sit up in a comfortable and safe position. To prevent choking, offer water only after they are fully awake, able to talk, and can swallow without discomfort.

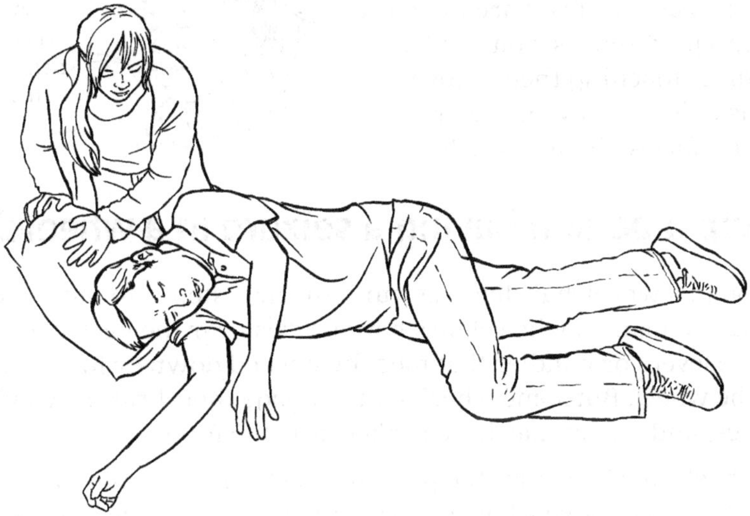

Tips for giving seizure first aid

Time the seizure. Note the start time and how long the seizure lasts. If a seizure lasts longer than 5 minutes, or if another seizure starts soon after, get medical help right away (see "Seizure emergencies," page 19). Use a watch or phone to measure how long the seizure lasts.

Taking videos. A video can help a doctor or other health worker identify a person's seizure type and offer treatment options. Only take a video after making sure the person is safe. Never let recording get in the way of helping. When recording video:

- show the whole body, not just the head.
- record any sounds.
- keep recording until the person starts to recover.

Ask the person if they would like a copy of the video to share with a doctor or other health worker. Always respect the person's privacy and dignity by deleting the video after you share it with them.

Touching a person during a seizure. In some cultures, physical touch, especially from a stranger or someone of the opposite gender, can be uncomfortable or even prohibited. If you know the person's background or preferences, do your best to honor them—step back and ask a friend or family member to assist. If you are in doubt about a person's preferences, you can keep them safe without touching them. Move any dangerous objects away and clear space. Offer comfort with kind words.

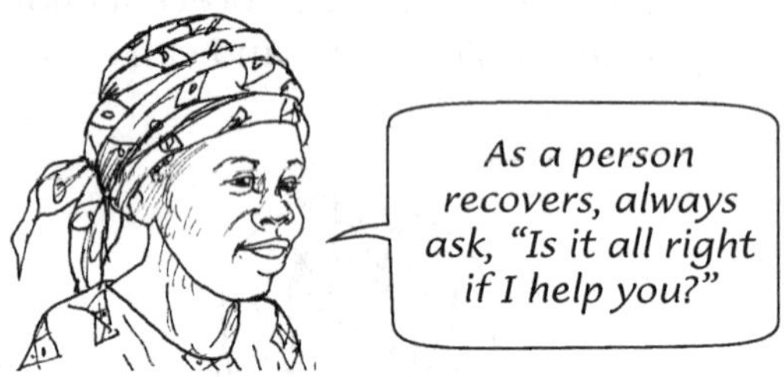
As a person recovers, always ask, "Is it all right if I help you?"

How to help a person having a seizure in a wheelchair

When a person in a wheelchair has a seizure, the first step is to put the wheelchair brakes on. Usually, manual wheelchairs have brakes near the back wheels. The brakes look like levers or handles that must be pushed down or forward until they lock against the wheel. But some wheelchairs engage their brakes by pulling the lever up or back, and others may have brakes near the footrest.

After the wheelchair is secure, the person can stay in the wheelchair during their seizure. Do not try to remove a harness or seatbelt if they are using one, but gently support their upper body to prevent them from falling out of the chair. It might help to gently turn their head to one side to help saliva drain from their mouth and keep their airway clear. Stay calm, do not put anything in their mouth, and remain with the person until the seizure ends and they are fully awake.

If the seizure lasts more than 5 minutes, it is a medical emergency—get help!

What not to do during a seizure

Do not put anything in the person's mouth.

Do not throw water on the person. This will not stop a seizure.

Do not make the person smell an onion, leather shoe, or other strong-smelling item. This will not bring a person back to consciousness and can worsen confusion.

Do not try to wake the person by slapping them or shouting. This will not stop a seizure and can increase confusion or cause injury.

Do not rub metal objects, keys, or other items on a person's hand. These actions will not stop a seizure and can distract from giving first aid that could help.

Do not try to "pull out" a spirit or a curse by using rituals that involve beating a person or making them breathe smoke. These will not stop a seizure and can cause injury and breathing problems. Seizures are not caused by spirits, curses, or demons.

Do not cover the person with blankets to "trap the spirit" or reduce shaking. This will not stop a seizure and can cause overheating and breathing problems.

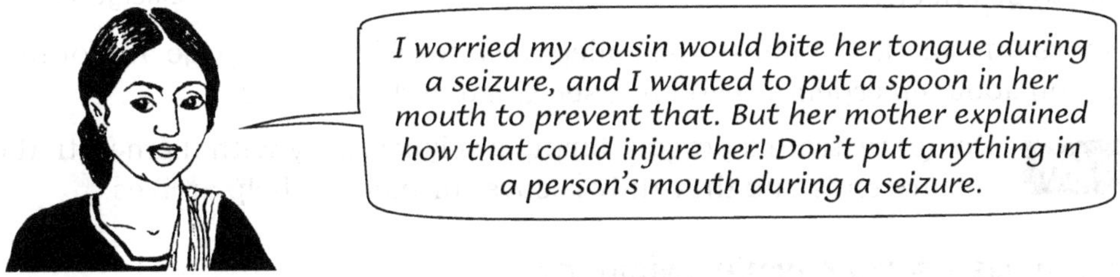

Seizure emergencies

Although most people who have epilepsy or seizures recover fully after just a few minutes, some seizures are medical emergencies. Medical help and emergency action are needed:

If a person has a seizure that lasts longer than 5 minutes (status epilepticus)

Status epilepticus is usually not one but many seizures with little or no recovery time between them.

If a seizure lasts longer than 5 minutes and the person cannot speak or respond, you need to look in their pocket or bag or backpack for emergency medicine or information. Tell others nearby that you are looking for instructions to help.

A person in status epilepticus needs emergency medicine. They often carry a medical ID card, bracelet, or necklace along with their emergency rescue medicine. Their emergency medical information should explain:

- the type and dose of rescue medicine to give.
- how and when to give it.
- when to call medical help or take the person to a clinic or hospital.

Rescue medicine is different from daily medicine a person takes for seizures. It is intended for use only in emergencies. It is commonly given in 2 ways:

By mouth. Some rescue medicines come as a pill that dissolves quickly under the tongue or between the cheek and gum. Do not attempt this if the person is actively convulsing and there is a risk they might choke on medicine or involuntarily bite you.

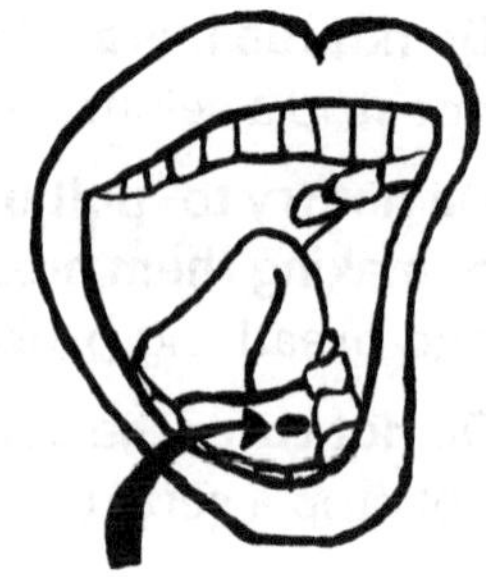

Emergency pill

As a nasal spray. Some rescue medicines come as a nasal spray. If you find this type of medicine, follow its instructions carefully. Usually you will spray the medicine into only one nostril. The person does not need to be awake for nasal spray medicine to be effective.

For more information about status epilepticus, see Chapter 3, page 57. For more information about emergency medicine, see Chapter 4, page 109.

IMPORTANT Do not restrain a person during a seizure. Stay with them until the seizure ends and they fully recover or medical help arrives.

If a person has a seizure while swimming

Get them out of the water as fast as you can and call for help if needed. If they are breathing, follow basic seizure first aid steps. If they are not breathing, and you know how, immediately start rescue breathing and chest compressions.

For information about how to do rescue breathing and chest compressions, see Hesperian's *Pocket Where There Is No Doctor: First Aid.*

If a person has a seizure in the bathroom

If a person has a seizure in the bathroom, first try to move them away from any water to prevent drowning. If you cannot move them, focus on keeping their head above water. If the bathroom door is locked and you suspect someone is having a seizure, you may need help to open the door. Once the person is safe from water, follow basic steps for seizure first aid (see page 16).

To avoid falling while bathing, it is safest to sit on a stool or chair. If heat is a seizure trigger, avoid using very hot water.

If a person falls from a height

If a person has a seizure and falls from a height, like down the stairs, off a ledge, or from a ladder or roof, they may get seriously injured and need emergency medical help.

Do not move the person unless they are in immediate danger, for example, from traffic or fire. If they have broken bones, especially in their head, neck, or back, moving them could make their injuries worse.

If they are breathing and safe where they are, stay close, keep them comfortable, and wait for medical help to arrive. If they are not breathing, immediately start rescue breathing and chest compressions if you know how.

If a person has difficulty breathing or stops breathing after a seizure

During a seizure, breathing may stop briefly but it should return after the seizure has passed. If the person does not start breathing again, call for help and, if you know how, immediately start rescue breathing and chest compressions.

For information about how to do rescue breathing and chest compressions, see Hesperian's *Pocket Where There Is No Doctor: First Aid.*

If a person does not regain consciousness after a seizure

If the person is not responsive after a seizure, immediately call for help.

If a person chokes on food or drink during a seizure

When a person has a seizure while eating or drinking, there is a small chance that food or liquids may get stuck in their throat or airway, blocking their breathing and making them choke.

Because breathing often stops briefly during a seizure, it may be difficult to know if breathing has stopped due to choking or due to the seizure itself. Breathing that stops due to a seizure will start again after the seizure has passed. But if breathing stops because of choking, it may not restart without action.

After the seizure ends, check if the person is breathing by looking for movement (their chest rising and falling) and listening to or feeling for air coming in or out of their mouth or nose. If the person has fallen, roll them onto their side to prevent any risk of swallowing food or vomit that can block breathing.

If the person is conscious but cannot breathe and you suspect they are choking, ask them to open their mouth so you can look inside to check for food. Use your small finger to sweep any food out of the mouth so it does not block the airway. **Only use a finger sweep if you can clearly see food or an object blocking the airway.**

IMPORTANT Do not push the food deeper into their throat. Also, be aware that the person's involuntary movements might lead them to bite your finger.

If breathing remains blocked, you can try giving abdominal thrusts (the Heimlich maneuver). For babies and pregnant people, give back blows instead.

HOW TO Give abdominal thrusts

If the person is on a bed or chair, move them onto their back on the floor. A floor is a solid, firm base upon which to do this rescue action. While kneeling beside their upper body:

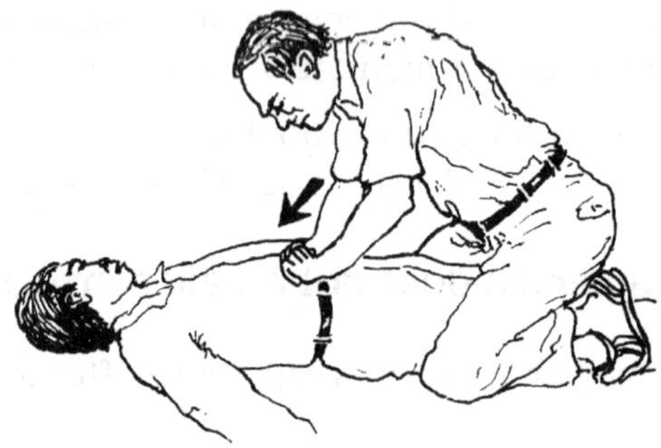

- Find the person's navel (belly button).
- Make a fist. Curl your fingers and tuck your thumb beneath the fingers, into the palm.
- Put your fist just above their navel but below their ribcage and hold it with your other hand on top.
- Use both hands to push toward the rib cage with a sudden jerk. Do this quickly, 3 to 5 times.
- Repeat this a few times to push increasing amounts of air through the person's lungs and windpipe to drive out whatever is blocking breathing.

Do not give abdominal thrusts to a person who is:

Unconscious. Abdominal thrusts work partly because they rely on a person's ability to forcefully cough out what is stuck in their airway. An unconscious person may not be able to do this.

Pregnant. Strong force applied during an abdominal thrust can injure the womb, threatening the life of the pregnant person and the baby. Instead, see "How to give back blows to a pregnant person lying down," page 23.

A baby. Abdominal thrusts are too strong for a baby's small, delicate body. Instead, see "How to give a back blow to a baby," page 23.

WHEN TO GET HELP If breathing does not start right away, call for help or take them to a nearby clinic or hospital immediately.

HOW TO **Give back blows**

How to give back blows to a pregnant person lying down. Turn the pregnant person on their side and place a cushion under their hip to tilt their body and the pregnancy slightly forward.

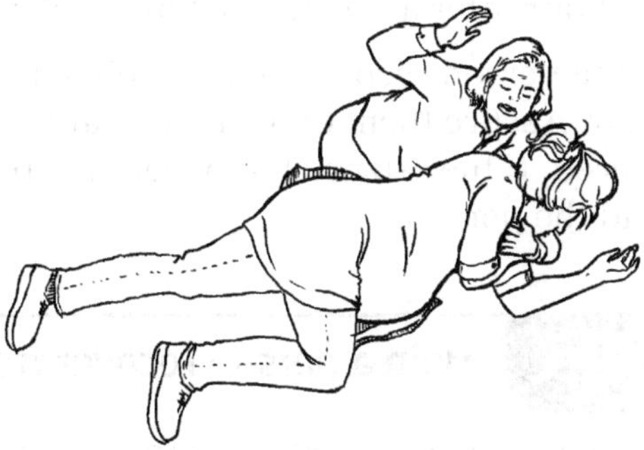

- Get on your knees behind the person's back.
- Gently hold their head in the palm of one of your hands.
- Use the bottom portion (the "heel") of your other hand to hit the person in the middle of their back, between the shoulder blades. Do not hit too hard.
- Repeat this 5 times or more until the food blocking the breathing is pushed out of the airway and mouth.

After recovery, the person should contact a midwife or doctor so they can check on other health issues related to pregnancy.

How to give back blows to a baby.

- Hold the baby face down with their head lower than their body.
- Use the bottom portion (the "heel") of your hand to give 5 firm blows between the shoulder blades.
- Repeat this 3 to 5 times or more until the baby breathes.
- If breathing does not return, try giving gentle chest thrusts with your fingers.

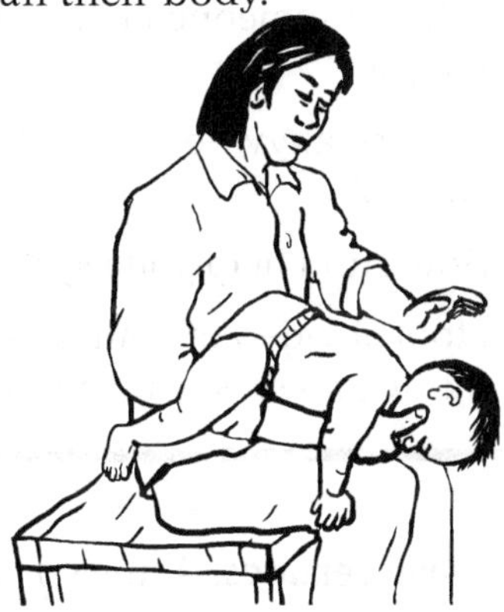

WHEN TO GET HELP If breathing does not start right away, call for help or take them to a nearby clinic or hospital immediately.

As soon as the person is breathing, encourage them to cough if food is still partially blocking their airway. Offer water after the airway is no longer blocked. If a person is not able to cough, it could be because food is still stuck and blocking their airway.

After the seizure

After a seizure, a person may need a few moments to come back to consciousness. They may feel confused, drowsy, or nauseous. They may vomit or have a headache. A person may feel this way for up to 30 minutes. If these signs continue for more than 1 hour after a seizure, get medical help.

As the person recovers from their seizure, introduce yourself and tell them what you saw. Assure them they are safe and offer to stay with them until they have recovered. If the seizure happened in a public place, prevent people from crowding around the person.

HOW TO Help a person recover from their seizure

As the person recovers from their seizure, you can ask:

- Are you feeling OK?
- Do you know what happened?
- Do you have any pain or feel hurt anywhere?
- Have you had a seizure before?
- Is there someone I can call for you?
- Is there anywhere I can help you go?
- How can I help you right now?
- I took a video of your seizure so you could share it with your doctor if you like. Can I send the video to you?

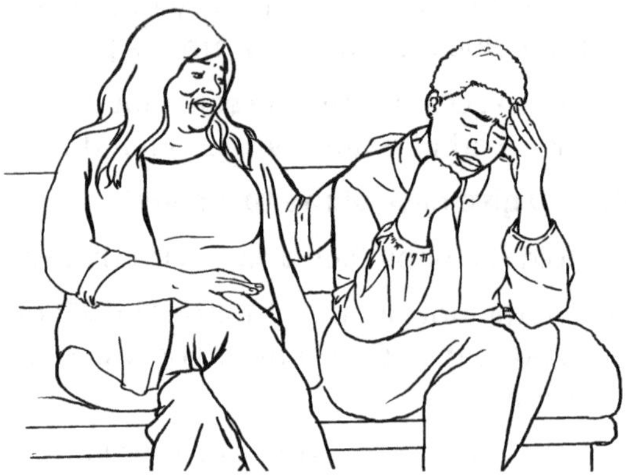

If you have seizures. After you recover from a seizure, it is helpful to let people who may have seen what happened know you are OK. Say something like, "I just had a seizure, but I am fine now," or "Thank you for helping me." Saying a few words helps ease worries others may be feeling for you.

If you need rest, you can say, "I need to sit down for a while." Ask for more help if you need it.

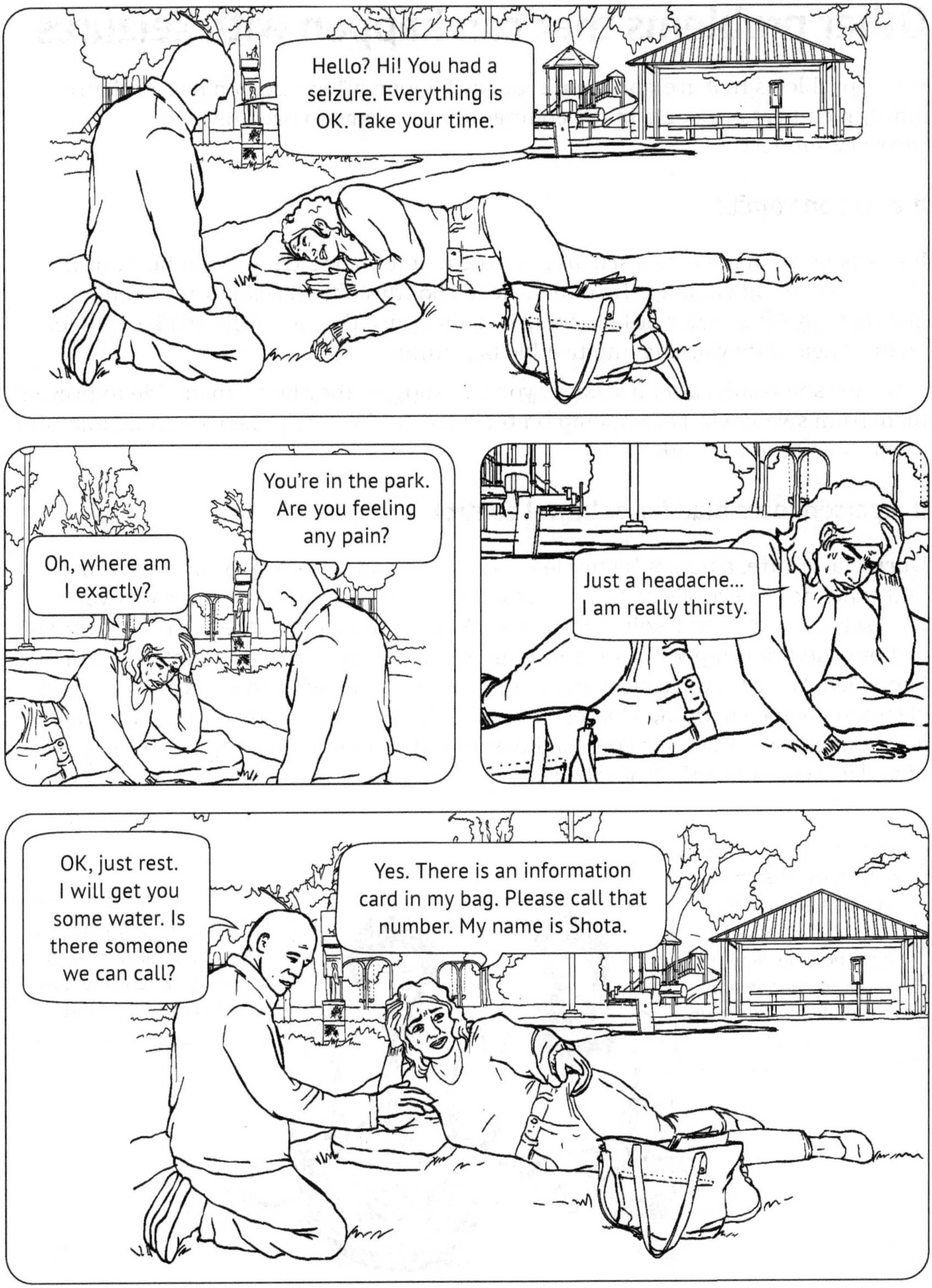
Hello? Hi! You had a seizure. Everything is OK. Take your time.
Oh, where am I exactly?
You're in the park. Are you feeling any pain?
Just a headache... I am really thirsty.
OK, just rest. I will get you some water. Is there someone we can call?
Yes. There is an information card in my bag. Please call that number. My name is Shota.

Other problems that can happen with seizures

When problems that are not an emergency happen after a person has a seizure, family members or people in the community can learn to provide basic recovery support.

If a person vomits

If a person vomits *during a seizure,* roll them onto their side to keep their airway clear and prevent choking. Turn their head slightly so fluids can drain from the mouth. Only offer water or help them clean up once they are fully awake. Call for medical help if they are having trouble breathing.

If a person vomits *after a seizure,* you can suggest they lie on their side to prevent them from swallowing or choking on their vomit. Then help them clean up and offer them something to drink.

If a person loses bladder or bowel control

During a seizure, a person's muscles may clench and unclench, or become tense and rigid, or loose and weak. This can cause them to accidentally urinate (wet themselves) or defecate (soil themselves). As they come out of the seizure, cover any wet or soiled clothing with something like a blanket or coat and calmly explain what happened. Once they are alert and able to move safely, offer them assistance with cleaning up and changing clothes, if needed. Let them know this is very common and happens without their control. Reassure them that it is nothing to be ashamed of and is a common effect of seizures.

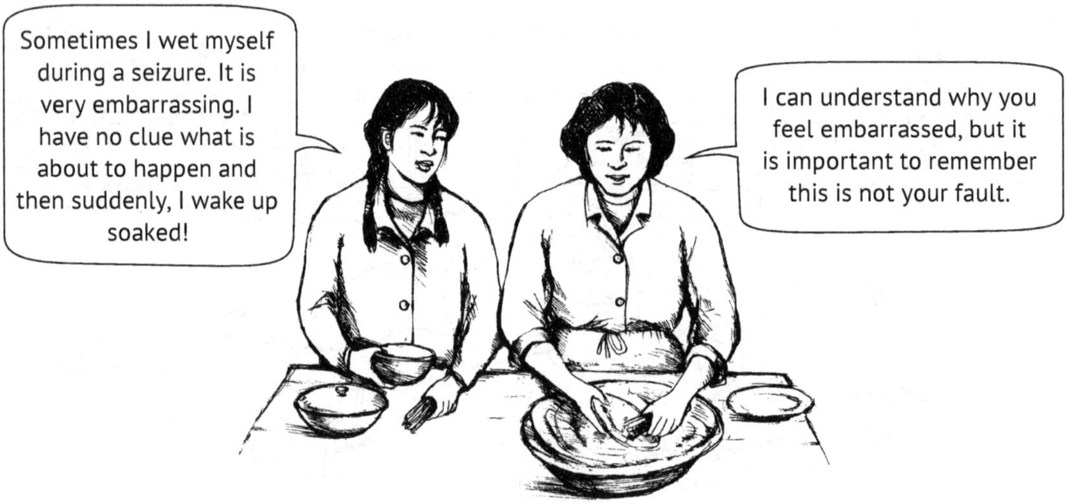
Sometimes I wet myself during a seizure. It is very embarrassing. I have no clue what is about to happen and then suddenly, I wake up soaked!
I can understand why you feel embarrassed, but it is important to remember this is not your fault.

If a person wants to sleep right away

Some people are very tired after a seizure and have difficulty staying awake. This is not a problem as long as they are breathing well and you do not see or suspect any injuries, especially to the head, back, or neck. You might roll them onto their side to prevent choking on saliva in case another seizure happens while they are resting.

If the person is wearing glasses, remove them so they do not break, as well as any large or unsafe items from their pockets.

If a person is injured or bleeding

Body injuries are common from seizures, especially if a person loses consciousness and falls. Because a person may not be able to feel injuries or talk immediately after a seizure, look carefully for any bumps, bruises, scrapes, or bleeding. Pay attention to areas most likely to be affected by a fall, such as the head, face, arms, and legs. If appropriate and the person agrees, check for tenderness or swelling by lightly touching exposed skin.

If a bone breaks during a fall, the person needs to go to a hospital or clinic. If they have broken bones in their head, neck, or back, bring medical help to them—moving them might worsen the injury.

If the person is bleeding, press a clean piece of cloth directly and firmly on the wound (even large, heavily bleeding wounds) and keep pressing until the bleeding stops. If the cloth gets soaked with blood, use another cloth on top of it rather than replacing it. For a large wound, keep pressure on for at least 15 minutes after the bleeding has stopped. If possible, keep the injured body part above the level of the person's heart.

For more information on broken bones, head or back injuries, or treating wounds, see Hesperian's *Pocket Where There Is No Doctor: First Aid.*

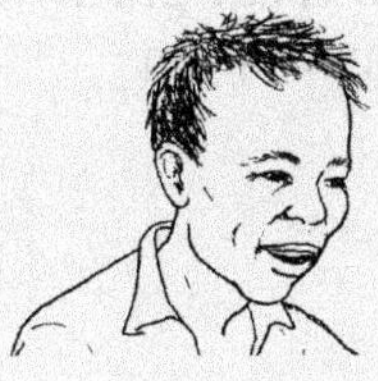

I attended a seizure first aid training in my community. A few days later, when my brother had a fall during a seizure, I knew exactly how to check and make sure he was not seriously injured.

If a person breaks or knocks out a tooth

If a person breaks or knocks out a tooth during a seizure, first help them rinse their mouth with warm salt water to keep the area clean and reduce the risk of infection. There will likely be bleeding in the gum around the tooth. If the tooth has come out, stop bleeding by placing a clean cloth, cotton, or gauze where it had been. Ask the person to bite down gently to maintain pressure and stop the bleeding. An ice pack on the cheek near the injury can reduce pain and swelling.

If the person can get to a dentist within an hour of the injury, it may be possible to save the tooth. Hold the tooth at the top and rinse it with milk or salt water. Be careful not to scrub or remove any tissue attached to the tooth. Place it in a container with milk, salt water, or even the person's saliva, or wrap it in a clean, wet cloth or gauze. Get to a dentist as quickly as possible.

If a person is burned

If a person has a seizure near a fire, flame, or hot surface, they may get burned. Burns can be minor or severe depending on how long and how much of a person's skin is involved.

What to do immediately

- **Stop the burning as soon as possible.** Move the person away from the hot surface or flame. Be careful not to get burned yourself.
- **Remove any jewelry, belts, or tight clothing near the burn.** Do not try to remove anything stuck to the skin.
- **Cool the burn with cool or lukewarm water for 20 minutes.** Cooling helps stop the burn from going deeper and reduces pain. If running water is not available, use a clean, cool, wet cloth or compress.
- **Do not put ice, grease, fat, animal hides or skins, coffee, herbs, or feces on a burn.** These will damage skin more.
- **Give aspirin, paracetamol (acetaminophen), or ibuprofen to treat pain.** Aspirin is not safe for children under 16 years. For information on pain medicines, see Chapter 4, page 115.

HOW TO Care for burns

Minor burns on hands, face, and feet. Cool the burn with running water as suggested above. Clean the burned area with soap and water. Use gloves or plastic bags on your hands to avoid touching blood or body fluids or anything touched by them. Gently cover the burn with sterile gauze or sterilized cloth. Secure with medical tape or bandages.

If the burn is on an arm or leg, keep it elevated to lessen swelling. If the burn is on hands or feet, separate fingers or toes with a clean cloth.

Give an antihistamine (such as diphenhydramine) if the burn itches as it heals. Small burns should heal by themselves in about 2 weeks.

See a health worker if the burn shows signs of infection: increased redness, swelling, pus or a bad smell, or if the person has a fever.

Severe burns. A burn is severe if it covers a large area, is deep and affects more than the top layer of skin, or is combined with other injuries. Burns in children are always considered severe and must be treated carefully. Get emergency medical help even if you are far from a clinic or hospital.

If you cannot reach a health center immediately, keep the burn area clean and dry. If the burn is dirty, gently rinse the surface with clean water. If you can, mix 1 part povidone iodine with 4 parts lukewarm water that is boiled, then cooled. Scrub gently so the burn does not bleed. Dry the area by blotting—not rubbing—with sterile gauze or sterilized cloth. Wearing sterile gloves, put one of the following directly on the burn to kill germs:

- Silver sulfadiazine: Use a thin layer. Do not use on eyelids, lips, or children less than 2 months old. —or—
- Honey: Use a thin layer. —or—
- Sugar: Pour granulated sugar over the burn to cover it. Throw away any sugar that does not stick but falls off. Do not put it back on wound.

Gently cover the burn with sterile gauze or sterilized cloth and secure this with tape or bandages.

Change the cloth or gauze covering daily and reapply the anti-germ treatment described above. Give pain medicine before cleaning or changing the dressing.

IMPORTANT If signs of infection appear—pus, bad smell, fever, or swollen lymph nodes—put an antibiotic ointment such as Polysporin on the burn and get medical help as soon as possible.

If a person is aggressive or shows unusual behaviors

Some seizures can cause a person to thrash, shout, swear, or strike out at people nearby. These actions are usually not done on purpose and the person often will not remember them after the seizure. Try to stay calm, give the person space, and keep them and those around them safe. Do not attempt to restrain the person or argue with them.

When to see a health worker

After a person recovers from a seizure, they are usually OK if they are awake, alert, and breathing normally. It is necessary to see a health worker afterwards when a person:

- does not regain consciousness (wake up) after or in between seizures.
- has their first seizure.
- has a single or a series of seizures lasting longer than 5 minutes (status epilepticus, see page 19).
- has a serious wound or injury, severe pain, or bleeding.
- has a fever.

Training the community in seizure first aid

If you learn seizure first aid skills and someone near you has a seizure, you will be able to help. Sharing these skills in community trainings ensures that if someone has a seizure anywhere in your community—at school, church, a park, a market, or on a bus—people will have the information they need to respond quickly and make injuries unlikely. This is especially important when medical centers are far away and emergency services like ambulances may not arrive quickly. In some places, advocacy groups train not only family members and neighbors, but also teachers, police officers, and community health workers.

Sharing information about epilepsy in a training also breaks the silence that surrounds epilepsy in many communities and helps fight stigma. Training prepares people to respond supportively instead of fearfully, and can help build empathy and respect throughout the community. When more people can recognize a seizure, offer help, and respond during an emergency, it creates a safer and more supportive environment for everyone in the community.

Purple Bench's community-driven approach to seizure first aid training

A persistent lack of awareness about epilepsy in their community motivated a daughter-mother team in Uganda to transform their personal struggle into community action. After Nina Mago was diagnosed with epilepsy, she and her mother Anita started the Purple Bench Initiative to create a supportive community space where people with epilepsy can openly share their experiences and challenges without fear of judgment.

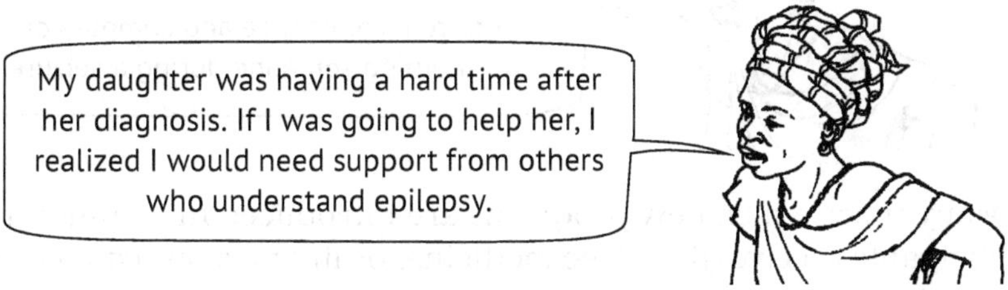

Nina and Anita chose the name Purple Bench because the color purple symbolizes epilepsy awareness, and a bench is a symbol for a place where people can pause, sit together, and discuss what is on their minds.

Purple Bench shares epilepsy facts through social media, creates support groups, and organizes seizure first aid trainings, especially in rural areas where there is little access to epilepsy information and care. They started by training 17 community members. Some they knew, others they had just met.

Anita transformed the information she had learned about seizure first aid into hands-on demonstrations, role-playing, and real-life situations.

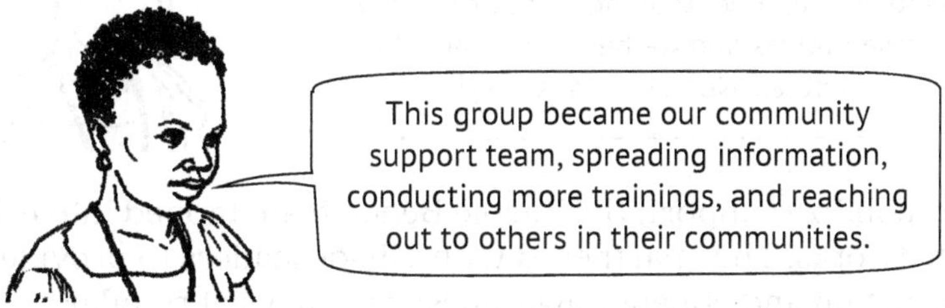

continues

Purple Bench's community-driven approach to seizure first aid training *(continued)*

To make the training more helpful to people in rural areas, Anita and Nina followed a simple truth: community members understand their own needs best. They trained local people to lead sessions in their own villages.

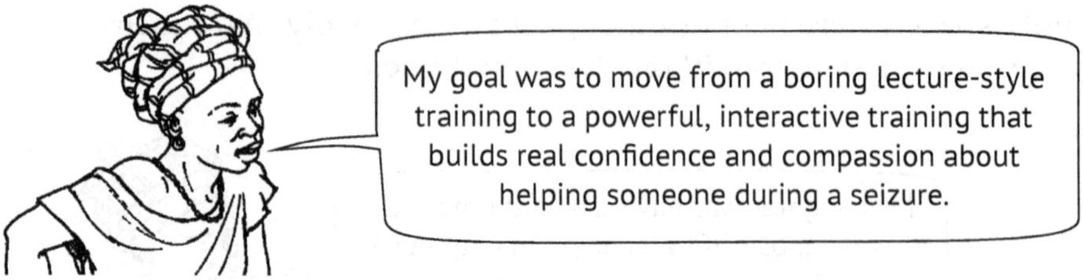

Many times, when new programs are introduced in communities, participants receive gifts, free medicine, or financial assistance. Anita and Nina made it clear from the very start that they were a small group and the only things they had to share were friendship, information about epilepsy, and trainings.

While not everyone trained went on to lead additional sessions, many of them did! They started with small trainings in people's homes, encouraging attendees to go out and share what they learned with others. In some villages, monthly trainings rotated among the homes of different hosts.

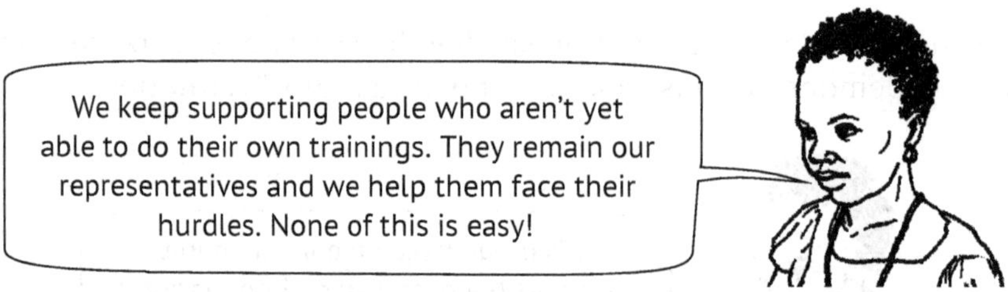

To further mobilize support, the Purple Bench team tapped into existing community networks. They partnered with village leaders to provide seizure first aid information and epilepsy awareness messages at regular village meetings. This helped reach people who were already meeting together, and it also increased their credibility.

continues

Purple Bench's community-driven approach to seizure first aid training *(continued)*

One dedicated youth coordinator worked with local youth to produce a skit presenting relatable characters and situations. The young actors brought the challenges of epilepsy to life through performance. Afterwards, the audience asked lots of questions, showing how drama can break barriers and start dialogue.

As more people share their experiences and learn about epilepsy through Purple Bench, there is greater acceptance and understanding in the community.

Because religion is often important in community life, Purple Bench also partners with spiritual leaders who can help counter common myths when they preach that "epilepsy is not contagious" and "epilepsy is not a punishment from God."

What is the Purple Bench commitment? Make Masaka, Uganda, an epilepsy-smart district!

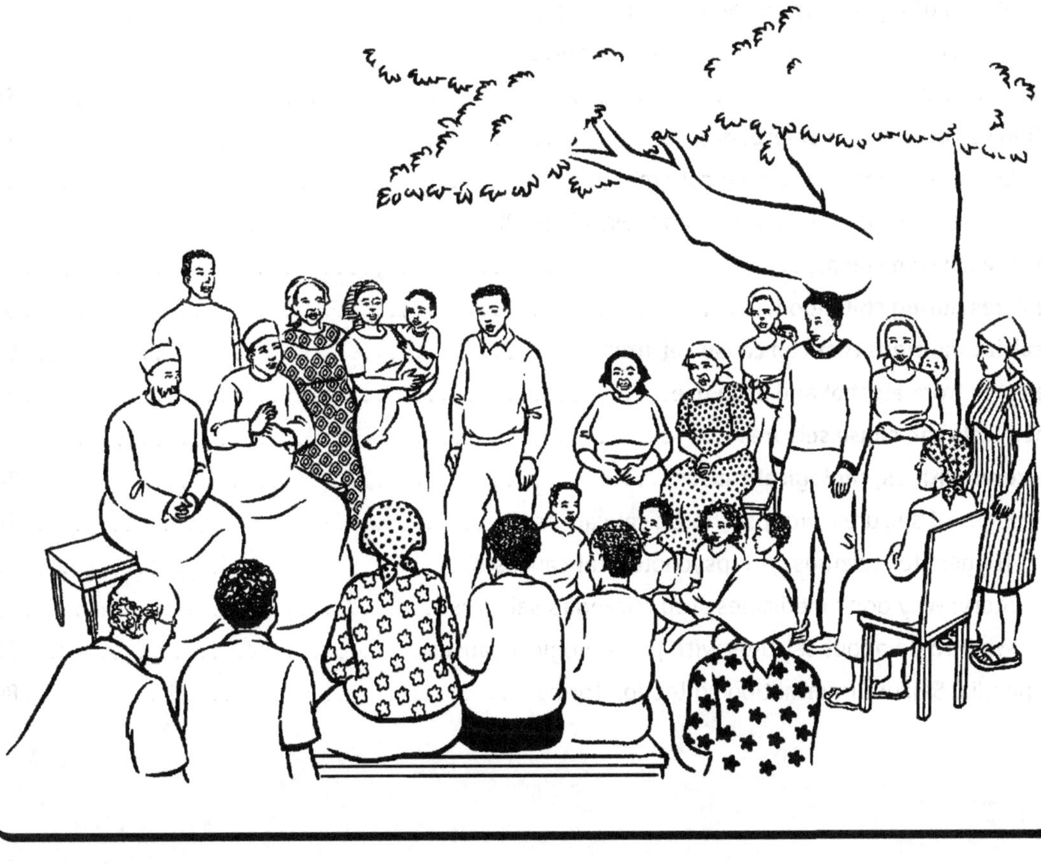

Chapter 3

In this chapter

There are many types of seizures **35**
Seizure experiences: Maya, Sharon, and Manuel 36
Find out what happened during a seizure 37
Questions to ask about seizures 38
For health workers: Asking about seizures 41
What Maya, Sharon, and Manuel learned about their seizures 42
Identifying types of seizures **45**
Identifying seizures by body movements 46
Generalized and focal seizures 47
Generalized tonic-clonic seizures 49
Stages of a generalized tonic-clonic seizure 51
Tonic, clonic, myoclonic, and atonic seizures 52
Absence seizures **56**
When seizures are an emergency **57**
Status epilepticus is a medical emergency! 57
Sudden unexpected death in epilepsy (SUDEP) 57
Seizures during sleep **58**
Seizures during childhood **59**
Health conditions that can cause seizures **61**
Seizures from alcohol and drug use **68**
Chemicals can cause seizures **69**
Seizures with psychological causes **70**
Signs of seizures with psychological causes 70
Triggers for seizures with psychological causes 72
Story: Why don't medicines stop Miranda's seizures? 75
What to do about seizures with psychological causes 77
Appendix: Seizure information collection form 80

Types of seizures and how to identify them

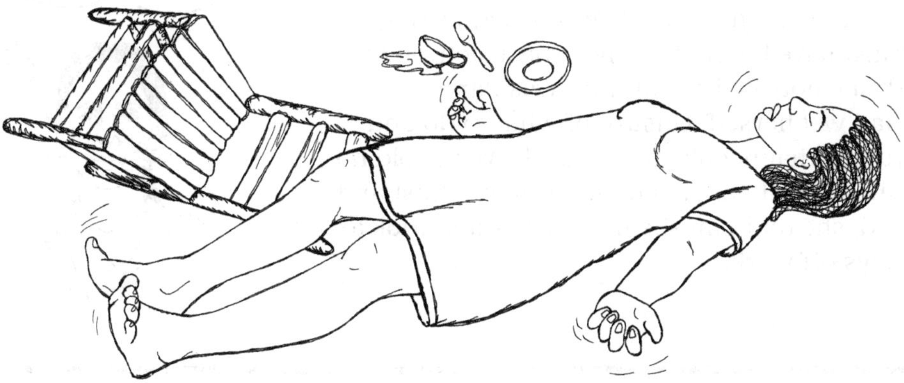

Identifying the type of seizures a person is having makes it possible to find out what treatment can control their seizures so they happen less often. For information about how to use medicines to manage different types of seizures, see Chapter 4.

Since not all seizures are caused by epilepsy—seizures may have psychological or other physical causes—looking carefully at and understanding the differences among them can provide clues to a seizure's cause.

There are many types of seizures

A seizure is a short-term change in the electrical activity of the brain that causes an interruption of consciousness. It may also cause movement of a single part or several parts of the body, or of the entire body. The variety of ways these mental and physical changes combine is how the different seizure types are identified. After a seizure, a person may know that something happened, but they may not be sure of **what happened** or **why it happened**. Let's follow the story of 3 people, Maya, Sharon, and Manuel, who each had a seizure for the first time. Each of them began to deal with—or ignore—their seizure in different ways.

Maya

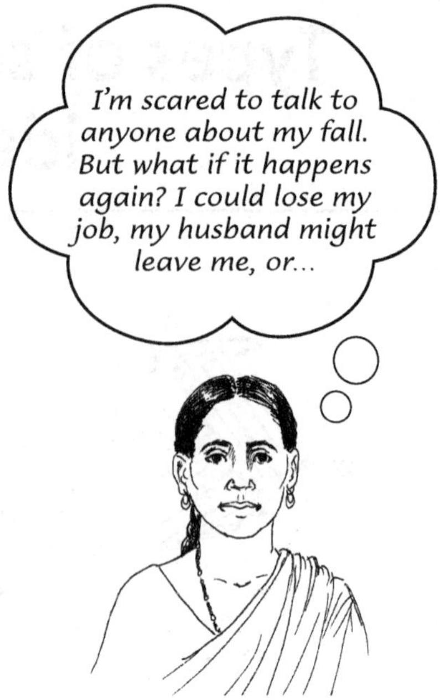
I'm scared to talk to anyone about my fall. But what if it happens again? I could lose my job, my husband might leave me, or...

Maya lives in a village in Kerala, India, where she manages a restaurant in a resort. One day, alone at the end of her shift, she began to feel dizzy. Then she fell to the ground. Her entire body stiffened and began jerking. Maya woke up confused. Why was she lying on the floor? She did not remember anything, including how she fell. Her tongue was bleeding, suggesting she must have bitten it. As her confusion slowly lifted, she noticed her clothing was damp. She had wet herself. Unsure of what to do and fearful of what people might think, Maya told no one about what happened, not even her husband. Instead, she told him she had a fever and took a few days off work.

Sharon

Sharon lives in Boyo, Cameroon. One day, when combing her hair after bathing, Sharon's right arm began to jerk open and closed at the elbow, making her drop the comb. Sharon remembered that the same thing had happened at school a few months earlier.

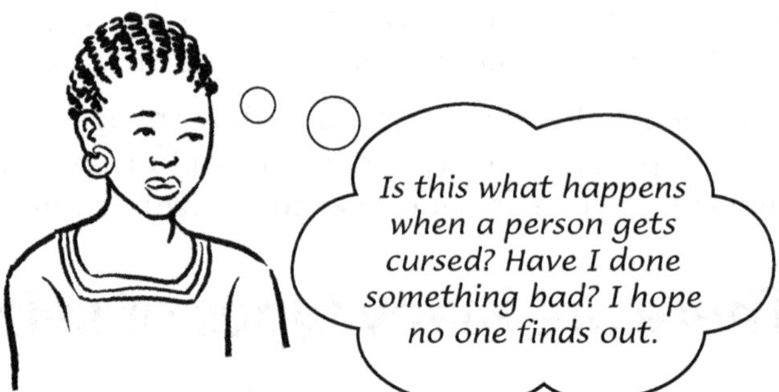
Is this what happens when a person gets cursed? Have I done something bad? I hope no one finds out.

Manuel

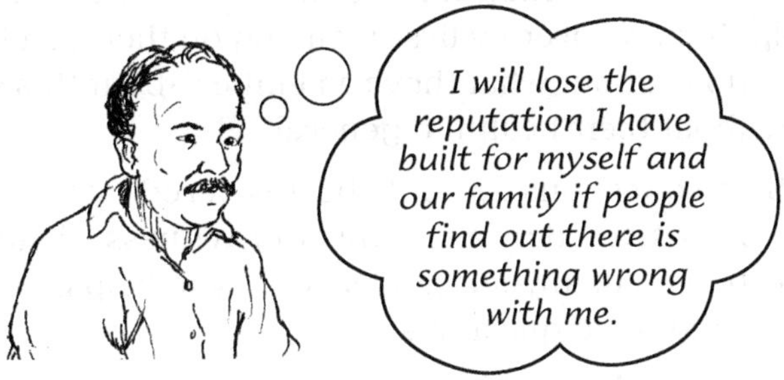
I will lose the reputation I have built for myself and our family if people find out there is something wrong with me.

Manuel and his wife Ana moved to a new neighborhood outside Santiago, Chile. Manuel is in his mid-60s and recently retired. He is having a hard time meeting new people and making friends in his new community. Manuel has started drinking more in the evenings, to relax and feel less lonely. One night, Ana noticed his body making jerking movements while he was asleep. After Ana described it to Manuel, he told her not to mention it to anyone.

Maya, Sharon, and Manuel's stories continue on pages 39 and 40.

Stigma makes getting help for seizures difficult

Although Maya, Sharon, and Manuel are of different ages and live in different parts of the world, their stories share 2 things:

- They do not know why their body is doing unusual things, moving in ways they cannot control.
- They do not want to talk to anyone about it.

Feelings of shame and fear of being judged and excluded from family, work, and community make it hard for a person to tell others about having a seizure or to decide to see a health worker. But without talking, it is impossible to ask for help, find out what is causing the seizures, and learn how to prevent them. See Chapter 5 for information about how to lessen epilepsy stigma so everyone in a community knows how to support people who have seizures.

Find out what happened during a seizure

By asking the right questions, you can help a person learn about their seizures and, eventually, how to prevent them from continuing. Detailed questions can help you find out:

- what type of seizure it is.
- whether the seizure is caused by epilepsy or by something else.
- what might trigger their seizures.
- what treatment might best control their seizure.

A person often feels confused after a seizure, for anywhere from a few moments to an hour. This may make it hard for the person to answer questions right away. Help them recover by first focusing on their safety and comfort, and then asking questions about what they remember about this seizure, about previous seizures, and about their health in general.

Some questions can only be answered by the person who had the seizure. Others can be answered by a caregiver or witness. Health workers are trained to ask questions, but anyone can learn how to help piece together what happened and why by asking good questions.

Tips for family and friends. Build on the trust you already have with the person. Choose a quiet moment and ask questions gently and kindly so the person knows you are there to listen and help, not to judge. Showing respect and promising confidentiality makes it easier for the person to feel safe talking about what happened.

Questions to ask about seizures

Ask the person who had a seizure:

- Have you experienced anything like this before or is this the first time?
- What do you remember about the seizure?
- Did you bite your tongue? Lose control of your bladder or bowel?
- What were you doing just before this happened?
- Have you seen a health worker or healer about this problem before?
- Have you tried any treatment?
- How do you feel now?
- Do you feel confused or unable to think clearly?
- Do you have a headache or any other pain or weakness in your body?
- Do you feel OK enough to go back to what you were doing or to go home?
- Do you think some other health problem you have might have caused this?

continues

Questions to ask about seizures *(continued)*

Ask caregivers or witnesses:

- How long did the seizure last?
- What exactly did you see? (Ask about movements, sounds, breathing, and behavior changes.)
- Did the person fall down?
- Did the person lose consciousness, or did they seem aware and responsive?
- Did you notice any cuts, bruises, or signs of head injury?
- Do you know if anyone in the family has a similar condition?

Ask everyone:

"Tell me everything that happened right before, during, and immediately after the seizure." This encourages people to share as much information as possible, including details that may get missed with more specific questions.

"What questions do you have?" Asking this before closing the conversation invites people to share concerns and learn what can be done. It also creates space for sharing anxieties, misunderstandings about seizures, and other challenges.

Maya, Sharon, and Manuel's stories continue from pages 36 and 37.

Maya

A few days after her seizure, Maya visited her sister. Maya admitted that she had been feeling low but did not share more. Her sister could tell something was wrong. She kept asking questions until Maya told her about the fall. Maya's sister suggested they go see Purnima, a health worker in their community. Maya agreed.

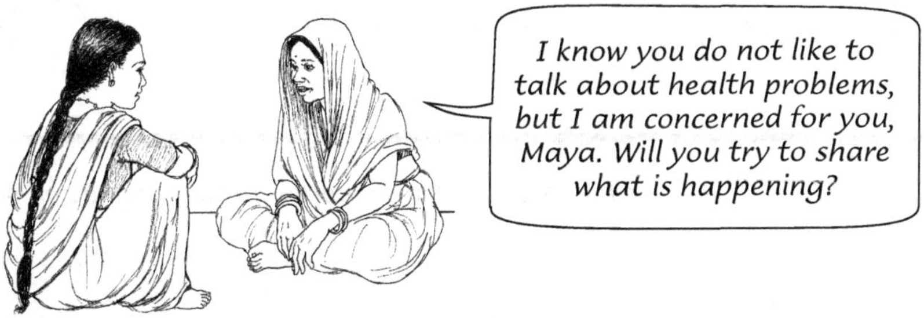
I know you do not like to talk about health problems, but I am concerned for you, Maya. Will you try to share what is happening?

Sharon

After her arm-jerking episode, Sharon was distracted and quiet. Her friend Neo observed something was on her mind. Neo asked Sharon what happened.

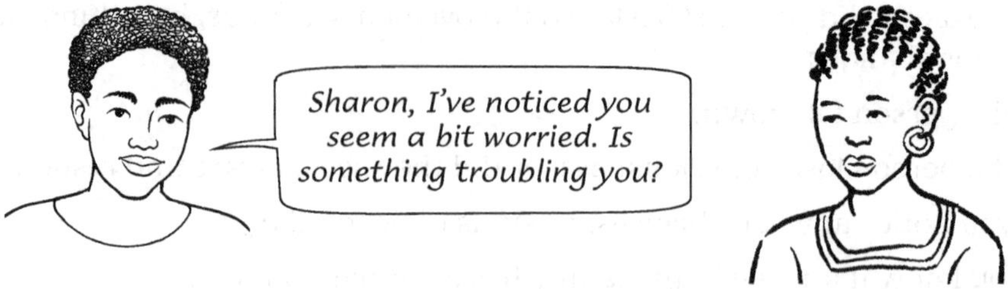

Sharon told Neo what happened and also shared how her arms jerked for a few seconds once when she was climbing stairs at their college. She paid no attention to it at the time, because it stopped quickly and she forgot about it. Neo encouraged Sharon to talk to a health worker. At first, Sharon hesitated. But finally, she agreed it was the best thing to do, and they made plans to go to the health center together the following day.

Manuel

A week after Ana told Manuel about the jerking movements during his sleep, Manuel was tending his garden. Suddenly he dropped the watering can and fell to the ground unconscious. When he woke up and told her what happened, Ana suggested that he visit a health worker.

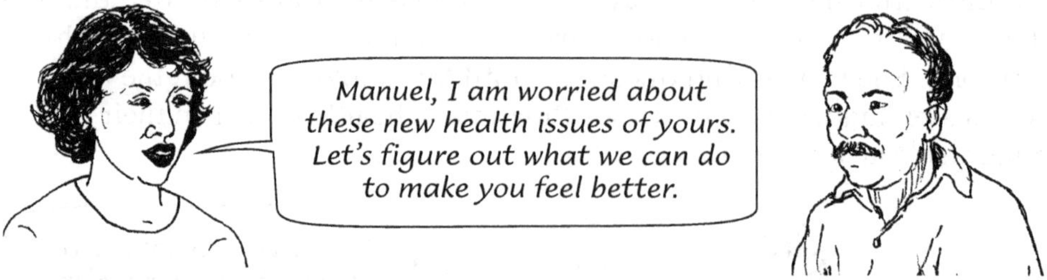

Maya, Sharon, and Manuel's stories further continue on pages 42, 43, and 44.

For health workers: Asking about seizures

As a health worker, you are used to talking about illness, but many people feel shame or fear when talking about health issues they are experiencing but do not understand. They may worry that sharing personal information could lead to losing work, relationships, or respect. To help a person feel safe, explain that you are asking questions so you can find ways to help. Be clear that you will keep their information private and only share it with their permission—and always keep that promise. If the person seems unsure, let them know that the more they share, the more you can help. Build trust by listening closely so the person feels truly heard and respected. Then write down their information on a form like the one at the end of this chapter (see page 80).

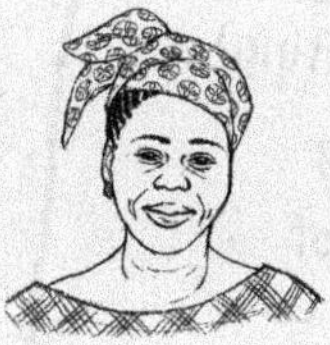

Your fall may have been due to a seizure. I would like to ask you some questions to find out if that is true. Is that OK?

Sometimes when jerking movements happen again and again, it can be epilepsy. It is a health condition that can usually be controlled with medicine.

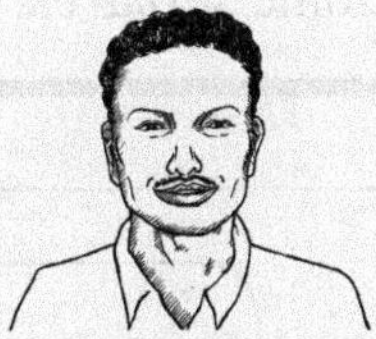

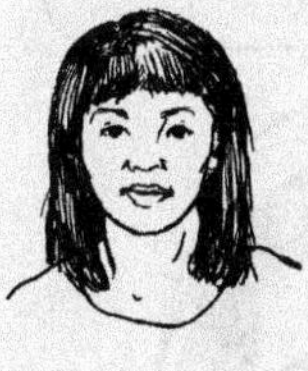

I will not share your health concerns with anyone without your agreement. It is part of my job to respect your privacy.

I am here to listen to all your concerns about your seizures. Answering your questions is just as important as finding the right medicine.

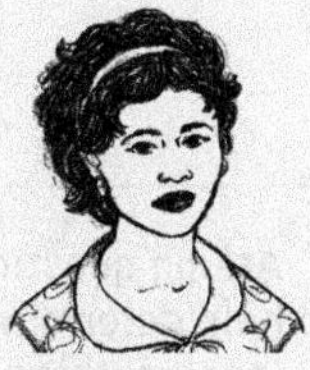

What Maya, Sharon, and Manuel learned about their seizures

Maya, Sharon, and Manuel's stories continue from pages 39 and 40.

Maya

At the clinic, health worker Purnima closed the door for privacy and asked Maya to describe what happened. She also asked Maya how she felt before and after.

After listening carefully, Purnima said, "From the way you describe it, it seems possible that you experienced what is called a generalized tonic-clonic seizure. If that's the case, there are medicines that can help keep it under control."

See page 49 for information about tonic-clonic seizures.

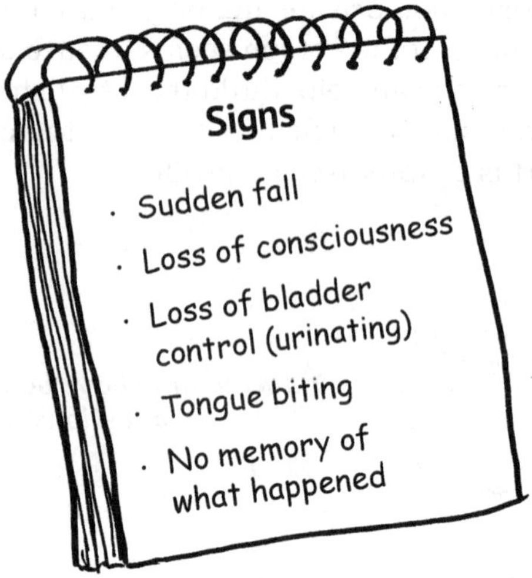
Signs
· Sudden fall
· Loss of consciousness
· Loss of bladder control (urinating)
· Tongue biting
· No memory of what happened

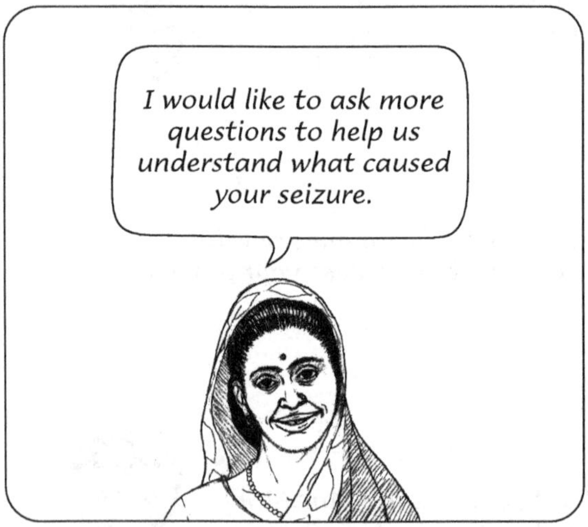
I would like to ask more questions to help us understand what caused your seizure.

Asking questions to collect medical history can help determine what health condition (epilepsy or something else) caused a seizure, and what type of seizure it was. See "Questions to ask about seizures," page 38.

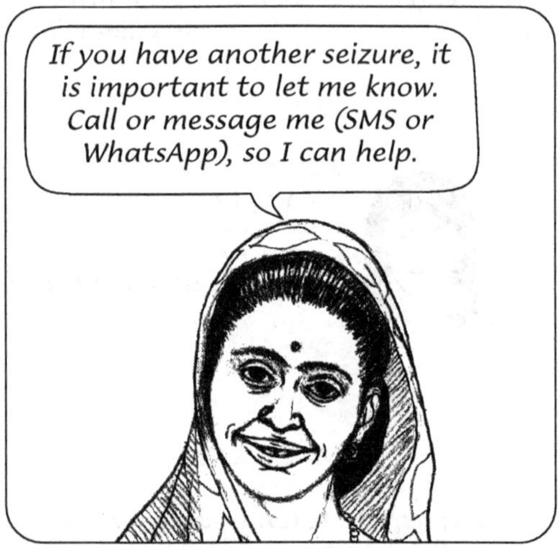
If you have another seizure, it is important to let me know. Call or message me (SMS or WhatsApp), so I can help.

A single seizure might be caused by a variety of issues, but repeated seizures are a strong sign of epilepsy.

Sharon

Sharon and Neo rode on Neo's motorcycle to get to the nearest clinic. In the waiting area, Sharon was afraid they would see someone from their neighborhood.

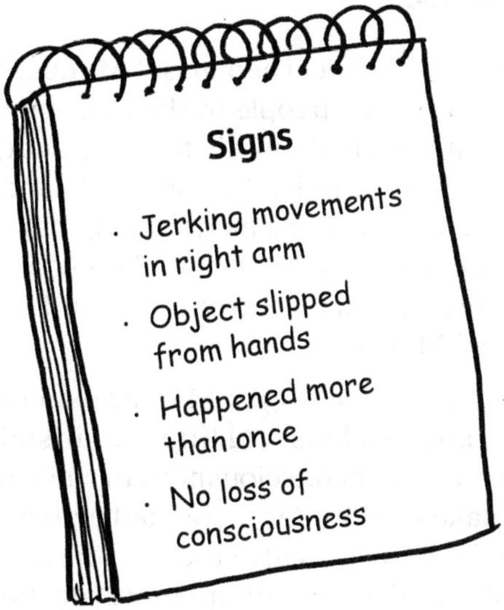

When Loyola, the health worker, called Sharon in, she began by introducing herself and assuring Sharon that everything they talked about would be kept private—she would not share any information with anyone else without first consulting Sharon. Sharon was still nervous and ashamed, but she told Loyola about her arm movement.

Loyola listened carefully and said, "From what you have described, this could possibly be a type of seizure called a focal seizure. These can happen to anyone. I'd like to gather more information and may recommend some tests. If that's what it is, there are medicines that can help manage it."

For information about focal seizures, see page 47.

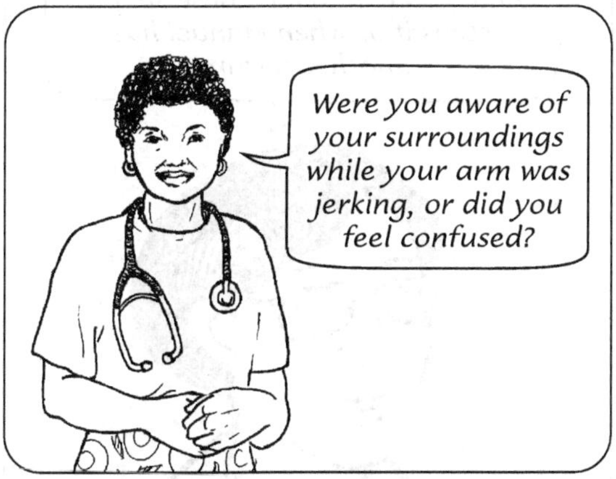

Finding out whether a person remembers the seizure happening and could respond to verbal cues helps tell if it was a focal seizure.

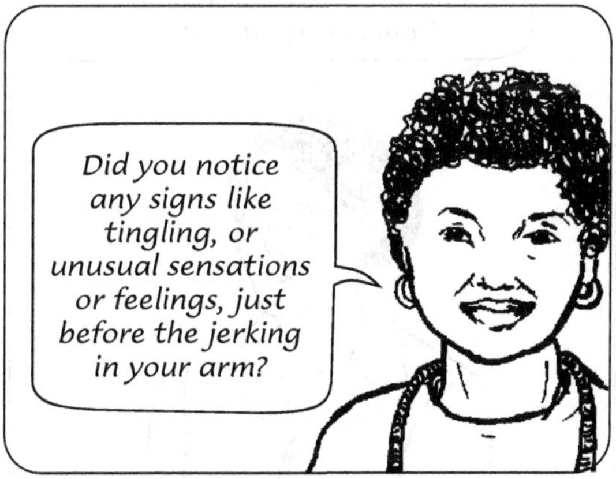

A person's description of sensations right before a seizure can point to the brain region where the seizure began and help clarify the type of seizure.

Manuel

Ana was concerned about Manuel's anxiety that people in their community might learn about his fall. She suggested they go see Luis, the son of a friend who was a doctor in a neighboring city. "If Luis talks to you at his home, then you can stop worrying that someone will find out," Ana told Manuel.

After listening to Manuel explain what happened, Luis told him, "Your sudden fall and loss of consciousness in the garden make me wonder if you had a generalized seizure, especially since you have been stressed and drinking more alcohol than usual. Let's talk about ways you can feel better about your move and transition."

For information about seizures and their link to alcohol use, see page 68.

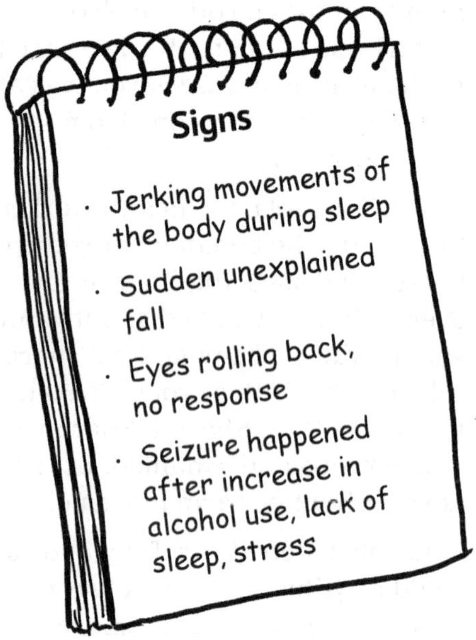

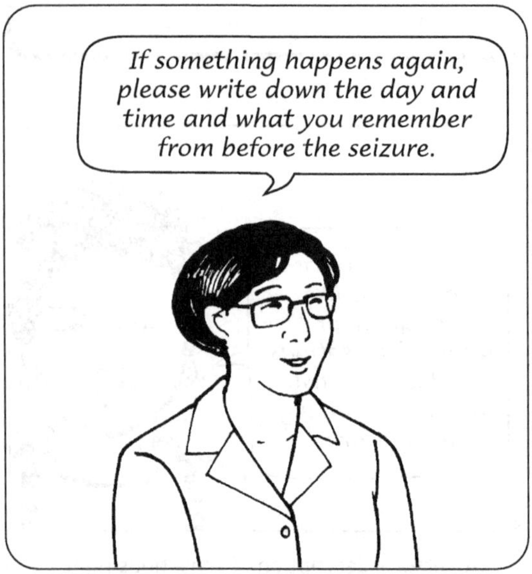
If something happens again, please write down the day and time and what you remember from before the seizure.

A seizure diary or calendar helps keep track of what happens and how often. It can help identify if epilepsy or another condition is causing seizures.

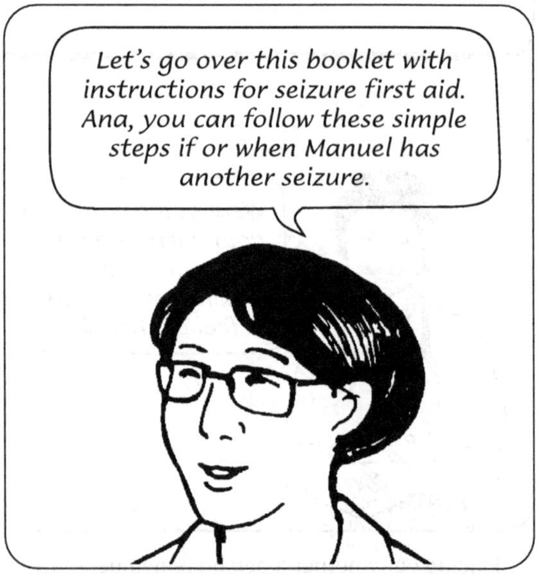
Let's go over this booklet with instructions for seizure first aid. Ana, you can follow these simple steps if or when Manuel has another seizure.

Learning about seizure first aid and training others can prevent injury and raise awareness. For more information, see Chapter 2.

Identifying types of seizures

When trying to identify the type of seizure a person has, first pay attention to what you see during their seizure, such as strong movements like the shaking or stiffening of body parts. Some seizures cause only small body movements, like the fluttering of eyelids, or happen with no movements, but only with staring or unusual feelings. These are harder to spot.

Seizure and epilepsy vocabulary

Medical words used to describe seizures are often unfamiliar and difficult to pronounce. But using them makes it easier to share information about what happens during different types of seizures and which medicines can manage them. Having a common vocabulary for seizures gives people living with epilepsy, their families, and caregivers a way to describe what is happening. This can help them get the support they need. That is why it is worth learning and using all the unfamiliar words.

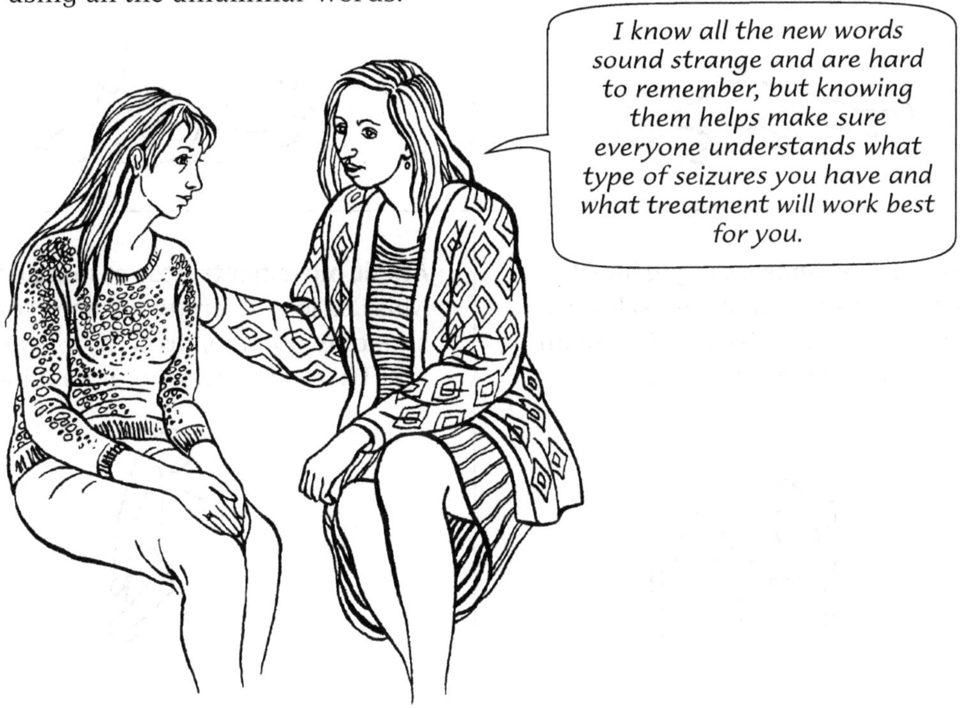
I know all the new words sound strange and are hard to remember, but knowing them helps make sure everyone understands what type of seizures you have and what treatment will work best for you.

Identifying seizures by body movements

The body movements that happen during a seizure can point to where the seizure started in the brain, and whether it might be spreading to other areas in the brain.

The most commonly recognized body movement that happens during a seizure is a convulsion. **Convulsions** are uncontrolled, repeated, and often jerking movements. They can be alarming and are often the reason people decide to get medical help after a seizure. Describing convulsions is important because it gives useful clues to identifying seizure type and treatment that can control it.

The different convulsions and body movements a person may have during seizures have different names:

Tonic convulsions (stiffness): Muscles suddenly stiffen and become tensed and inflexible, especially the arms and legs. A person may fall.

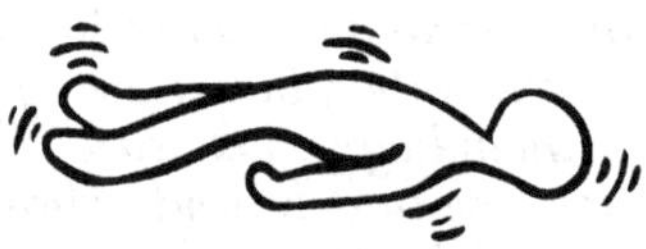

Clonic convulsions (rhythmic jerks): Muscles, especially in arms and legs, rhythmically jerk or twitch, often on both sides of the body. Jerking movements can cause person to fall.

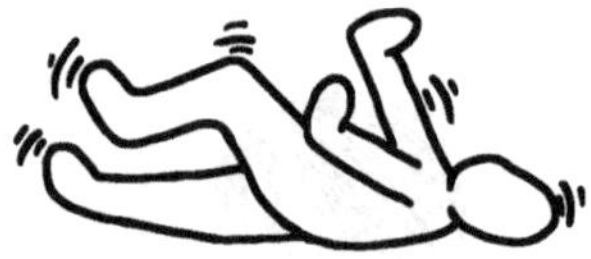

Myoclonic movements (rapid jerks): Sudden, rapid jerks of a muscle or a group of muscles, like a twitch of an arm, hand, or leg, or the face.

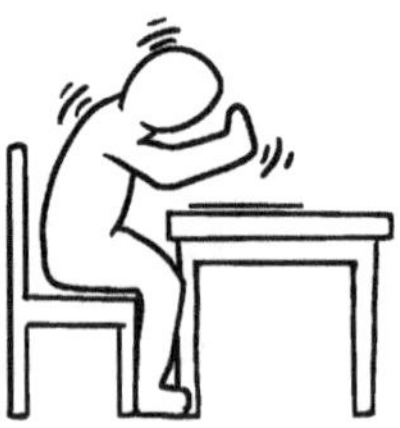

Atonic movements (loss of muscle tone): Muscles lose strength, so a person may suddenly go limp, drop their head, or fall. There is no jerking or shaking.

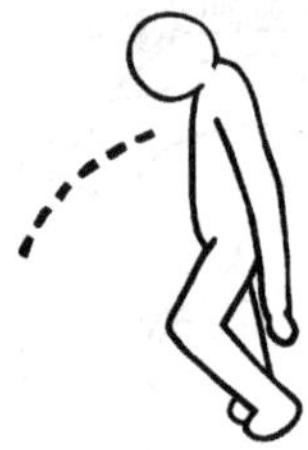

Not all seizures include convulsions. Some seizures may cause other body movements, or only affect a person's alertness, awareness, and attention, causing changes in mood and behavior. It can be harder to know a seizure is happening if it does not cause convulsions.

Generalized and focal seizures

Generalized seizures affect both sides of the brain, and usually both sides of the body at the same time. **Focal seizures** occur in just one part of the brain and cause movements or sensations on only one side of the body. A focal seizure sometimes spreads to involve the whole brain, turning into a generalized seizure.

Both generalized and focal seizures can be caused by epilepsy or by other health conditions. Keeping track of seizure details—which parts of the body are affected and when, what kinds of movements happen, what the person feels or does before and after the seizure—can help determine what treatment will best control the seizures. Use the form on page 80 to gather seizure information and details.

Generalized seizure (Big: starts in, or spreads to, entire brain)

Types of convulsions or other movements:

- Tonic: sudden stiffening of muscles in the entire body
- Clonic: rhythmic jerking in the entire body
- Tonic-clonic: arm and leg muscles become stiff and jerk repeatedly
- Myoclonic: brief, muscle jerks in specific areas of both sides of the body
- Atonic: loss of muscle tone in the entire body
- No movement or very minor movement: see "Absence seizures," page 56

Some possible causes:

- Epilepsy
- Brain injury, tumor
- Recent brain surgery
- Stroke
- Tapeworm infection in brain (neurocysticercosis)
- Tick- or mosquito-borne brain diseases (encephalitis, malaria, others)
- High fever, especially in children
- Withdrawal from or heavy use of alcohol or other drugs
- Low blood sugar or low sodium

Focal seizure (Small: occurs in one part of the brain)

Types of convulsions or other movements, feelings, or sensations:

- Tonic: sudden stiffening in one part of the body, like an arm, leg, or face
- Clonic: rhythmic jerking in one area, like one arm or side of the face
- Myoclonic: brief, shock-like muscle jerks in one area, like a finger, hand, or part of the face
- Atonic: loss of muscle tone in just one part of the body
- Lip smacking, chewing, swallowing, or repetitive hand movements
- Intense feelings and emotions such as fear, anger, others
- Unusual sensations such as tingling, crawling, burning, "butterflies" in the stomach
- Unusual smells, tastes, or visuals (seeing things that aren't there)
- Feeling too hot or too cold, or hot then cold

Some possible causes:

- Epilepsy
- Brain injury, tumor
- Stroke
- High fever, especially in children
- Withdrawal from or heavy use of alcohol or other drugs
- Low blood sugar or low sodium
- Low or high blood pressure

Generalized tonic-clonic seizures

A generalized tonic-clonic seizure affects the entire brain and body. It causes loss of consciousness, falls, and noticeable convulsions. The generalized tonic-clonic seizure is often the most dramatic and most recognized type of seizure.

Generalized tonic-clonic seizures are sometimes called "grand mal" seizures, which means "big illness" in French. It's better to call it a generalized tonic-clonic seizure because it clearly describes what happens—both sides of the brain are involved (generalized) and the seizure has both stiffening (tonic) and jerking (clonic) movements.

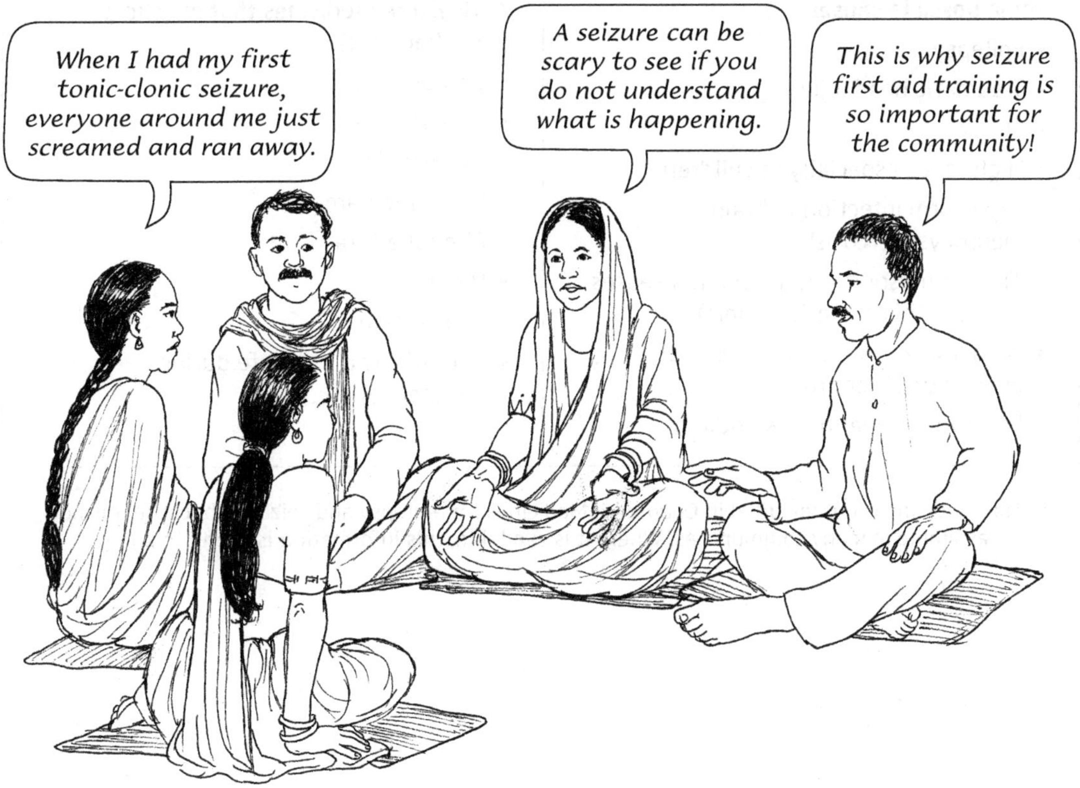
When I had my first tonic-clonic seizure, everyone around me just screamed and ran away.
A seizure can be scary to see if you do not understand what is happening.
This is why seizure first aid training is so important for the community!

If you are not used to seeing people lose control of their body movements, it can be disturbing to see someone have a generalized tonic-clonic seizure. Do not let that stop you from helping them to prevent injury during the seizure. For information about how to give seizure first aid, see Chapter 2.

Generalized tonic-clonic seizure (grand mal seizure)

Description:

- Tonic-clonic convulsions (arm and leg muscles become stiff and jerk repeatedly)
- Loss of consciousness, often causing a fall
- Tongue-biting
- Saliva or bubbles coming from the mouth
- Passing urine or stool during the seizure
- Movements usually last around 2 minutes

Some possible causes:

- Epilepsy
- Traumatic head injury
- Stroke
- High fever, especially in children
- Tapeworm infection in brain (neurocysticercosis)
- Tick- or mosquito-borne brain diseases (encephalitis, malaria, others)
- Withdrawal from or heavy use of alcohol or other drugs
- Low blood sugar or low sodium

Antiseizure medicines that may help (see Chapter 4):

- Carbamazepine
- Lacosamide*
- Lamotrigine
- Levetiracetam
- Phenobarbital
- Phenytoin
- Topiramate
- Valproic acid (not safe during pregnancy)

*This medicine is not included in Chapter 4: Medicines for epilepsy and seizures, because it is not available in many communities. Where it is available, this information is useful to know.

Stages of a generalized tonic-clonic seizure

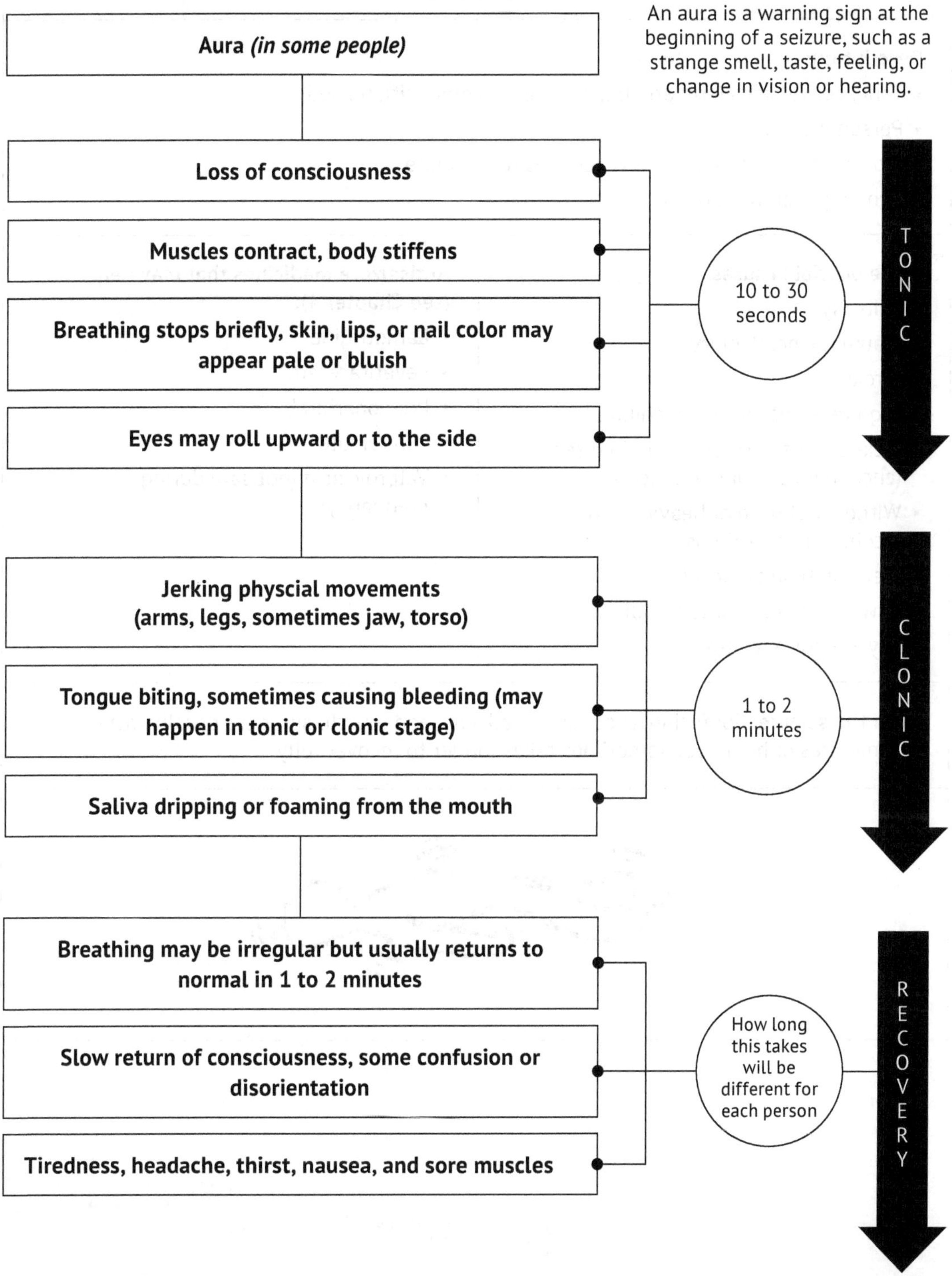

Tonic seizure

Description:

- Tonic convulsions (arm and leg muscles become stiff, tensed)
- Person may fall
- Movements usually last a few seconds to 1 minute
- Can be generalized or focal

Some possible causes:

- Epilepsy
- Traumatic head injury
- Stroke
- High fever, especially in children
- Tick- or mosquito-borne brain diseases (encephalitis, malaria, others)
- Withdrawal from or heavy use of alcohol or other drugs
- Electrolyte imbalances
- Low blood sugar or low sodium
- Psychological causes

Antiseizure medicines that may help (see Chapter 4):

- Lamotrigine
- Levetiracetam
- Phenobarbital
- Topiramate
- Valproic acid (not safe during pregnancy)

After the seizure: Confusion, tiredness, headache, and muscle soreness usually lasts for a few minutes or hours but sometimes takes longer to recover fully

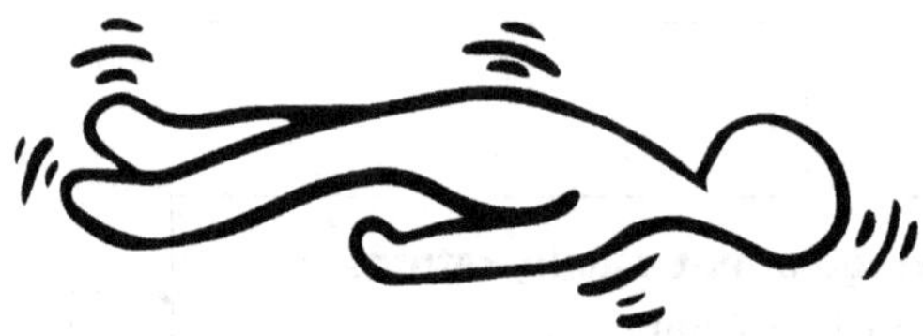

Clonic seizure

Description:

- Clonic convulsions (legs and arms jerk repeatedly)
- Movements can be on one or both sides of the body
- Person may fall
- Movements usually last 1 to 2 minutes
- Can be generalized or focal

Some possible causes:

- Epilepsy
- Head injury
- Tick- or mosquito-borne brain diseases (encephalitis, malaria, others)
- Withdrawal from or heavy use of alcohol or other drugs
- Electrolyte imbalances
- Low blood sugar or low sodium
- Psychological causes

Antiseizure medicines that may help (see Chapter 4):

- Lamotrigine
- Levetiracetam
- Phenobarbital
- Topiramate
- Valproic acid (not safe during pregnancy)

After the seizure: Confusion, tiredness, headache, and muscle soreness can last for a few minutes or hours but sometimes takes longer to recover fully

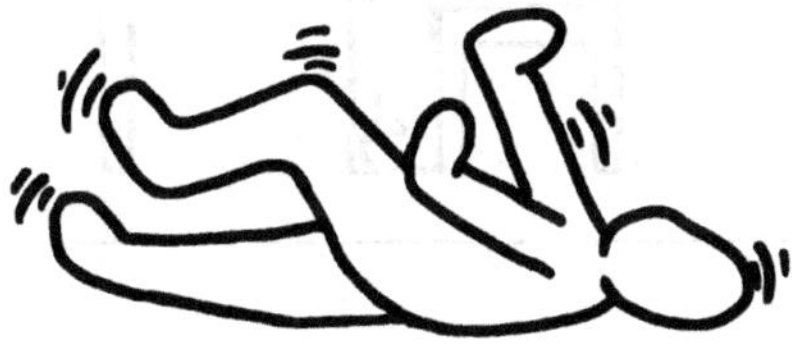

Myoclonic seizure

Description:

- Usually begin between 3 to 13 years of age, may continue into adulthood
- Myoclonic body movements (one or both arms suddenly and rapidly jerk), often causing the person to drop things
- Sometimes affects only the fingers or shoulders
- Each jerk typically lasts 1 to 2 seconds, episodes often happen while falling asleep or just after waking up
- Can be generalized or focal

Possible causes:

- Epilepsy, especially childhood epilepsy syndromes (see page 60)

Antiseizure medicines that may help (see Chapter 4):

- Levetiracetam
- Valproic acid (not safe during pregnancy)

After the seizure: Very rapid recovery

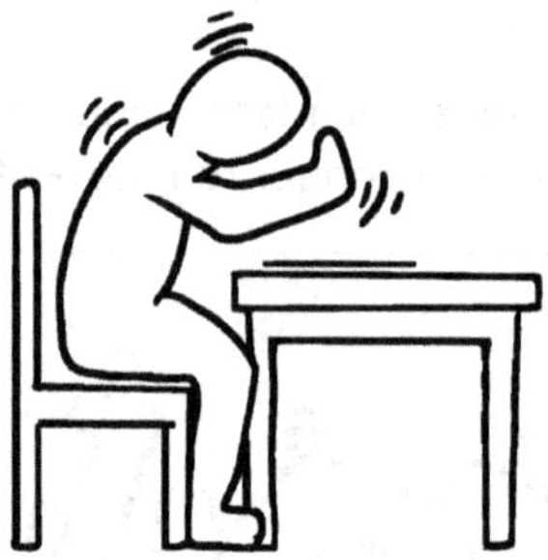

Atonic seizure

Description:

- Usually begins between 2 and 5 years of age, but can happen at other ages
- Atonic body movements (sudden loss of muscle strength), causing person to go limp, drop their head, or collapse
- Often called "drop attacks" because the person falls suddenly
- Usually lasts between 1 and 5 seconds
- Can be generalized or focal

Possible causes:	Antiseizure medicines that may help (see Chapter 4):
• Epilepsy, especially childhood epilepsy syndromes (see page 60)	• Lamotrigine • Valproic acid (not safe during pregnancy)

After the seizure: Very rapid recovery, but risk of injury from sudden fall

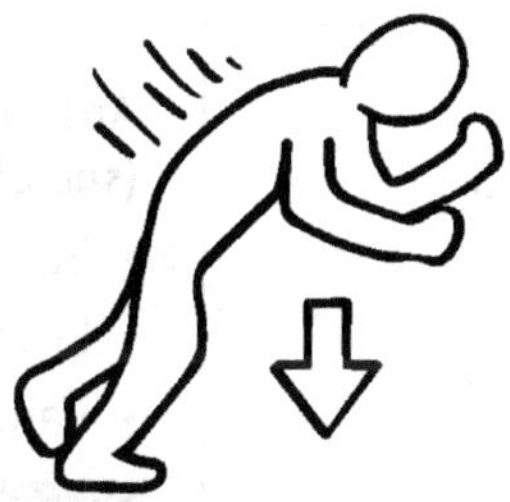

Absence seizures

Absence seizures do not involve convulsions or other body movements. Instead, an absence seizure will cause a brief break in awareness, perhaps with a short period of staring or blinking. Absence seizures are most common in children and often last just a few seconds.

<table>
<tr><th colspan="2">Absence seizure</th></tr>
<tr><td colspan="2">Description:
• Usually begin between 3 to 13 years of age and usually stop during adolescence but may continue into adulthood
• Rarely begin in adulthood
• Blank, empty look on face, appears as if child is daydreaming or not paying attention
• All activity suddenly stops, and restarts after seizure stops
• No response to talking or touching
• Sometimes blinking, fluttering, or trembling eyelids
• Typically lasts up to 20 seconds, can happen many times a day
• Generalized (in rare cases begins as focal)</td></tr>
<tr><td>Some possible causes:
• Epilepsy (especially in children)
• Psychological causes</td><td>Antiseizure medicines that may help (see Chapter 4):
• Ethosuximide
• Levetiracetam
• Valproic acid
IMPORTANT Do not use carbamazepine, it will worsen absence seizures</td></tr>
<tr><td colspan="2">After the seizure: Awareness and attention return, person will likely continue speaking or other activities where they had left off</td></tr>
</table>

When seizures are an emergency

Status epilepticus is a medical emergency!

Status epilepticus is the name for a seizure that lasts longer than 5 minutes. It is usually not one but many seizures with little or no recovery time between them. To someone watching, though, status epilepticus may look like one long seizure. Status epilepticus is a medical emergency that needs to be treated immediately with rescue medicine.

A person in status epilepticus may or may not have convulsions or other body movements. A lack of convulsions can make status epilepticus difficult to recognize. When a person has uninterrupted absence seizures for more than 10 to 15 minutes, this is also a form of status epilepticus.

IMPORTANT Status epilepticus can continue for up to 30 minutes (for generalized tonic-clonic seizures) or 60 minutes (for focal seizures), even after giving emergency medicine. This can cause brain injury and may even lead to death. To learn how to help, see Chapter 2, page 19.

Sudden unexpected death in epilepsy (SUDEP)

When people with epilepsy have access to the medicines and support they need, many injuries and risks to health can be avoided. But even when people know how to stay safe and do everything right, there is still a possibility they may fall victim to a condition called SUDEP.

SUDEP stands for sudden unexpected death in epilepsy. As the name suggests, death from SUDEP happens quickly and without warning. It can shock and traumatize families who are often unaware of its existence until it happens. Thankfully, SUDEP is relatively rare.

Little is known about what causes SUDEP. It can affect people with all types of seizures, but it seems to affect those with tonic-clonic seizures more. Since access to medicine and care seems to lower the risk of SUDEP, preventing it requires community action. More research into the causes of SUDEP is desperately needed.

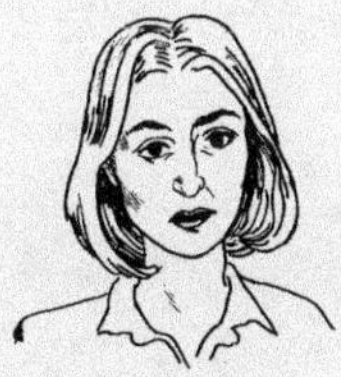

My son was a loving, joyful child, healthy and full of life. Then everything changed in an instant! He died from SUDEP after a nighttime seizure. We had never even heard of this, let alone imagined it could take our child's life. I want more attention to SUDEP, more research, more community awareness.

Seizures during sleep

Seizures during sleep can be hard to notice because the person feels them differently than they would if they were awake and may not notice them at all. If a person having sleep seizures lives with others, their seizures might go unnoticed because they happen while everyone else is also sleeping. Clues to having sleep seizures include waking up with a headache, feeling very tired after sleeping, falling out of bed while asleep, and mood changes.

Talk to a health worker if you worry that something unusual is happening while you sleep. Since all these signs can have causes other than seizures, a health worker will need information from you and anyone who has seen you sleep to figure out what is causing your sleep problems.

<table>
<tr><th colspan="2">Seizures during sleep</th></tr>
<tr><td colspan="2">Description
• Usually begin during adolescence, may continue into adulthood
• Typically happen within 1 to 2 hours of falling asleep or upon waking up
• Can involve convulsions or other body movements
• Can be generalized or focal</td></tr>
<tr><td>Some possible causes:
• Epilepsy
• Brain injury or infection
• Stroke
• Disrupted sleep patterns</td><td>Antiseizure medicines that may help (see Chapter 4):
• Carbamazepine
• Levetiracetam</td></tr>
<tr><td colspan="2">After the seizure: May wake up confused, disoriented, tired, or with unexplained injuries</td></tr>
</table>

For more information about sleep seizures, see Chapter 6, page 194.

Seizures during childhood

During the first 3 years, children's bodies develop quickly as new connections form in the brain, and between the brain and the rest of the body. Puberty, which begins between 8 and 14 years of age, is another time when change happens quickly and new hormones (chemicals that control growth) affect the brain's electrical activity. All this rapid change makes seizures most common during these years. Childhood seizures may be caused by a variety of conditions, including fever and epilepsy.

Fever seizures

The most common seizures in children—fever seizures—are not epilepsy. However, in rare cases, fever seizures can increase the risk that a child will develop epilepsy.

<table>
<tr><th colspan="2">Fever seizure (also called "febrile seizure")</th></tr>
<tr><td colspan="2">Description:
• Happens between 3 months and 6 years of age, most commonly between 6 and 18 months, and rarely during adulthood
• Triggered by a fever above 38.3°C (101°F) from sore throat, ear infection, bad cold, or other cause
• Can be generalized or focal, with tonic-clonic convulsions (arm and leg muscles stiffen, and legs and arms jerk repeatedly) or only tonic (stiffness) or clonic (rhythmic jerks)
• Loss of bladder or bowel control
• Seizure lasts less than 5 minutes, sometimes happens as a group of seizures</td></tr>
<tr><td colspan="2">How to know if it's a fever seizure:
• Age: If the child is younger than 3 months or older than 6 years, fever may not be the cause.
• Previous fever seizures: Children who have fever seizures once may have them again when they have a high fever.
• Fever seizures in the family: If a child's siblings have had fever seizures, they may too.
• Health problems that can cause high fevers and seizures: Diarrhea, viral infection with cold and cough, infection in the lungs or skin, malaria, meningitis, and others.</td></tr>
<tr><td>Medicines: Medicines to lower fever and medicines to treat condition causing it are both needed (see Chapter 4). Antiseizure medicines will not help.</td><td>After the seizure: Child quickly recovers, can breastfeed and eat. Seizures will likely stop when health condition causing fever is treated.</td></tr>
</table>

Childhood epilepsy syndromes

An "epilepsy syndrome" is a collection of signs, symptoms, and seizure types that usually start around a specific age or under certain conditions. Recognizing and treating a syndrome early is important. More than 30 different syndromes affect children and adolescents. Most require care and management for a person's entire life.

Dravet syndrome begins in early childhood, often during the first year of life. A child with Dravet syndrome can have tonic, clonic, tonic-clonic, myoclonic, fever, and absence seizures.

Lennox-Gastaut syndrome (LGS) begins before age 4. A child with LGS may have atonic, tonic, or absence seizures that are slightly different from the typical absence seizure. Typical absence seizures usually involve only a blank stare, but absence seizures with LGS may include muscle movements, such as blinking eyes, smacking lips, or rubbing of the fingers or hands.

West syndrome or infantile spasms (also called "baby spasms") can happen between 3 and 18 months of age, most commonly starting at 6 months. Arms and legs open and close suddenly and the body bends forward. Babies may cry during or after these seizures. Seizures last only a second to 10 seconds, but they can happen close together in a series.

Seizures caused by Dravet syndrome, LGS, and West syndrome can be managed with medicines, but treatment can be complicated. If seizures are uncontrolled, children are at risk for status epilepticus, behavior and mood changes, and delays in learning and development.

A doctor with experience in epilepsy can use brain scans, blood tests, and the child's and family's health histories to find out if seizures are caused by one of these rare forms of epilepsy in children.

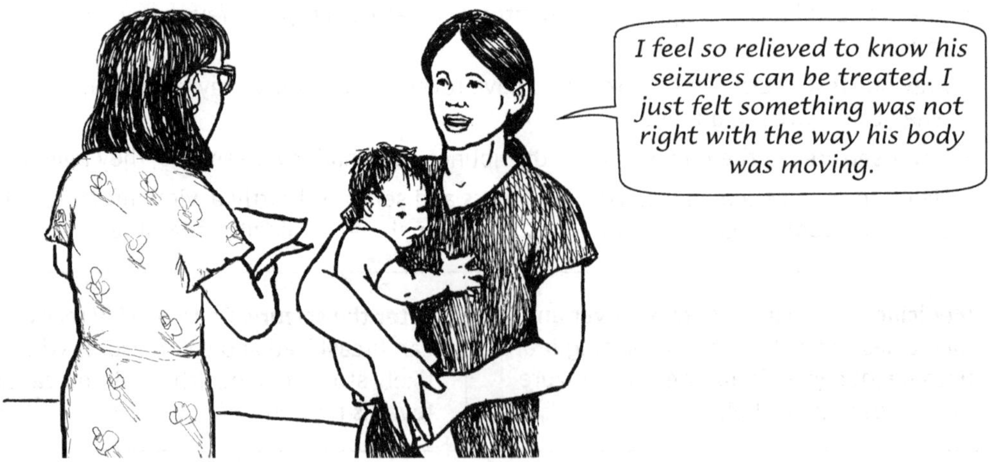
I feel so relieved to know his seizures can be treated. I just felt something was not right with the way his body was moving.

Health conditions that can cause seizures

Seizures can be caused by a variety of health conditions other than epilepsy, including head injury, tapeworm infection, and mosquito- or tick-borne diseases such as malaria, encephalitis, and others. All too often, health workers mistakenly identify epilepsy as the cause of these seizures and give antiseizure medicines that fail to either control the seizures or treat the underlying health condition. If these conditions are not properly treated, a person's illness and seizures may continue, which can increase their risk of developing epilepsy in the future.

See Hesperian's *Where There Is No Doctor* or search the Hesperian HealthWiki: en.hesperian.org/hhg/HealthWiki for more information on the conditions described below.

Seizures after head injury

Falls, vehicle accidents, sports injuries, and physical violence can all cause head injury. Sometimes a head injury may result in bleeding inside the skull, loss of consciousness, and seizures. Not every head injury causes these problems, but they are signs that a head injury has also injured the brain.

Repeated seizures from a head injury need medical attention. Watch a person for 24 hours after the injury and get medical help if they:

- show continuing signs of confusion.
- have a headache that gets worse.
- have seizures.

SIGNS Mild brain injury (also called "concussion")

- Temporary confusion or loss of consciousness
- Not remembering what happened
- Temporary blurry vision or "seeing stars"
- Dilated pupils
- Nausea or vomiting
- Headache, dizziness, or tiredness

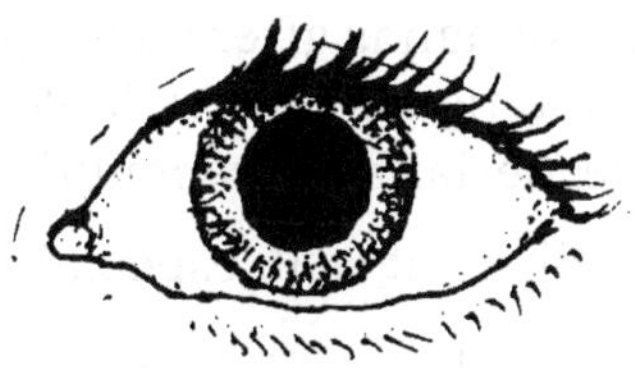

dilated pupil

Rest is important for recovery from a head or brain injury, and the injured person needs sleep. If their pupils are dilated (very large) or if they are confused or unsteady on their feet, wake them every few hours during the first 24 hours to make sure they can think clearly and answer simple questions.

Get medical help if these signs do not improve or become worse. If signs are mild and nothing new develops, the person can return to their normal sleep routine.

Seizures caused by untreated tapeworm infection

Usually, tapeworms infect the intestines. But sometimes they move to the brain, where their eggs cause an infection called neurocysticercosis. This can cause seizures and, if not treated, can lead to epilepsy.

Tapeworms in raw meat (most common in pork) are usually killed when the meat is cooked. When someone eats meat that is not cooked enough, the worms can survive and lay eggs in the person's intestines. The eggs then come out in the person's stool. If the person does not wash their hands properly, these eggs can spread to and contaminate food, drinking water, and water used for irrigation, allowing others to accidentally swallow the eggs. Pigs can also get infected from these sources.

Neurocysticercosis happens when tapeworm eggs inside the intestines hatch into baby worms that enter a person's bloodstream and travel to their brain, where cysts (fluid-filled sacs) develop. These cysts harden over time. Hardened cysts can cause disturbances in brain activity and seizures.

In some people, seizures go away after neurocysticercosis is treated with medicine that destroys the cysts. But in other people, if there are many cysts, if the cysts leave scars in the brain, or if the infection isn't fully treated, then seizures may continue or return. They can be managed with antiseizure medicine.

Prevent infection and seizures from tapeworms

- Wash hands after passing stool and before handling food. If safe water or sanitation is not available, join with your community to find solutions (see Hesperian's *A Community Guide to Environmental Health*, chapters 6 and 7).
- Cook meat well, especially pork, to kill tapeworms and eggs.
- Do not feed raw meat or feces to pigs. Infection can follow.
- Keep pigs away from homes and community water sources.
- Keep fingernails short so tapeworms and eggs don't lodge under them and get into food.
- Wash dishes, cutting surfaces, and cooking utensils with clean water and soap.
- Wash vegetables before cooking them.

Seizures caused by tick- and mosquito-borne diseases

Encelphalitis

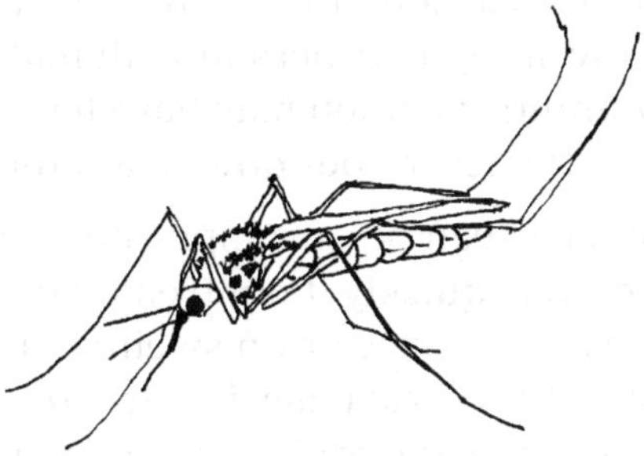

Encephalitis is an inflammation of the brain that is often caused by viruses spread by mosquitoes and ticks. Seizures from encephalitis need medical attention fast. Encephalitis can cause loss of consciousness and brain injury, and can lead to epilepsy even after the person recovers.

Some people with encephalitis may only have a few mild symptoms. Others get seriously ill.

Medical treatment can help a person with encephalitis recover, but prevention is best. Vaccination can prevent tick-borne and Japanese encephalitis. It is also important to avoid insect bites and keep mosquitoes from breeding (see Hesperian's *A Community Guide to Environmental Health,* chapter 8).

SIGNS Encephalitis

Mild encephalitis

- Fever
- Headache
- Tiredness or fatigue
- Nausea, vomiting, lack of appetite
- Mild confusion or irritability

Serious encephalitis

- Severe confusion
- Severe headache that does not go away
- Loss of consciousness
- Seizures
- Difficulty speaking

Take a person with signs of serious encephalitis to a medical center or hospital quickly.

Malaria

Malaria is a blood infection caused by a parasite that spreads by mosquito bites, usually at night. A person with malaria will have cycles of fever and chills. In the beginning, a person may have fever every day. After a while, the person begins to sweat, the fever goes down, and they feel weak.

Malaria can be uncomplicated (mild or regular) or severe. It can become dangerous quickly if not treated or not treated soon enough. Sometimes, severe malaria can cause brain swelling, blocking the flow of blood and oxygen to the brain (signs of cerebral malaria). Seizures, confusion, and loss of consciousness are signs of malaria in the brain. Treatment in a hospital or clinic is needed to prevent death.

In regions with malaria, people with unexplained fevers should get tested and start treatment right away. Even if testing is not available, start treatment if a person has signs of malaria. Because different medicines work in different places, use malaria medicines recommended by your local health authorities.

Prevent malaria by avoiding mosquito bites and draining standing water where mosquitoes breed. Sleeping under an insecticide-treated bednet is a good way to avoid mosquito bites.

SIGNS Malaria

Uncomplicated malaria

- High fever of 39°C (102°F) or more
- Chills and sweats
- Headaches and body aches
- Nausea, vomiting, lack of appetite
- Mild jaundice (yellow in white part of the eyes)

Severe malaria—the above signs plus

- Too weak to sit or stand
- Mental confusion, seizures, or loss of consciousness
- Repeated vomiting
- Rapid breathing or difficulty breathing

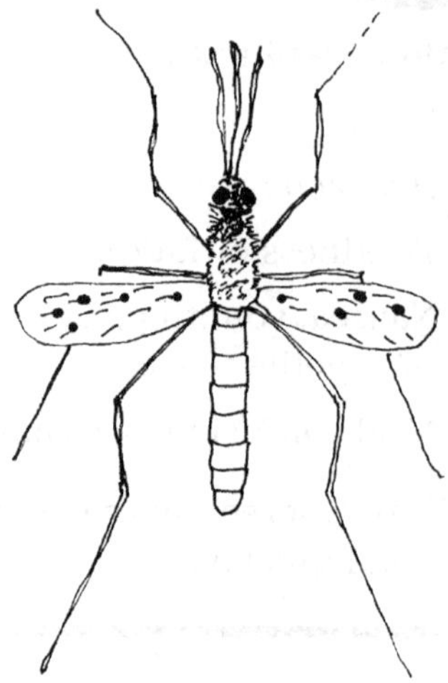

The malaria mosquito may have spotted wings.

Take a person with signs of severe malaria to a medical center or hospital quickly.

Seizures caused by meningitis

Meningitis is a rare but dangerous infection around the brain and spinal cord. It can result from another illness, such as tuberculosis, measles, or mumps, but often it has no clear cause.

A high fever is the first sign of meningitis. It can cause a seizure and loss of consciousness.

Meningitis needs medical attention fast. Treatment involves a combination of antibiotics. If meningitis is caused by another illness, that infection will also need to be treated. Seizures from meningitis can be controlled with antiseizure medicine.

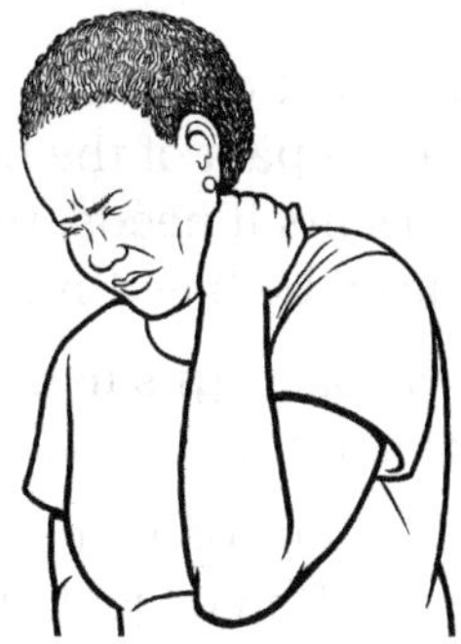

Get medical help as soon you can for meningitis.

SIGNS Meningitis

- Fever
- Vomiting and headache
- Stiff neck
- Sensitivity to touch and light
- Irritable and upset
- Very tired and sleepy

Other physical causes of seizures

- Severe infections that cause blood infections, called “sepsis”
- Very low blood sugar
- Very low sodium
- Severe dehydration (see page 183)

Seizures after a stroke

The most common type of stroke (ischemic stroke) happens when blood cannot reach a part of the brain. When that part of the brain does not get the oxygen and nutrients it needs, the brain is harmed, affecting its activity. Strokes can also be caused by bleeding in the brain (hemorrhagic stroke).

Stroke signs usually start suddenly and can last more than 24 hours, even when mild:

- Numbness or weakness in the face, arm, or leg, often on just one side of the body
- Confusion, difficulty speaking or understanding another person
- Inability to see clearly in one or both eyes
- Loss of balance, difficulty walking
- Face may droop on one side

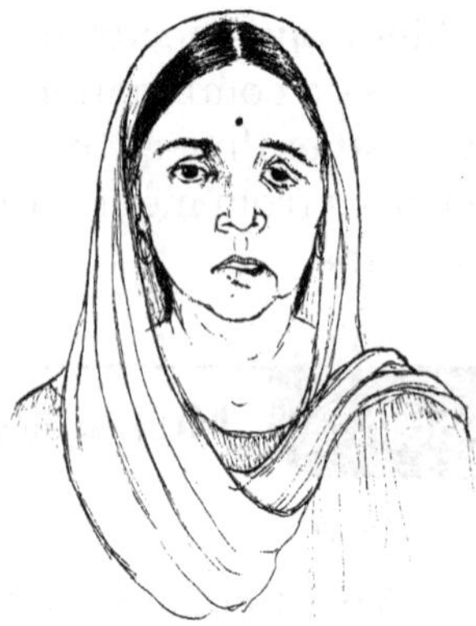

A severe stroke happens when a blood vessel bursts in the brain causing bleeding.

SIGNS Severe stroke

- Severe headache
- Nausea and vomiting
- Stiffness and pain in the neck and shoulders
- Loss of consciousness, fainting, or feeling sleepy

A person who has a stroke needs medical attention quickly. Get emergency help right away.

Not everyone who has a stroke will have a seizure, but it is not uncommon, especially in elders. Different types of seizures may happen. Some people feel confused or have unusual sensations. Others have generalized tonic-clonic seizures where their body shakes, muscles jerk, and they lose consciousness and fall.

Seizures can happen within the first few days after a stroke. As more time passes, the chances of having a seizure are less, but they can happen months or even years after a stroke.

People who recover from stroke without having had a seizure, or who had only 1 seizure, are at low risk for epilepsy. If epilepsy is caused by stroke, seizures can be managed with antiseizure medicine.

Seizures and cerebral palsy

Cerebral palsy means "brain paralysis." It is a common disability among children, caused by brain injury that happened before, during, or soon after birth. The brain injury can affect how the child is able to use parts of their body. The same brain injuries can also cause epilepsy.

Seizures are an early sign of cerebral palsy. Ways to tell if a child's seizures are due to cerebral palsy, not epilepsy, include:

- When you see movement in the child's arm or leg, gently lay your hand on the moving part. If your touch reduces or stops the movement, it is likely caused by cerebral palsy, not epilepsy.
- When you see a twisting or jerking body movement, change the child's position or give them a gentle hug. If this stops the twisting or jerking, it is likely caused by cerebral palsy, not epilepsy.

While brain injury cannot be reversed, antiseizure medicine can prevent further injury. A child with cerebral palsy can learn to use unaffected parts of their body to become as independent as possible.

SIGNS Cerebral palsy

- Limp and floppy body at birth (often, not always)
- Takes longer than other children to hold head up, sit, or move
- Muscle stiffness causes difficulty learning to feed, dress, or bathe
- More than usual crying or irritability, or very often quiet, passive, rarely crying or smiling

Eclampsia seizures

A dangerous condition called eclampsia can cause seizures during pregnancy or shortly after giving birth. Signs of eclampsia are high blood pressure and protein in the urine during pregnancy. If not treated right away, eclampsia seizures can increase the risk of brain injury that, in rare cases, can lead to epilepsy. For information about signs, prevention, and treatment of pre-eclampsia and eclampsia, see Chapter 7, pages 216 to 218.

Seizures from alcohol and drug use

When a person regularly uses alcohol or other drugs, their mind and body can become addicted. Addiction is when a person feels an overpowering desire for something. An addicted brain is unable to control alcohol or drug use, even when it is harming the person's health. Their body feels ill without it, and they may have seizures if they are using very high levels of alcohol or drugs or if they stop using suddenly.

Withdrawal seizures. When a person stops drinking or using another addictive drug, they may go through a period of withdrawal. Physical signs of withdrawal include sweating, nausea, vomiting, stomach pain, and tremors. Withdrawal can also cause generalized tonic-clonic seizures (see page 49), usually during the first 2 days after drinking stops.

Not all people in withdrawal from alcohol and other addictive drugs have seizures. Seizures can happen anytime during the first week of withdrawal, usually within 48 hours of last use of alcohol or drugs. People who have gone through withdrawal before are more likely to have withdrawal seizures.

Addictive drugs that can cause withdrawal seizures when their use is stopped include:

- alcohol.
- opiates, including oxycodone, heroin, and opium.
- stimulants, including cocaine and amphetamines.
- anti-anxiety, pain, sleep, and muscle-relaxing medicines, including diazepam, alprazolam (*Xanax*), and quaaludes.

To prevent withdrawal seizures, reduce the use of alcohol or other drugs gradually instead of stopping all at once. Drinking water to stay hydrated and eating nutritious foods can relieve some of the stress on the body caused by withdrawal. A health worker may be able to provide medicines that lessen the physical effects of withdrawal. See a health worker if withdrawal signs do not go away or get worse.

While withdrawal seizures are not epilepsy, a person with epilepsy who is also physically addicted to alcohol or other drugs is more likely to have withdrawal seizures when they stop using. A health worker can offer help on how to continue taking antiseizure medicine through the withdrawal process. The amount or type of antiseizure medicine being used may need to change.

People quit using alcohol and other drugs in different ways. Some quit at home. Others go to a treatment center. Some rely only on friends, family, and peers for support. Others seek support from counselors or treatment programs. Spending time with people who support your desire to stop using can help you talk about how you are feeling during withdrawal.

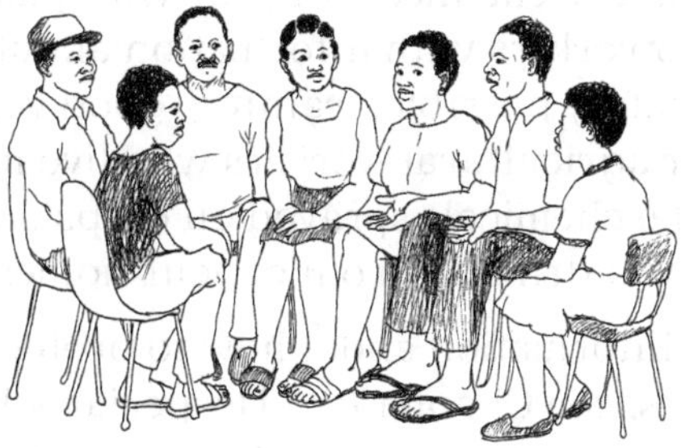
Groups like Alcoholics Anonymous are safe, accessible places to find support.

Chemicals can cause seizures

Some chemicals that get into the body affect the brain and nervous system. They may be breathed into the lungs, absorbed into the skin or eyes, or in food you eat or water you drink. Among the many health problems they can cause are seizures. Although these may look like epileptic seizures, unlike seizures caused by epilepsy, these seizures usually stop after the person stops being exposed to the chemicals.

Chemicals that can cause seizures are ingredients in some solvents, paints or coatings, agricultural chemicals, and cleaning products, and include heavy metals such as lead or mercury. For some people with epilepsy, exposure to chemicals is a seizure trigger. Long-term exposure to chemicals—for instance, to pesticides in agricultural areas—increases a person's risk of epilepsy.

The best way not to be affected by a harmful chemical is not to use it, and to use a safer chemical (or no chemicals) instead. If you must work with chemicals that may be harmful, try to follow the instructions that explain how to use them safely: outdoors or with good ventilation, pouring or mixing carefully, limiting the amount of time you use them, wearing necessary protective equipment (gloves, masks or respirators, long sleeves, boots, etc.), and cleaning up afterwards. Clean yourself, your equipment, your clothing, and your body—especially washing hands and face before eating or drinking.

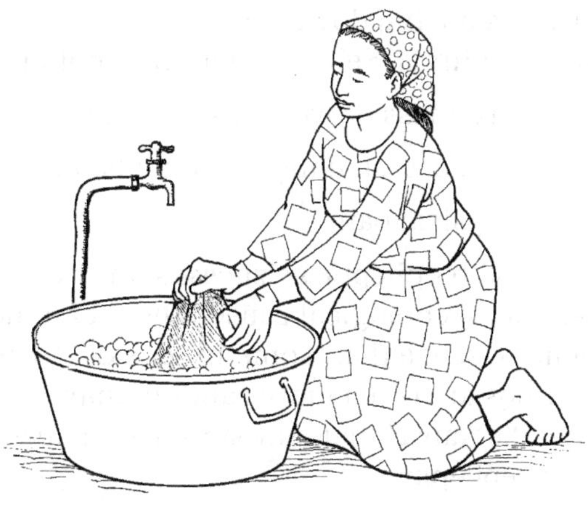
Do not bring chemicals on your clothing home to make your family sick.

If you use chemicals in your workplace, your employer should provide you and your coworkers with information about how to work safely and the conditions that make safety possible: training, good ventilation, protective gear, and a place to wash up. For agricultural workers who live near their fields, it can be more difficult to keep the chemicals sprayed on crops out of the air you and your family breathe, the water you drink, and out of your homes.

For information about how to protect workers from chemicals that could cause seizures, see Chapter 8 of Hesperian's *Workers' Guide to Health and Safety.* To learn about how to protect people in agricultural areas from chemicals that could cause seizures, see Chapter 14 of Hesperian's *A Community Guide to Environmental Health*.

Seizures with psychological causes

Not all seizures are caused by epilepsy or other physical health conditions. Sometimes seizures have psychological or emotional causes. Thoughts, feelings, or memories about painful or difficult life experiences can lead to seizures that may look like epileptic seizures but are not.

Seizures with psychological causes can be reduced or cured by improving a person's emotional and psychological wellbeing, including by changing the conditions causing their stress. Antiseizure medicines that treat epilepsy will not help control these seizures.

Signs of seizures with psychological causes

People who have seizures with psychological causes often describe feeling spacey or "zoned out," having difficulty remembering things or concentrating, or their brain "shutting down." Some people feel disconnected from themselves or their surroundings. Seizures with psychological causes can also have physical signs:

- tiredness or weakness in the limbs
- tremors, shaking, or convulsions
- physical pain

As with epileptic seizures, some people may feel a warning sign before a seizure with a psychological cause. These can include feelings of anxiety, discomfort, or a general sense that "something is off." These feelings are often more random than the specific "aura" that may signal a seizure from epilepsy.

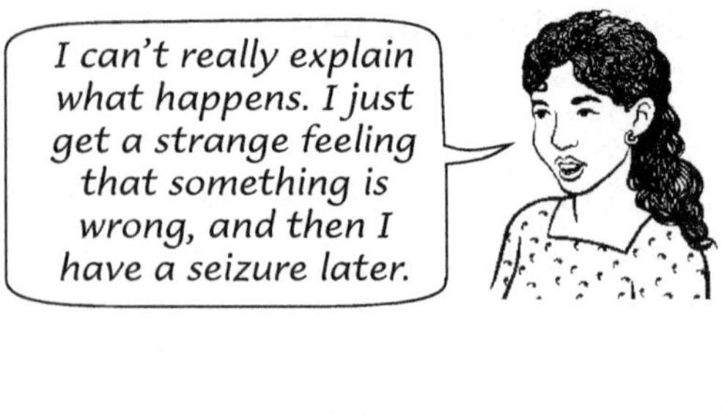
I can't really explain what happens. I just get a strange feeling that something is wrong, and then I have a seizure later.

Differences between seizures with psychological causes and epilepsy seizures

Seizures with psychological causes can look a lot like seizures from epilepsy. Here are some ways to tell them apart.

Seizures from psychological causes	Seizures from epilepsy
Physical effects may differ from one seizure to another	Physical effects are identical from one seizure to another
Emotional trigger common	Physical or no specific trigger
Seizure progresses slowly	Seizure happens suddenly, progresses quickly
Seizure can last longer than 2 minutes	Seizure usually lasts a few seconds to 2 minutes
Person usually conscious during seizure	Person loses consciousness partially or completely during seizure
Seizure rarely causes injury, tongue-biting, or loss of bladder or bowel control	Seizure may cause injury, tongue-biting, or loss of bladder or bowel control
Convulsions or other movements rarely cause arm to hit face	Convulsions or other movements may cause arm to hit face
Eyelids may be held closed or eyes stare without moving	Eyelids not tightly closed, eyes may move irregularly
Person can follow commands, respond, or talk during seizure	Person cannot follow commands or talk during seizure
Brain scan (EEG) will show no seizure activity	Brain scan (EEG) will show seizure activity

Names for seizures with psychological causes

Several names are used to describe seizures caused by psychological or emotional distress, including:

- psychogenic non-epileptic seizures (PNES)
- non-epileptic seizures
- functional dissociative seizures
- conversion disorder

Some health workers avoid using the word "seizure" to put seizures from psychological causes in a different category than epileptic seizures. Instead, they call them "dissociative attacks" or "episodes." No matter what name is used, non-epileptic seizures and the emotional and psychological distress that causes them are real. They are a mental health challenge that can be treated.

Triggers for seizures with psychological causes

Many psychologically-caused seizures are triggered by high levels of stress. Everyone has stress in their lives—from work, illness, family, and life in general. Most of the time, we resolve our stresses without paying much attention. But sometimes, they pile up and become too much for us. Unresolved stress can lead to mental health issues like anxiety and depression. If left untreated, these may contribute to or cause non-epileptic seizures. These seizures can also be a response to a past or continuing trauma. Sometimes, a cause for non-epileptic seizures cannot be identified.

Anxiety and Depression

A person with **anxiety** may be always worried, with no specific situation causing their worry. They may feel a constant dread or fear that something awful will happen.

The worry may come with other signs:

- feeling tense, restless, or nervous
- difficulty thinking clearly
- difficulty sleeping
- sweating, headaches, muscle aches, stomach aches, or unexplained pains that get worse when upset

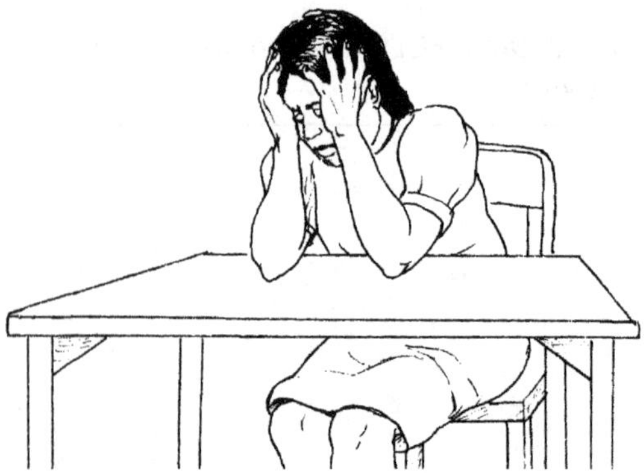

A person with **depression** can be taken over by constant feelings of sadness, hopelessness, or numbness. These feelings last for weeks or months and can be so strong that the person does not leave home or even get out of bed. Different from sadness that follows a difficult event or feelings of distress about the state of their life or the world, depression may feel like a fog in which nothing seems important.

Depression may have other signs, such as:

- sleeping too much or difficulty sleeping.
- loss of interest in activities, such as eating, spending time with others, or sex.

Anxiety and depression not only affect how we feel and think, they affect our bodies. One effect can be non-epileptic seizures triggered by stress and emotional harm. Not everyone with anxiety or depression will have non-epileptic seizures. They usually happen when the stress of these conditions is severe and unresolved.

Of course, anxiety and depression can also affect people with epilepsy. For example, anxiety itself may be a seizure trigger, and if anxiety prevents a person from sleeping, that may also trigger an epileptic seizure. The same may be true for depression.

People with anxiety and depression may need mental health support to help them recover, just as someone with a physical health problem may need help to get better. Encourage and help them find a group or an individual with counseling experience.

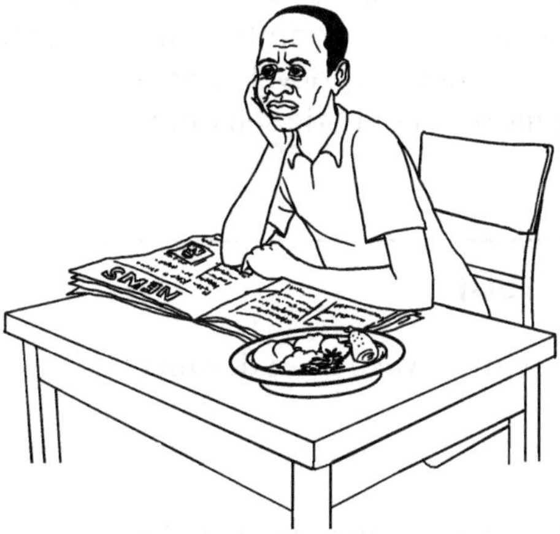

Anxiety and depression can take the joy out of life.

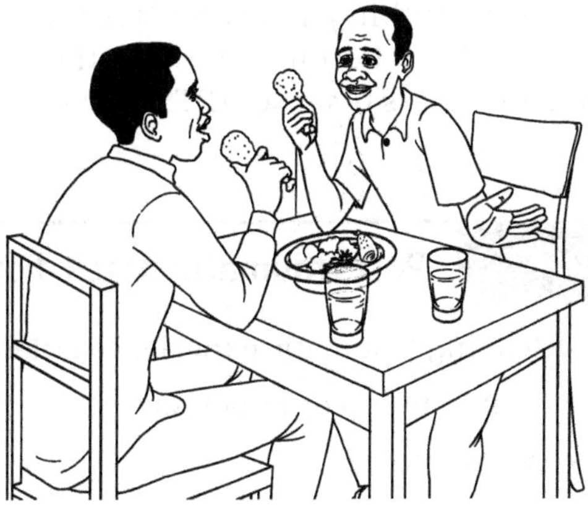

But you don't have to face them alone.

Trauma

Trauma is an emotional or physical response to a terrible event a person saw or experienced in the past or is going through now that feels life-threatening to them or others. Events or situations that can cause trauma include:

- war, or social and political unrest.
- police, mob, and gang violence.
- abuse or bullying.
- physical, sexual, or emotional violence.
- unexpected injury, illness, or death of a friend, caregiver, or family member.
- disasters like flood, cyclones, earthquakes, and fires.
- car crashes or other accidents.
- severe untreated pain due to physical illness or injury.
- sudden loss of basic income or housing.

Trauma can follow:

- a single incident, like a dog bite.
- a horrific event affecting many people, like a mass shooting or war.
- events taking place over a long time, like growing up with abuse in the home.

Trauma can make a person feel unsafe, insecure, helpless, and unable to trust anyone or anything. Instead of feeling better over time, their condition may become so severe that it becomes hard for them to function. They may develop post-traumatic stress disorder (PTSD) which can trigger non-epileptic seizures.

SIGNS **Post-traumatic stress disorder (PTSD)**

- Reliving traumatic experiences (flashbacks) while awake or in dreams
- Feeling numb or hopeless
- Severe anxiety
- Always being watchful and alert to danger, overreacting when startled
- Feeling disconnected from thoughts, feelings, memories, or one's body or identity

Anxiety, depression, trauma, PTSD, and other mental health challenges can also be caused by structural violence: when social conditions harm people because of their identity (race, gender, sexual orientation, class, caste, religion, language, disability, or another characteristic). Structural violence has a greater effect on people with less control over their lives and can put them at risk of harms that cause epilepsy and seizures. See Chapter 9 for information about how preventing violence can prevent epilepsy.

Why don't medicines stop Miranda's seizures?

Miranda worked as a nanny for the Santos family, caring for baby Sophie. She liked it—good pay, reasonable hours, and Sophie was adorable!

Then Sophie's parents started fighting. Miranda tried her best to ignore it, focusing on keeping Sophie happy and healthy. Finally, Mr. Santos left home with a suitcase and did not come back. Both Sophie and Mrs. Santos cried a lot and the house became gloomy. Suddenly Miranda felt she had to care for the family's emotional health.

Then Mrs. Santos started seeing Lucas. When he moved in, Miranda was hopeful he would bring happiness and stability back to the household. But Lucas's behavior toward Miranda quickly worried her. He made unwanted comments about her body and tried to touch her in a sexual way whenever Mrs. Santos was not around.

At first, Miranda just tried to avoid him. She was scared Mrs. Santos would fire her if she said anything. But Lucas didn't stop. One day he grabbed her from behind as she was putting Sophie down for a nap. She got away from him and ran out of the house, deciding never to return.

Miranda began looking for a new job, but because she could not show references from Mrs. Santos, no one would hire her. Low on money and worried she would never find a job, Miranda began having nightmares. In her dreams, she was a child again, being touched by a man and powerless to stop him. The dreams were so real and so upsetting. They kept coming back, night after night.

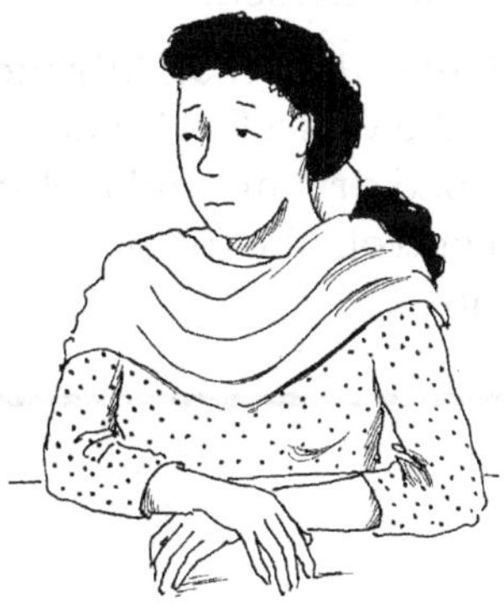

Miranda didn't tell anyone about her dreams, not her parents and not her friends. She just kept being upset by them.

continues

Why don't medicines stop Miranda's seizures? *(continued)*

One night, Miranda woke up from another scary dream. When she got out of bed and walked to the bathroom, the bathroom light seemed brighter than usual, and she felt dizzy. Miranda suddenly found herself lying on the floor beside the toilet with no idea how she had gotten there. She pulled herself up and went back to bed. The experience frightened her enough that she went to a health clinic in the morning.

A health worker listened to Miranda describe waking up on the floor and told her she had a seizure because of epilepsy. She gave her a prescription for an antiseizure medicine and told Miranda to start taking it the next morning and every morning after that.

Miranda took the medicine but continued to have seizures—she had 2 more in the month after starting the medicine. During a follow-up visit, the health worker said that if Miranda really was taking the medicine every day but was still having seizures, it must be because her epilepsy was "drug resistant." (For information about drug-resistant epilepsy, see page 98.)

Miranda wondered if she really had epilepsy, or if she had some other problem. But whatever it was, she had to find a job and support herself. She thought about how the lights got brighter before her seizures. From now on, she would sit down when that happened, so she would not fall and hurt herself.

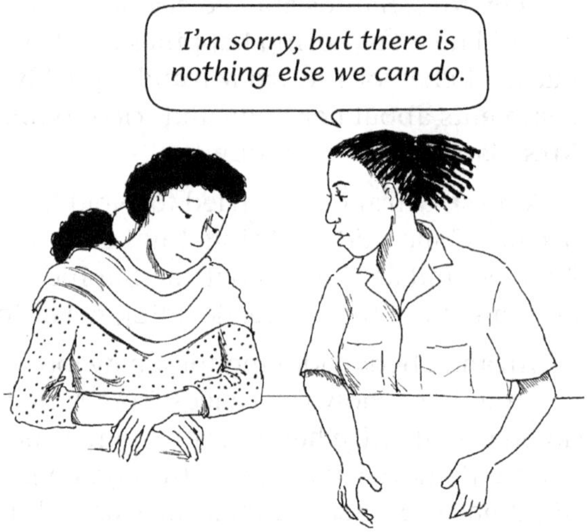
I'm sorry, but there is nothing else we can do.

Other than that, Miranda felt like she was left with nothing but her bad dreams and feeling out of control. She did not know what to do.

Misunderstanding Miranda's seizures

The health worker's failure to try to learn more about Miranda's life and the onset of her seizures did not help Miranda and did not help solve her health problem. Since Miranda quit a job where she experienced sexual harassment and abuse that triggered memories of childhood trauma, her seizures could likely be caused by the unresolved stress and anxiety of these events. This is why epilepsy seizure medicines did not work for Miranda.

If the health worker believed Miranda's seizures were caused by epilepsy, she should have tried another medicine after the first one did not work. Typically, a health worker needs to try at least 2 different antiseizure medicines and be as certain as possible about a person's seizure type before calling their epilepsy "drug resistant."

What to do about seizures with psychological causes

While seizures caused by epilepsy are typically managed with antiseizure medicines, seizures with psychological causes need different treatments, and antiseizure medicines will probably not affect them. But because stopping antiseizure medicine suddenly may make a person feel worse, it is important to talk with a doctor or other health worker about how to safely reduce and stop using any antiseizure medicine. For more information, see "How to stop taking medicine," page 123.

A mental health worker or experienced counselor can help someone try to understand what is causing these seizures and support them to deal with anxiety, depression, trauma, or other mental health challenges. When a person feels better emotionally, their seizures often happen less or stop completely.

Paying attention to the body can also help a person heal. For example, in situations that make you anxious, learning to slow your breathing might help you become calm. But speaking with a counselor or participating in a mental health support group can help uncover the root of the problem causing the seizures. Where the cause of anxiety is related to larger injustices, it is especially helpful to share experiences with others.

For anxiety, depression, and trauma, finding support and treatment that works is key. Talk therapy is useful, and many find that massage, yoga, prayer, and artistic expression help as well. Sometimes, anti-depressant medicines are combined with other types of therapy. Everyone is different. The main point is to get support to get better.

Asking questions about mental health

Signs of anxiety, depression, trauma, and other mental health challenges may not be visible to a health worker. A person may be living with these challenges for a long time before a non-epileptic seizure occurs. Often, it is not until someone has a chance to discuss their emotional wellbeing that connections can be made between seizures and mental health challenges.

Just as you would when asking questions about a person's physical health, show compassion, empathy, and patience, and listen more than talk to help a person speak freely. Taking time to build trust can make someone comfortable enough to talk about their emotional pain.

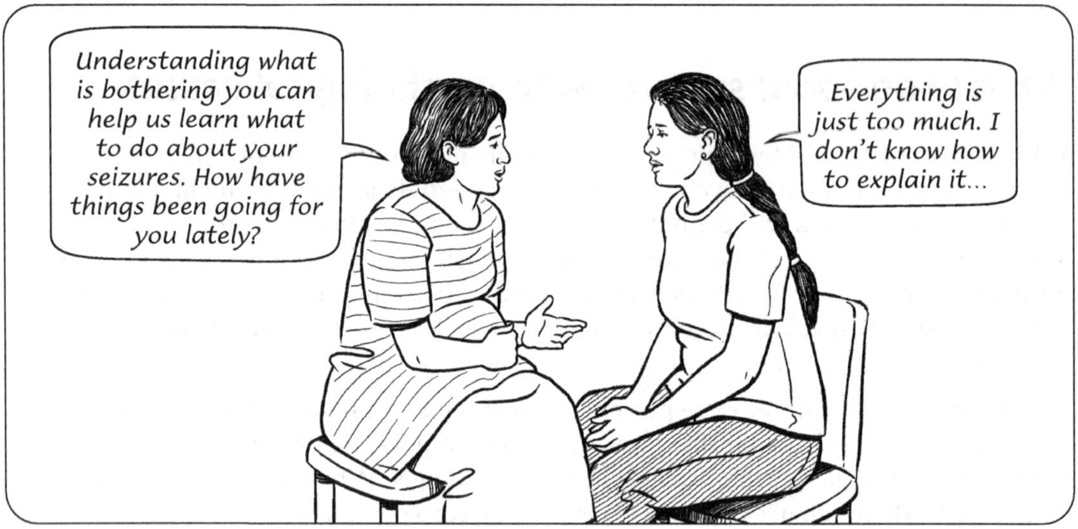
Understanding what is bothering you can help us learn what to do about your seizures. How have things been going for you lately?
Everything is just too much. I don't know how to explain it...

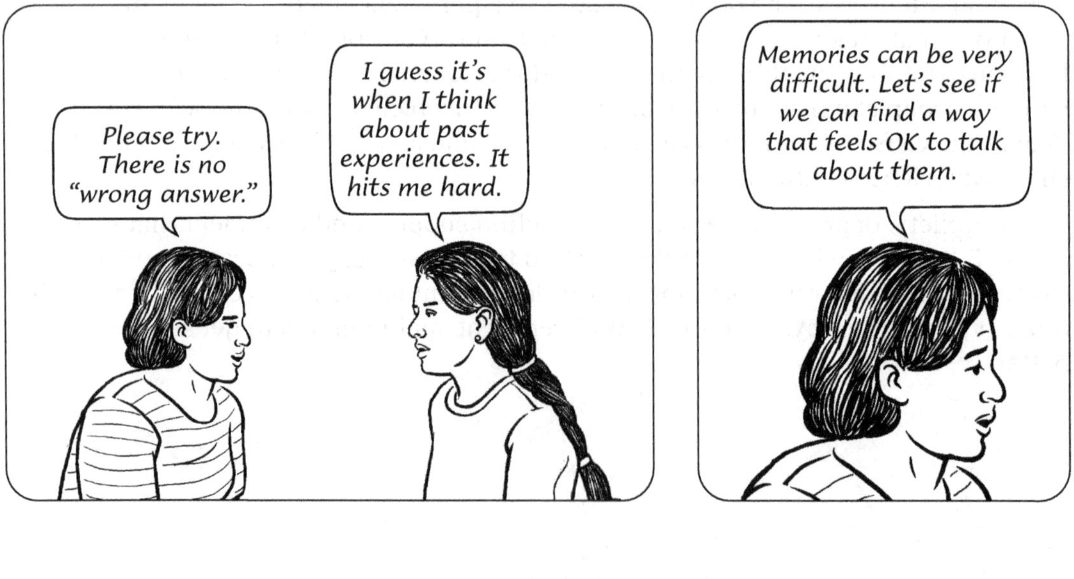
Please try. There is no "wrong answer."
I guess it's when I think about past experiences. It hits me hard.
Memories can be very difficult. Let's see if we can find a way that feels OK to talk about them.

Challenges of promoting mental health

In general, most health workers receive little training about either epilepsy or mental health. As a result, both seizures caused by epilepsy and seizures with psychological causes are often misunderstood. Some people think seizures are caused by God, ghosts, or magic. Even when non-epileptic seizures are understood to be a mental health issue, a person may still be met with ridicule, discrimination, and fear, making it harder to get the help they need. For information about support groups to help with stigma no matter what the cause, see Chapter 5, page 136.

A health worker may not always find the cause of a person's non-epileptic seizures. Emotional and psychological problems can be hard to understand. But by taking an interest in a person's situation, the health worker can offer ideas about how to cope with distress and make appropriate referrals to other services in the community.

For information on ways to manage and treat anxiety, depression, and trauma, as well as ideas to create community support for people with mental health challenges, see Hesperian's *Promoting Community Mental Health*.

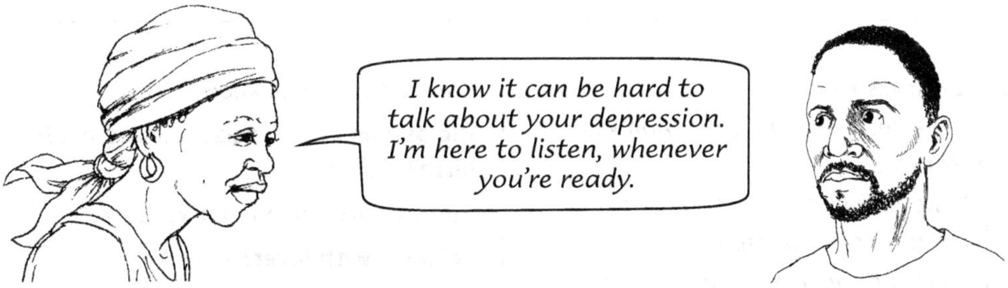

Seizure information collection form

Collect information about seizures on this sample form or add to it, change it, or use it as a guide to asking questions. If some questions cannot be answered, that is OK. Just try to gather as much information as possible. The answers can help identify seizure type, cause, and treatment options.

PERSON HAVING SEIZURE

Name: ______________________

Age: ______________________

Mobile Number: ______________________

Community/Neighborhood: ______________________

Occupation: ______________________

SEIZURE DESCRIPTION

Aura: *Yes • No*

Aura description:

____

Convulsions: *Yes • No*

If yes: *Whole body • Right • Left • Arm • Leg*

Falling: *Yes • No*

Consciousness: *Fully aware • Confused • Responds to voice • No response*

Convulsion type: *Jerking • Stiffness • Both*

Mouth: *Dry • Drool • Foam • Tongue bite • Don't know*

Urinating or passing stool: *Yes • No*

Talking: *Normal • Mixing up words • • Nonsense words • Unable to talk*

Blank Staring: *Yes • No*

Fever: *Yes • No* **Temperature:**

Other signs: ______________________

____

Triggers (list any possible): ______________________

____

KEY SUPPORT PERSON
(spouse, parent, sibling, other family, friend, other)

Name: ______________________

Relationship: ______________________

Mobile Number: ______________________

Other contact information: ______________________

EPILEPSY-RELATED QUESTIONS

Person in family has epilepsy: *Yes • No*

If yes, who:

____

Cause: *Known • Unknown*

Did person having seizures have a difficult birth? *Yes • No*

Seizures after head injury? *Yes • No*

Seizures with fever? *Yes • No*

Seizures from stopping alcohol or other drug? *Yes • No*

Mental health history:

____

____

More information on possible cause:

____

____

____

____

Chapter 4

In this chapter

Getting antiseizure medicines 84
Where can you get antiseizure medicines? 84
Try not to run out of medicine. 85
Using antiseizure medicines 86
Measuring medicines 86
How often and when to take medicine 87
Taking medicine on a full or empty stomach 89
What to do about missed doses 89
How to remember to take antiseizure medicines. 90
Starting medicine for epilepsy 92
Finding the right dose: Dosing by body weight 94
Finding the right dose: Dosing in a range 95
Splitting daily doses into smaller doses 95
Add-on therapy 96
Follow-up visits 96
Changing antiseizure medicines. 97
Changing medicines for pregnancy or breastfeeding 97
Drug-resistant epilepsy. 98
Common antiseizure medicines 98
Rescue medicines for status epilepticus 109
Medicines to lower fever 114
Side effects of antiseizure medicines 116
Common side effects and what to do about them 116
When and how to stop antiseizure medicines 122

Medicines for epilepsy and seizures

Antiseizure medicines can help manage or control seizures caused by epilepsy or other health conditions by preventing seizures from happening as often or stopping them completely. Unfortunately, there are not yet any medicines that cure epilepsy. Antiseizure medicines work by slowing down and balancing the electrical activity in the brain that causes seizures.

Antiseizure medicines mostly come as pills or capsules taken by mouth, and some are available as liquids for children. Most emergency antiseizure medicines are injected into a vein (intravenous, or IV).

Different antiseizure medicines at different doses control different types of seizures. That is one reason why learning to identify different types of seizures is important (see Chapter 3). It can take time to find the right medicine and dose for each person. The best medicine, or medicine combination, for a person with epilepsy will:

- prevent seizures.
- work at the lowest possible dose for that person.
- have few side effects.
- be compatible with other medicines they may be taking.
- be easy for them to get.
- be free of charge or affordable.

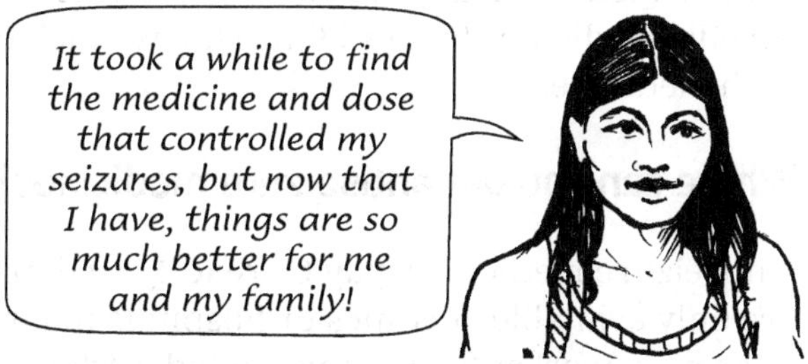
It took a while to find the medicine and dose that controlled my seizures, but now that I have, things are so much better for me and my family!

Antiseizure medicines can help people feel better and give them more control over their lives. For children with epilepsy or other health conditions that cause seizures, antiseizure medicines can help them learn well, participate in everyday activities, and prevent other problems that may be caused by seizures.

A seizure can be caused by a health condition other than epilepsy, such as meningitis, malaria in the brain, or others. The medicines used to treat those conditions are different than the medicines for epilepsy and are not all discussed in this chapter. High fever in very young children can also cause seizures (see page 59).

Medicines are not the only way to treat seizures and epilepsy. See Chapter 6 to learn about how getting enough sleep, eating healthy foods, exercising, and avoiding things that trigger seizures can improve health and make medicines work better. Sometimes a special diet will help control seizures, even when medicines do not (see "Drug-resistant epilepsy," page 98).

Getting antiseizure medicines

For many years, only a few antiseizure medicines were available. Research in the past few decades has led to the development of many new medicines. These provide more treatment options and may have fewer side effects or be easier to combine with other medicines.

Unfortunately, newer medicines may not be available everywhere or may cost more than most people can afford. Making sure antiseizure medicines are available to everyone who needs them is one of the greatest challenges facing people with epilepsy worldwide.

Medicine names

Medicines usually have at least 2 names. The generic (or scientific or chemical) name is almost always the same all over the world. Companies that make medicines often give each medicine they make a brand name. The same medicine made by 2 different companies will have 2 different brand names. In this book, we use generic names. Although they contain the same ingredients and their quality is just as good, generic medicines usually cost less than brand name medicines. In the boxes about specific medicines (pages 99 to 115), we include examples of brand names for each medicine.

Where can you get antiseizure medicines?

Antiseizure medicines may be readily available where you live. But often, they are only available at clinics or hospitals in large towns or cities. A health worker, pharmacy worker (sometimes called a "chemist"), or a person with epilepsy can help you learn whether the antiseizure medicine you need is available in your area, either as a generic or a brand name medicine.

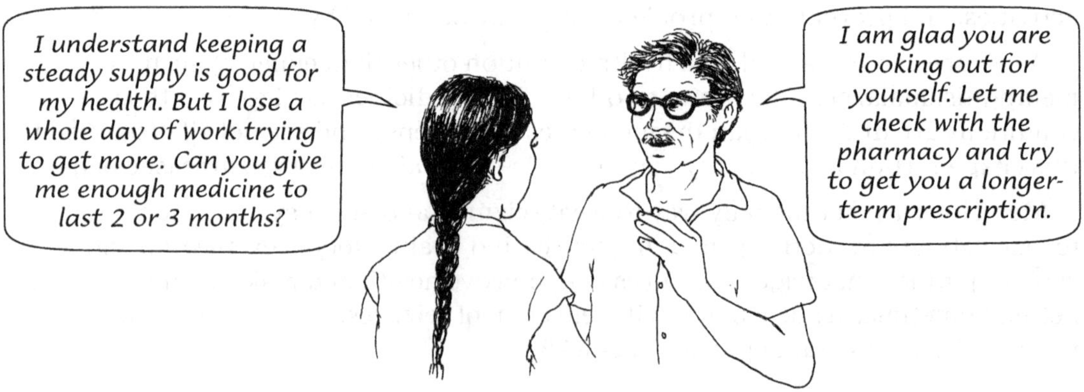

Try not to run out of medicine

Because most antiseizure medicines must be taken every day, it is important to have a steady supply. If someone misses a dose or suddenly stops taking their medicine, it can cause them to have seizures again. Talk to a pharmacist or other health worker to know if the medicine you need is regularly available in your community. If it is sometimes not available or is only available at places difficult for you to get to, find out if you can get larger refills or where you can get more if local supplies run out. If possible, keep enough medicine on hand for a month. For information about what to do about missed doses, see page 89.

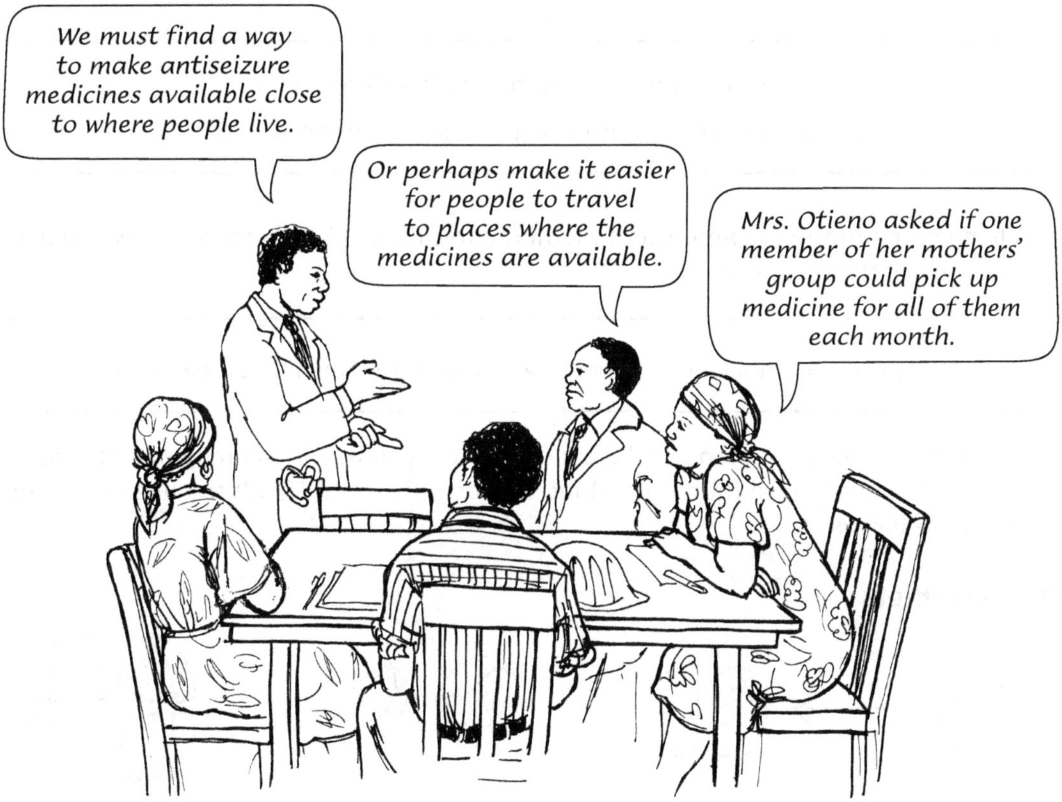
We must find a way to make antiseizure medicines available close to where people live.
Or perhaps make it easier for people to travel to places where the medicines are available.
Mrs. Otieno asked if one member of her mothers' group could pick up medicine for all of them each month.

Do not share medicine

People with epilepsy control their seizures with different doses of different antiseizure medicines. This makes safely sharing antiseizure medicine with another person difficult and maybe even dangerous. Talk to a health worker if your medicine supply is running out and medicine is not available or affordable.

Using antiseizure medicines

Measuring medicines

Medicines come as tablets, capsules, powders, or liquids. The amount of medicine in a tablet, capsule, or liquid is important to know so the correct dose can be given. The amount is indicated on the label or on a sticker on the medicine packet. Look closely—it may be in small print! The amount of medicine contained in each tablet or capsule is commonly given in grams (g), milligrams (mg), or micrograms (mcg). For information about measuring liquids, see page 87.

1g = 1000 mg (1 gram has 1000 milligrams)

1 mg = 1000 mcg (1 milligram has 1000 micrograms)

When you combine the amount of medicine to take with how many times a day to take it, you get the daily dose.

Daily dose = amount of medicine × number of times taken each day

If a medicine does not come in the exact amount you need, you may need to take pieces of a tablet or more than one tablet. It is usually too difficult to cut a tablet into more than 4 pieces.

Cutting tablets

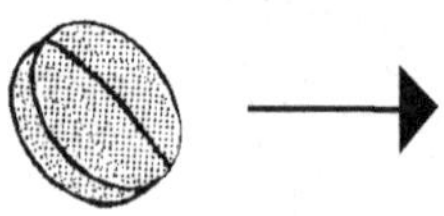

1 tablet
(one whole tablet)

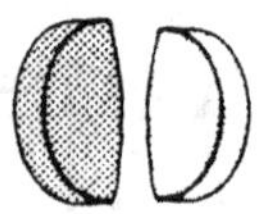

½ tablet
(half of a tablet)

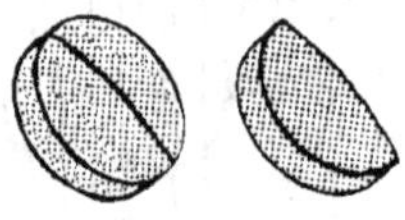

1 ½ tablet
(one and one-half tablets)

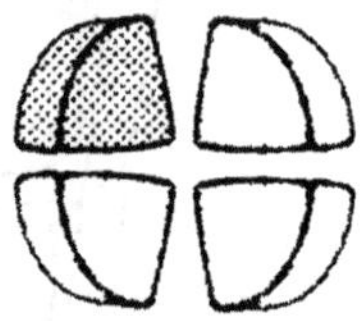

¼ tablet
(one quarter or one-fourth of a tablet)

If you need to cut tablets regularly, find out if you can purchase a small, inexpensive, pill-cutting tool to use at home.

Measuring liquid medicines

Doses for syrups, suspensions, injections in liquid form, or liquids taken by mouth will note how much medicine is to be taken, for example: 10 ml (milliliters) or 10 cc (cubic centimeters). A cubic centimeter is the same as a milliliter. Household spoons come in all different sizes and cannot be depended on as accurate measures. If a liquid medicine does not come with a special measuring spoon or dropper, take it to the pharmacy and ask them to measure exactly how much your spoon or small glass or container holds. Try as best you can to measure the exact dose of medicine.

1 tablespoon (Tbsp) = 15 ml

1 teaspoon (tsp) = 5 ml

1 Tbsp = 3 tsp

When instructions for a medicine say: Take 1 tsp, this means: Take 5 ml.

How often and when to take medicine

Different antiseizure medicines are effective in the body for different lengths of time. Some have effects that are longer-lasting, while others have effects that wear off more quickly. By taking antiseizure medicine at the same time every day, you are better able to keep a constant level of medicine in your body, which helps the medicine work best.

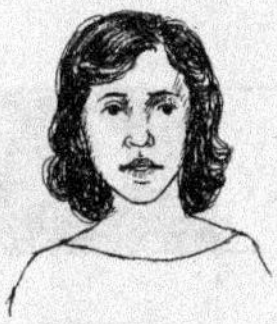

When I discuss taking antiseizure medicine, I talk with the person about how taking medicine at specific times helps to keep the level of medicine constant in the body. This is key to managing and controlling seizures.

Taking a dose of antiseizure medicine more often or in a larger amount than recommended may make you feel sleepy, dizzy, nauseous, or slow. It may give you a headache or make you feel distant or uninterested in things. But these may also be side effects of a correct dose of antiseizure medicine. If your medicine is causing these reactions and they are difficult to manage, talk to a health worker.

If you take medicine once a day, get in the habit of taking it before going to bed or when you get up in the morning. Unless the instructions specify a certain time, find a time that works for you that you will remember.

If a medicine needs to be taken two times a day, take it in the morning and 12 hours later in the evening.

If a medicine needs to be taken three times a day, take it 8 hours apart throughout the day. This may mean taking the first dose early in the morning or the third dose late at night.

If you are writing a note for someone about how much medicine to take each day and when to take it, pictures can be helpful. Draw instructions like these and explain that 2 times means 12 hours between doses, and 3 times means 8 hours between doses. Use the spaces under the pictures showing sunrise, daytime, and nighttime to show how much medicine to take. Explain carefully. For example:

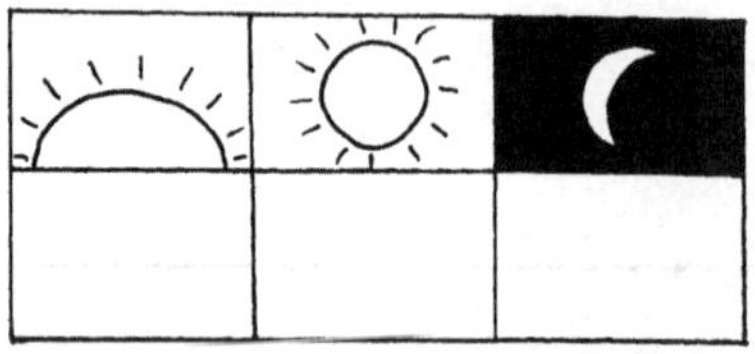

This means take 1 tablet 2 times a day. Take 1 tablet in the morning, and then another tablet 12 hours later in the evening.

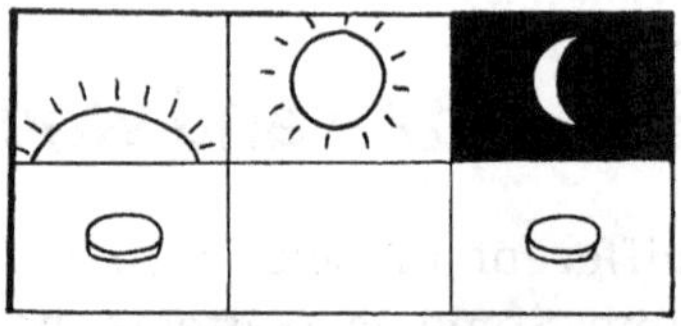

This means take ½ (one-half) tablet 3 times a day. Take ½ tablet in the morning, ½ tablet 8 hours later during the day, and ½ tablet 8 hours later at night.

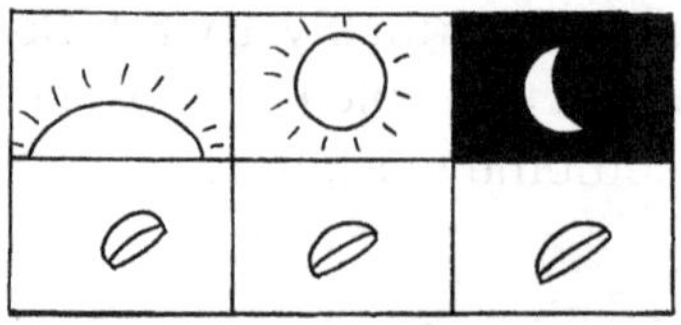

This means take 1 capsule 3 times a day. Take 1 capsule in the morning, 1 capsule 8 hours later during the day, and 1 capsule 8 hours later at night.

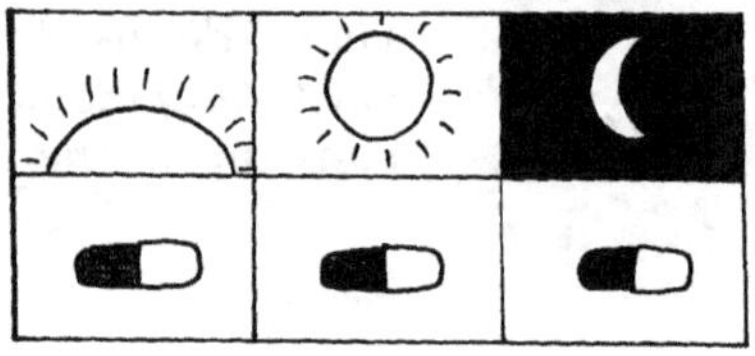

Remember: Taking more medicine, or taking it more often, may not be better for your seizure control. But it will make you run out of medicine faster.

Swallowing whole tablets or crushing them

When taking antiseizure medicines as tablets, swallowing whole tablets with water is often recommended. Some tablets can be safely crushed and taken mixed in water. Others must not be crushed because it can affect how the medicine is absorbed in the body. Check with your doctor or health worker about whether a medicine is "crushable" and how best to do so.

Crushed tablets may taste unpleasant. Bad taste can be masked by eating something sweet, like jam or honey, immediately after taking the medicine.

Especially for children and others who have difficulty swallowing tablets and capsules, it helps to sit up or stand when taking medicine and also to drink some water immediately after. Avoid chewing or biting into tablets and capsules.

Taking medicine on a full or empty stomach

Some medicines are more comfortable to digest if taken with food, and others are better taken without food. Check the instructions or ask your health worker if it makes a difference for each medicine.

If the antiseizure medicine works best when taken on an empty stomach, take it:

- at least 1 hour before a meal, or
- at least 2 hours after finishing a meal.

If the antiseizure medicine works better with food, to help reduce stomach upset and diarrhea, take it:

- with a meal or right after.

Try to stick to the same routine daily to help keep medicine levels constant in the body. Listen to your body and pay attention to how your stomach feels. If you have stomach upset or diarrhea, talk to a health worker to see if there are changes to how you take your medicine that might help you feel better.

What to do about missed doses

Sometimes missing a dose of medicine cannot be helped. But when doses are missed regularly, the medicines may stop controlling seizures. If a medicine is missed after the body has gotten used to it, it can trigger a "breakthrough seizure."

For some people, epilepsy causes memory problems that make it difficult to remember to take medicine. Ask friends or family members to remind you to take your medicine at the right times each day.

If for whatever reason you did not take your medicine, do not take twice as much for your next dose. If it is 6 hours or more until your next dose, take the missed dose as soon as possible. Otherwise, wait to take your next dose as scheduled and continue with the following doses on your regular schedule.

HOW TO Remember to take antiseizure medicines

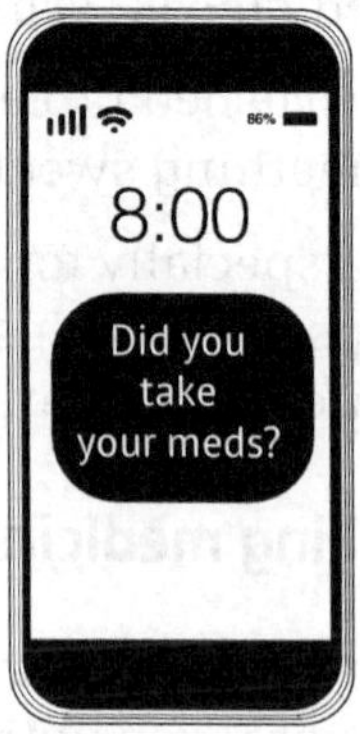

Some people use meals, tea or coffee time, or bedtime as reminders to take their medicine. Others use charts, calendars, phone alarms, mobile phone apps, or weekly pill organizers, or they place the medicine in a spot they see every day. Family members and caregivers can support and encourage people with seizures to keep track of when to take their antiseizure medicine.

Use a weekly pill organizer

Many people use a pill organizer with 7 sections, 1 for each day of the week.

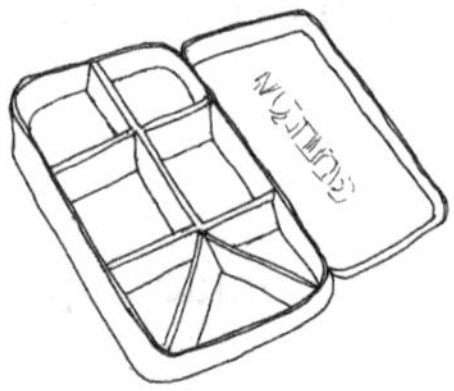

They fill it on the same day each week. This way they know what medicine to take each day and can see if they took their medicines. Pill organizers can be made using wood, plastic, cardboard, or very heavy paper to make dividers in a metal tin. Each week, fill the 7 compartments with the pills you need for each day.

Link taking antiseizure medicine with a daily activity

Connect taking medicine with any activity you always do at the same time, such as:

- after brushing your teeth or bathing in the morning,
- when you hear a morning or evening call to prayer, or
- when a favorite television or radio show begins.

continues

HOW TO Remember to take antiseizure medicines *(continued)*

Turn the bottle upside down

If you take medicine in the morning, turn the pill bottle upside down before going to bed and place it where you will see it when you wake up. Seeing the bottle upside down will remind you to take your medicine. Then turn the bottle right side up so you know that you took it.

Use a calendar to track medicine

Find or make a calendar that shows each day of the week. Mark it when you take your medicine. A health worker might give you a chart to track your medicine use. You can show and discuss your chart with them during your follow-up visits.

Name: Abel
Month: April

Medicine/Dose: 1 tablet, carbamazepine 200 mg (*Tegretol*) at 8 am. 1 tablet at 8 pm.

	Sun	Mon	Tue	Wed	Thur	Fri	Sat
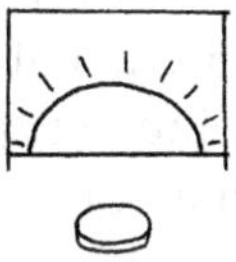 8 am	√	√		√	√	√	√
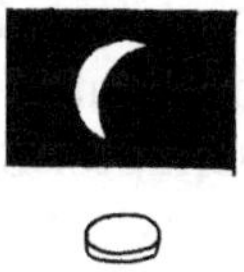 8 pm	√	√	√	√	√	√	√

Using technology to help people remember to take antiseizure medicine

In Kenya, the Kenya Association for the Welfare of People with Epilepsy (KAWE) has a mobile messaging service that sends reminders as SMS messages to remind people with epilepsy to take their antiseizure medicine. The program has enrolled 1,200 people with epilepsy. KAWE is trying out different SMS strategies to see what works best—some people get texts only, others receive only a picture, and some get both.

To keep it simple, they limit message length to 120 to 140 characters. Sometimes the message includes words of support or motivation. All graphics are hand-drawn by a local artist and the picture files work on all mobile phone types.

The program not only reminds people to take their medicine each day—the regular, positive messages help people with epilepsy and their caregivers develop strong habits that support better seizure control and safety.

Starting medicine for epilepsy

People start medicines for epilepsy when 2 or more seizures happen more than 24 hours apart and it is clear that no other condition is causing the seizures. A doctor may suggest starting antiseizure medicines after only one seizure, especially for very young children. This may be because the danger from seizures can be greater than the potential side effects of antiseizure medicines, or because the seizure type and person's health history suggest they have epilepsy or an increased risk for repeated seizures.

Health workers who regularly treat seizures and epilepsy will ask many questions to identify the seizure type and what is causing seizures. This helps them determine the best treatment and medicine for a person's seizures. For information about questions that health workers may ask about epilepsy and seizures, see Chapter 3, page 38.

A seizure can be caused by a health condition other than epilepsy, such as meningitis, malaria in the brain, or others. High fever in very young children can also cause seizures. The medicines used to treat these conditions are different than the medicines for epilepsy and are not all discussed in this chapter.

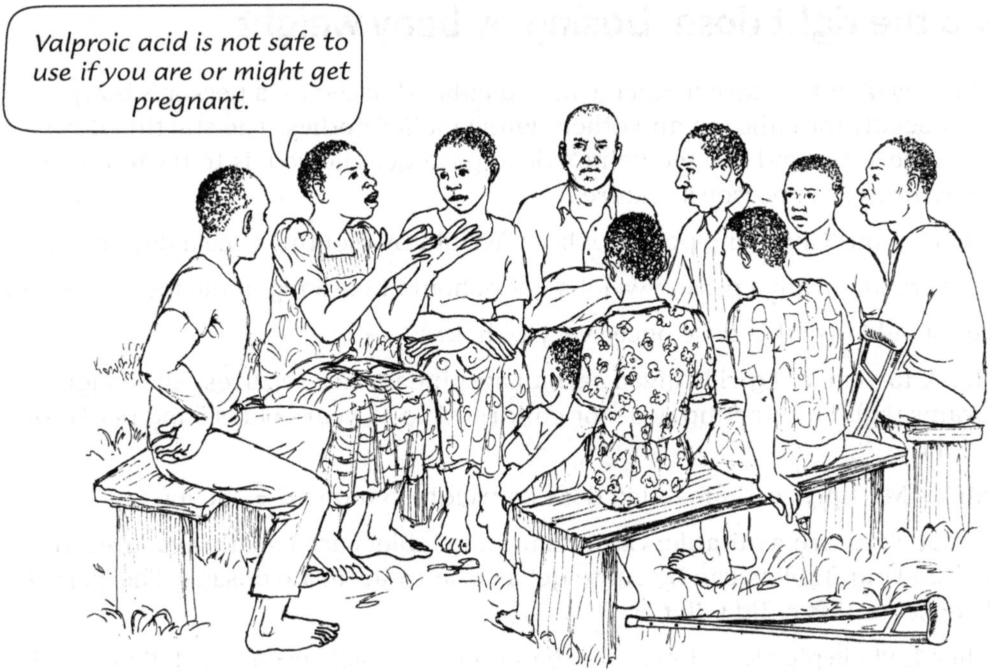
Valproic acid is not safe to use if you are or might get pregnant.

Sharing information about medicines helps educate entire communities about ways to treat epilepsy with the least amount of risk.

Tell the health worker if you are:

- **taking any other medicines.** Medicines that are safe and effective can sometimes not work well or cause harm when taken with another medicine, for instance, some birth control pills.
- **pregnant or breastfeeding.** Antiseizure medicines can pass to the baby during pregnancy or through breast milk. For information about the safety of medicines during pregnancy and breastfeeding, see Chapter 7.

Once you and your healthcare team decide on a medicine, you will start using a standard dose. Typically, a dose starts low and is slowly increased until seizures are controlled. If the medicine does not stop your seizures or if it causes discomfort or other problems, the doctor may adjust the dose or give you a different medicine to try. Finding the best medicine and the best dose can take time.

If the medicine you start taking does not work at all or does not work well enough, you may have a different type of seizure disorder and need a different antiseizure medicine.

For example, juvenile myoclonic seizures look a lot like generalized tonic-clonic seizures. But instead of treating them with carbamazepine, they respond to valproic acid or lamotrigine.

Finding the right dose: Dosing by body weight

The first doses of antiseizure medicine are calculated based on a person's body weight, especially for children and others with smaller bodies. The starting dose is typically at the lower end of a medicine's dosing range. The goal is to try to find a dose that will stop the person's seizures.

The instruction "Give 5 mg per kg of body weight by mouth 1 time a day" means:

- for every kilogram a person weighs, they should take 5 mg of the medicine, and
- they should take this dose once every 24 hours.

Example: A 10-year-old girl is given carbamazepine for her seizures. She weighs 32 kilograms (kg). The starting dose for children 1 to 11 years old is 5 mg per kg of body weight.

Calculation: Multiply recommended dose by weight: 5 mg × 32 = 160 mg

What tablet sizes are available: Carbamazepine tablets are usually available in 100 mg or 200 mg. Tablets can be cut to get a close-to-accurate dosage. The closest possible dose for this child will be:

- either 1 whole plus ½ of 100 mg carbamazepine tablets each day (150 mg total), or
- ¾ of a 200 mg tablet each day (150 mg total).

For information about splitting doses, see page 95. For information about measuring medicine in tablet and liquid form, see page 86.

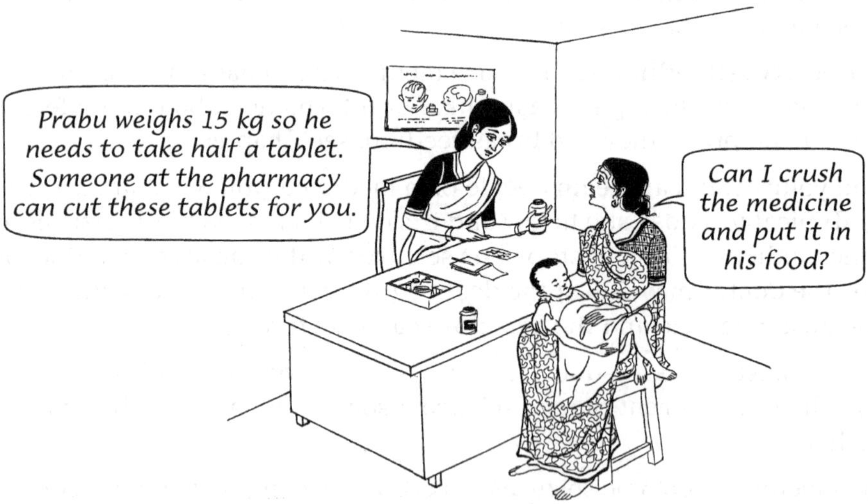
Prabu weighs 15 kg so he needs to take half a tablet. Someone at the pharmacy can cut these tablets for you.
Can I crush the medicine and put it in his food?

Find out how often to give the medicine, if it is easier to take before or after eating, and answers to any other questions you may have.

Finding the right dose: Dosing in a range

Antiseizure medicines are often recommended in dose ranges. This allows medicine amounts to be adjusted to meet individual needs because different people's bodies absorb and process medicines differently.

When dosing within a range, you usually start with a low dose and increase it slowly over 6 to 12 weeks until you reach the right dose. The right dose is one that will stop the seizures and cause the fewest side effects. If seizures stop with the first amount, you might then lower the dose to see if that stops seizures as well. Each medicine has a maximum dose. Increasing the dose above that amount is not safe and will not stop the seizures.

Having more severe seizures does not always mean that you need a larger dose.

Example: The dose of carbamazepine for children 12 years and older is: 100 to 200 mg by mouth 1 time a day, or 50 to 100 mg by mouth 2 times a day, with a maximum dose of 1800 mg per day. That range means you might start with a dose of 100 mg of carbamazepine and then add more each week until the seizures stop or the maximum dose of 1800 mg is reached.

Splitting daily doses into smaller doses

It is common to split a daily dose of antiseizure medicine into 2 or 3 smaller doses to be taken at different times during the day. Splitting a dose can be helpful because it keeps the amount of medicine in a person's body more constant at all times. Side effects of a medicine may be less intense with smaller doses than with a single large dose. Check with a health worker who has experience with antiseizure medicines to find out if splitting a dose might be helpful for you.

If splitting involves cutting a larger tablet into smaller pieces, ask the clinic or pharmacy to cut them for you. Pharmacy workers (or chemists) have tools that cut pills accurately, making sure each part has the right amount of medicine (see "Measuring medicines," page 86).

Of course, splitting doses also gives a person more chances to forget or miss a dose. Take this into account as well and help the person find ways to remember to take their medicine.

Add-on therapy

Sometimes a new medicine is added to supplement an antiseizure medicine that is not completely controlling seizures. This is called "add-on therapy." Follow add-on therapy instructions carefully.

There are several reasons for using an add-on therapy. When one antiseizure medicine is not completely controlling a person's seizures, a different antiseizure medicine that affects the brain differently might be added to see if by working together both medicines can stop the seizures. In combination, the effects of each medicine are sometimes increased. Also, add-on therapy may allow smaller doses of each medicine to be used, reducing side effects.

Adding on lamotrigine to valproic acid can result in a lower dose of valproic acid. Levetiracetam is added on to other antiseizure medicines to better control several seizure types. For more add-on therapy information, see the specific medicine boxes between pages 100 and 107.

Follow-up visits

The health worker who started you on medicine will want to see you several times after you start. During follow-up visits, they will ask about how well the medicine is controlling your seizures, or about side effects or allergic reactions, and they may adjust your dose or change the medicine so it works best for you.

Try not to miss follow-up visits. If it is difficult for you to go, maybe the health worker can come to you where you live, or connect over a phone or video call. If there is a health center that is closer for you, ask your health worker for a referral note with their name, phone number, and any important instructions for a different health center. Ask about mobile health clinics or epilepsy camps that provide epilepsy screening, access to antiseizure medicines, and tips to live well with epilepsy.

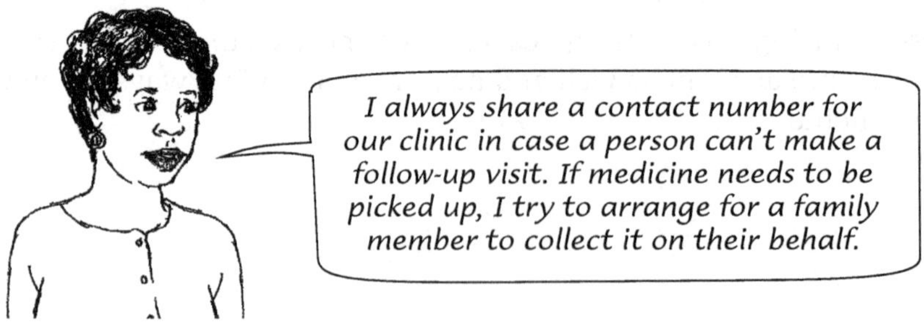

Changing antiseizure medicines

There are many reasons to change from one antiseizure medicine to another, and also reasons not to make a change. These reasons often have as much to do with the social conditions of where you live as they do with the kind of epilepsy you have.

Reasons to change medicines:

- You want to be or are pregnant.
- A new or different medicine might work better or can be taken less often.
- The side effects of the medicine are troubling and not getting better.
- The medicine seems to be working less well than it had.
- The medicine costs too much.
- The medicine supply is unreliable—it is always running out.
- You have another health condition the medicine negatively affects.

Reasons not to change medicines:

- The new medicine costs too much.
- The supply of the new medicine is unreliable or is hard to find.
- You are comfortable with the medicine you are using.
- You do not want to go through the process of stopping your medicine and starting a new one.

If you change your medicine, an experienced health worker or epilepsy specialist's advice can help you do so safely and comfortably. The dose of your old medicine may be slowly lowered. Your body may need time to get used to the new medicine.

Changing medicines for pregnancy or breastfeeding

Some antiseizure medicines are dangerous for a developing baby or newborn. If your antiseizure medicine is not safe during pregnancy or breastfeeding, talk to a health worker about changing it or adjusting your dose. For information about pregnancy and breastfeeding, see Chapter 7.

Medicines that are not safe during pregnancy or breastfeeding are marked in the medicine boxes in the following pages with these signs:

CAUTION

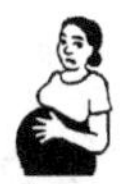

Use carefully if you are pregnant.

CAUTION

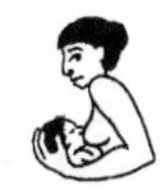

Use carefully if you are breastfeeding.

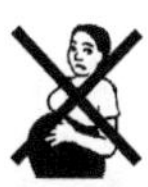

Do not take if pregnant.

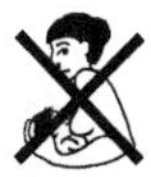

Do not take if breastfeeding.

Drug-resistant epilepsy

While medicines can help control most seizures, they do not work for everyone. After trying various doses, if one antiseizure medicine is not working, your health worker will try a different medicine or combination of medicines. If a person's seizures are not controlled after trying at least 2 medicines, their epilepsy is considered "drug resistant."

Having drug-resistant epilepsy does not mean that your seizures cannot be controlled, it just means that antiseizure medicines may not control them. With drug-resistant epilepsy, it is more important than ever to try to control seizures with the variety of activities and practices, including special diets, avoiding seizure triggers, getting more rest, and others options discussed in Chapter 6. It is also important to make sure your seizure type is correctly identified and that your seizures are caused by epilepsy and not another health condition. For information about seizure types and causes, see Chapter 3.

Common antiseizure medicines

Information about epilepsy medicines is often hard to find or written only for people with high levels of medical training. By sharing it here, we hope to make it more accessible to health workers (especially those who do not often treat epilepsy), and people with epilepsy everywhere. We also hope the information will help people with epilepsy and seizures have conversations with health workers about their treatment options and be aware of how to use medicines safely. **The information is meant to support, not replace, the guidance of a trained health worker.** Finally, we also hope it will support advocacy to make antiseizure medicines more available to all who need them.

We describe many of the antiseizure medicines that are widely available, but not all medicines used around the world. Some medicines used in your area—such as gabapentin, lacosamide, or vigabatrin—may not be included here. To learn about them, talk to a health worker.

Carbamazepine *(Carbatol, Mazetol, Tegretol, Tegrital, Zeptol)* CAUTION

Carbamazepine is a common antiseizure medicine and the first choice for several seizure types. Do not use for absence seizures. Monitor side effects carefully.

In what forms does this medicine come?

Tablet (100 mg, 200 mg, 400 mg)

Oral liquid (100 mg in 5 ml)

How to use

For generalized tonic-clonic or focal seizures:

For children 1 month to 11 years, give 5 mg per kg of body weight by mouth 1 time each day, or 2.5 mg per kg 2 times a day. Increase this daily dose by 2.5 to 5 mg per kg each week as needed, up to 5 mg per kg 2 to 3 times a day. Do not give more than 20 mg per kg total in 1 day.

For children 12 years and older, give 100 to 200 mg by mouth 1 time each day, or 50 to 100 mg 2 times a day. Increase this daily dose by 100 to 200 mg each week as needed, up to 200 to 400 mg 2 to 3 times a day. Do not give more than 1800 mg total in 1 day.

For adults, give 100 to 200 mg by mouth 1 time each day, or 50 to 100 mg by mouth 2 times a day. Increase this daily dose by 100 to 200 mg each week as needed, up to 400 mg 2 to 3 times a day. Do not give more than 2000 mg total in 1 day.

Commonly used for these seizures:

- Focal
- Focal that becomes generalized
- Generalized tonic-clonic

Important

To lessen stomach upset or diarrhea, give medicine with food. Even just a piece of fruit or bread can help.

If there is skin rash after a few weeks of using medicine, reduce dose. Change medicine if rash becomes severe and spreads fast. Use carefully if operating heavy machinery or driving. Not effective against fever seizures in children.

Carbamazepine may have harmful effects in pregnancy. It is best not to start this medicine in the first 3 months of pregnancy. If medicine started before pregnancy, do not stop suddenly. Lower dose little by little before stopping or changing to another medicine. Avoid or use with caution during breastfeeding.

Side effects

Feeling tired, dizziness, stomach upset or diarrhea, skin rash, feeling sad and worried, or memory, thinking, and attention problems

Warning Do not drink alcohol while using carbamazepine.

Clobazam *(Frisium, Sympazan)*

CAUTION

Clobazam is a benzodiazepine medicine. It is used to treat several types of seizures, by itself and as add-on therapy.

In what forms does this medicine come?

Tablet (10 mg, 20 mg)

Oral liquid (2.5 mg in 1 ml)

How to use

For Lennox-Gastaut syndrome (LGS):

For children 2 years or older and 30 kg or under, give 5 mg by mouth 1 time each day at bedtime for 1 week or longer. Then increase to 5 mg 2 times a day for 1 week or longer. Then increase to 10 mg 2 times a day.

For children 2 years or older and over 30 kg, give 5 mg by mouth 2 times a day for 1 week or longer. Then increase to 10 mg 2 times a day for 1 week or longer. Then increase to 20 mg 2 times a day.

For add-on therapy of LGS:

For adults, give 5 mg by mouth 2 times a day for 1 week or longer. Then increase to 10 mg 2 times a day for 1 week or longer. Then increase to 20 mg 2 times a day.

Commonly used for these seizures:

- Lennox-Gastaut syndrome (by itself in children, as add-on therapy in adults)

Important

Adjust dosages when giving to people with liver problems.

How this drug affects a developing pregnancy and newborn babies is not clear. Use with caution during pregnancy and breastfeeding.

All benzodiazepine medicines such as clobazam can be addictive, may need to be increased over time, and can cause withdrawal seizures if stopped suddenly.

Do not use with alcohol.

Side effects

Feeling tired, behavior changes, drooling, trouble speaking, constipation

Ethosuximide *(Zarontin)*

CAUTION

Ethosuximide is used to manage and prevent absence seizures.

In what forms does this medicine come?

Capsule (250 mg)

Oral liquid (250 mg in 5 ml)

Commonly used for these seizures:

- Absence

Important

Reduce dose if skin rash develops a week after starting medicine. Change to a different medicine if rash becomes severe and spreads fast. Always slowly reduce the dose rather than stopping abruptly.

How to use

For absence seizures:

For children 1 month to 5 years, give 5 mg per kg of body weight by mouth 2 times a day. Increase this daily dose by 5 to 10 mg per kg each week as needed, up to 10 to 20 mg per kg 2 times a day. Do not give more than 1500 mg total in 1 day.

For children 6 to 17 years, give 250 mg by mouth 2 times a day. Increase this daily dose by 250 mg each week as needed, up to 500 to 750 mg 2 times a day. Do not give more than 1500 mg total in 1 day.

For adults, give 500 mg by mouth 1 time each day, or 250 mg 2 times a day. Increase this daily dose by 250 mg each week as needed, up to 1500 mg divided into 2 doses per day. Do not give more than 1500 mg total in 1 day.

Side effects

Feeling tired, weight loss, dizziness, sudden stomach upset, diarrhea, hiccups, headache

Lamotrigine *(Lamictal, Lamotrix, Lamotrigina)*

Lamotrigine manages different types of seizures, often when used together with another medicine. Talk to a health worker when using it as an add-on therapy, as the combination affects dosing. Lamotrigine is safe during pregnancy and breastfeeding.

In what forms does this medicine come?

Tablet (25 mg, 50 mg, 100 mg, 150 mg, 200 mg)

Commonly used for these seizures:

- Focal
- Lennox-Gastaut syndrome
- Generalized tonic-clonic (as add-on therapy)

How to use

For focal seizures and Lennox-Gastaut syndrome (LGS):

For children 12 to 17 years and adults, give 25 mg by mouth 1 time each day for 2 weeks. Then give 50 mg 1 time each day for 2 weeks. Then increase this by 50 mg per day every 1 to 2 weeks as needed, up to 100 to 200 mg a day.

For add-on therapy of LGS, generalized tonic-clonic seizures, or focal seizures in people taking valproic acid:

For children younger than 2 years, give 0.15 mg per kg of body weight by mouth in 1 or 2 doses each day for 2 weeks. Then increase the dose to 0.3 mg per kg in 1 or 2 divided doses each day if needed. After the fourth week, increase the dose by up to 0.3 mg per kg per day each week up to 1 to 5 mg per kg per day in 3 divided doses. Do not give more than 200 mg total in 1 day.

For children 2 to 12 years old, round doses down to the nearest whole tablet. Give 0.15 mg per kg of body weight by mouth in 1 or 2 doses each day for 2 weeks. (For children in this age group who weigh 6.7 to 14 kg, give 2 mg every other day.) After 2 weeks, increase the dose to 0.3 mg per kg of body weight in 1 or 2 divided doses each day if needed. After the fourth week, increase the dose by 0.3 mg per kg per day each week up to 1 to 5 mg per kg per day in 1 or 2 divided doses. Do not give more than 200 mg total in 1 day.

For adults, give 12.5 to 25 mg by mouth 1 time every other day for 2 weeks. Then increase the dose to 25 mg 1 time each day for 2 weeks. After the fourth week, increase the dose by 25 to 50 mg per day every 1 to 2 weeks as needed up to 100 to 200 mg per day divided in 2 doses.

For add-on therapy of LGS, generalized tonic-clonic seizures, or focal seizures in people taking carbamazepine, phenobarbital, phenytoin, or another medication that decreases lamotrigine in the body* (but not valproic acid):

For children younger than 2 years, give 0.6 mg per kg of body weight by mouth in 1 or 2 doses each day for 2 weeks. Then increase the dose to 1.2 mg per kg in 1 or 2 divided doses each day if needed. After the fourth week, increase the dose by up to 1.2 mg per kg per day each week up to 15.6 mg per kg per day divided in 3 doses. Do not give more than 400 mg total in 1 day.

For children 2 to 12 years old, round doses down to the nearest whole tablet. Give 0.6 mg per kg of body weight by mouth divided in 2 doses each day for 2 weeks. After 2 weeks, increase the dose to 1.2 mg per kg divided in 2 doses each day. After the fourth week, increase the dose by 1.2 mg per kg per day each week up to 5 to 15 mg per kg per day divided in 2 doses. Do not give more than 400 mg total in 1 day.

For adults, give 50 mg by mouth in 1 or 2 doses each day for 2 weeks. Then increase the dose to 100 mg in 1 or 2 doses each day for 2 weeks. After the fourth week, increase the dose by 100 mg per day every 1 to 2 weeks as needed up to 300 to 500 mg per day divided in 2 doses.

**Other medicines that decrease lamotrigine in the body include rifampin (rifampicin) taken for tuberculosis, and atazanavir (ATV), lopinavir/ritonavir (LPV/r), and ritonavir (RTV) taken for HIV.*

continues

Lamotrigine *(continued)*

Important	Side effects
Read medicine instructions carefully to find out if you can cut tablets for dosing. If not, you may have to round doses up or down to the nearest whole tablet. See instructions on this above for each seizure type and age group. Raise the dose of this medicine very slowly to avoid skin rash. If there is skin rash after a few weeks of using medicine, reduce dose. Change to a different medicine if rash becomes severe and spreads fast. Always slowly reduce the dose rather than stopping medicine abruptly. Lamotrigine can make your mouth very dry, which can lead to tooth decay. Pay attention to dental hygiene.	Feeling tired, dizziness, upset stomach and diarrhea, severe skin rash (Stevens-Johnson syndrome), feeling sad and worried

Levetiracetam *(Keppra, Torleva)*

CAUTION

Levetiracetam treats several types of seizures. The dosing here is for "immediate release" levetiracetam, which is most common. There is also an "extended release" or "XR" version of this medicine which is absorbed more slowly by the body, so it lasts longer. That dosing is different from the information here.

In what forms does this medicine come?

Tablet (250 mg, 500 mg, 750 mg, 1000 mg)

Oral liquid (500 mg in 5 ml)

How to use

For generalized tonic-clonic, focal, or absence seizures:

For children 1 to 5 months, give 7 mg per kg of body weight by mouth 1 time each day for 2 weeks. Then increase to 7 mg per kg 2 times a day for 2 weeks. If seizures continue, increase each dose by 7 mg per kg every 2 weeks, up to 21 mg per kg 2 times a day.

For children 6 months to 17 years, give 10 mg per kg of body weight by mouth 1 time each day for 2 weeks. Then increase to 10 mg per kg 2 times a day for 2 weeks. If seizures continue, increase each dose by 10 mg per kg every 2 weeks, up to 30 mg per kg 2 times a day.

For adults, give 250 mg by mouth 2 times a day for 2 to 4 weeks. Then increase to 500 mg 2 times a day for 2 to 4 weeks. If seizures continue, increase each dose to 1000 mg for 2 to 4 weeks, and then, if needed, increase to 1500 mg 2 times a day.

For myoclonic seizures:

For adults, give 250 to 500 mg by mouth 2 times a day for 2 weeks. Then increase by 1g (1000 mg) a day every 2 weeks as needed, up to 2 g (2000 mg) 2 times a day.

For add-on therapy of myoclonic seizures:

For children 12 years and over, give 500 mg by mouth 2 times a day for 2 weeks. Then increase each dose by 500 mg every 2 weeks, up to 1500 mg 2 times a day.

Commonly used for these seizures:

- Focal
- Focal that becomes generalized
- Generalized tonic-clonic
- Absence
- Myoclonic (as add-on therapy in children, by itself in adults)

Important

How this drug affects a developing pregnancy and newborn babies is not clear. Use with caution during pregnancy and breastfeeding. Sometimes this medicine harms the kidneys. Talk to a health worker if you are passing very little urine or have swollen legs, ankles, or feet after starting the medicine.

Carefully monitor children with absence seizures who are beginning use of this drug. Sometimes it can make these seizures worse.

Side effects

Feeling tired, trouble sleeping, headache, dizziness, stomach upset or diarrhea, skin rash, feeling sad and worried, aggressive behavior

For behavioral or mood-related side effects, taking vitamin B6 may help. For more information about this, talk to a health worker.

Warning

Use with caution if you have heart or kidney problems such as acute kidney injury, frequent urinary tract infections, or kidney stones.

Phenobarbital

(Epitan, Fenirol, Fenobarb, Gardenal, Luminal, Phenobarb, Phenoleptil, Solfoton)

Phenobarbital is a sedative in the barbiturate family of medicines and is one of the oldest medicines used to control seizures.

In what forms does this medicine come?

Tablet (15 mg, 30 mg, 60 mg, 100 mg)

Oral liquid (15 mg in 5 ml)

How to use

For generalized tonic-clonic or focal seizures:

For children 1 month to 11 years, give 2 to 3 mg per kg of body weight by mouth 1 time each day at bedtime or 1 to 1.5 mg per kg 2 times a day for 2 weeks. Then increase this daily dose by 1 to 2 mg per kg each week as needed, up to 2 to 6 mg per kg 1 time each day.

For children 12 years and older and adults, give 1 mg per kg of body weight by mouth 1 time each day at bedtime for 2 weeks. Then increase this daily dose by 15 to 30 mg each week as needed, up to 3 mg per kg per day. Do not give more than 180 mg in 1 day.

Commonly used for these seizures:

- Focal
- Focal that becomes generalized
- Generalized tonic-clonic

Important

If used regularly, the dose must be increased over time to keep working.

Side effects

Stomach upset or diarrhea, difficulty breathing, tiredness, sadness and worry, memory or thinking problems, cognitive delay in children

Warning

Do not use during pregnancy or breastfeeding, or when trying to get pregnant unless there is no other option.

Do not use with alcohol.

Phenobarbital is habit-forming (addictive). If this medicine is used for a long time, suddenly stopping or lowering the dose can cause severe and possibly life-threatening medical reactions, including seizures. To avoid this, work with a health worker to gradually reduce the amount of medicine you take if you change or stop using this medicine.

Phenobarbital slows the functioning of several body systems and can make you sleepy. Be careful when driving or operating machinery while using this medicine.

Phenytoin *(Dilantin, Epanutin, Epsolin, Eptoin, Fenidantoin, Diphantoine)*

Phenytoin is among the oldest antiseizure medicines.

In what forms does this medicine come?

Tablet (50 mg, 100 mg, 300 mg)
Capsule (50 mg, 100 mg)

Commonly used for these seizures:

- Focal
- Focal that becomes generalized
- Generalized tonic-clonic

How to use

For generalized tonic-clonic or focal seizures:

For children 1 month to 11 years, give 1.5 to 2.5 mg per kg of body weight by mouth 2 times a day for 2 weeks. Then increase this dose by 5 mg per kg per day every 1 to 2 weeks as needed, up to 2.5 to 5 mg per kg 2 times a day. Do not give more than 300 mg in 1 day.

For children 12 to 17 years, give 75 to 150 mg by mouth 2 times a day for 2 weeks. Then increase this dose by 25 mg a day every 1 to 2 weeks as needed, up to 150 to 200 mg 2 times a day. Do not give more than 300 mg 2 times a day.

For adults, give 150 to 300 mg by mouth in 1 or 2 doses each day for 2 weeks. Then increase this dose by 50 mg a day every 1 to 2 weeks as needed, up to 200 to 400 mg 1 time each day or 100 to 250 mg 2 times a day. Do not give more than 400 mg 1 time a day or 300 mg 2 times a day.

Important

Some people get painfully swollen and enlarged gums that may bleed. If this happens, medicine may need to be changed.

Side effects

Feeling tired, dizziness, stomach upset and diarrhea, blurred vision, skin rash, swollen gums, feeling sad or worried, memory and thinking problems, excess hair growth on any area of the body

Warning

Do not use during pregnancy or breastfeeding, or when trying to get pregnant unless there is no other option.

Use carefully with children.

Topiramate *(Topamax)*

CAUTION

Topiramate is used for different seizure types.

In what forms does this medicine come?

Tablet (25 mg, 50 mg, 100 mg, 200 mg)
Capsule (15 mg, 25 mg)

Commonly used for these seizures:

- Focal
- Focal that becomes generalized
- Generalized tonic-clonic
- Lennox-Gastaut syndrome (as add-on therapy)

How to use

For generalized tonic-clonic or focal seizures:

For children 2 to 10 years, give 25 mg by mouth 1 time each day at bedtime for 1 week. Then increase this dose to 25 mg by mouth 2 times a day for 1 week. Then increase this dose by 25 to 50 mg a day every week as needed for 5 to 7 weeks, up to 150 to 400 mg in 2 doses per day.

For children 10 years or older, give 25 mg by mouth 2 times a day for 1 week. Then increase this dose by 50 mg a day every week as needed, up to 100 mg 2 times a day. This dose can be increased further by 100 mg a day every week as needed, up to 200 mg 2 times a day.

For adults, give 25 mg by mouth 2 times a day for 1 week. Then increase this dose by 50 mg a day every week as needed, up to 200 mg in 1 or 2 doses each day. This dose can be increased further by 100 mg a day every week as needed, up to 400 mg in 1 or 2 doses per day.

For add-on therapy of Lennox-Gastaut syndrome (LGS), generalized tonic-clonic seizures, or focal seizures:

For children 2 to 16 years, give 1 to 3 mg per kg of body weight by mouth 1 time each day at bedtime for 1 week. Then increase this dose by 1 to 3 mg per kg per day every 1 to 2 weeks, up to 400 mg in 2 doses per day.

For adults, give 25 to 50 mg by mouth 1 time each day for 1 week. Then increase this dose by 25 to 50 mg a day every 1 to 2 weeks as needed, up to 400 mg in 1 or 2 doses per day.

Important

These tablets taste very bitter, so it is best not to crush, break, or chew them. A capsule that can be opened and sprinkled on food may be available.

Use with caution during breastfeeding. Avoid use during pregnancy or when trying to get pregnant because there is a risk of the baby developing cleft palate. Speak with your health worker to find out if another medicine is available.

People with glaucoma or kidney or liver problems should avoid using topiramate or use with careful monitoring.

Side effects

Weight loss, feeling very tired, memory and thinking problems, tingling or prickly feeling in arms, hands, legs, or feet, dizziness

Valproic acid *(Depakote, Depakene)*

Valproic acid is a common treatment for different types of seizures.

In what forms does this medicine come?

Tablet (100 mg, 200 mg, 500 mg)

Oral liquid (200 mg in 5 ml)

Commonly used for these seizures:

- Focal
- Focal that becomes generalized
- Generalized tonic-clonic
- Absence
- Myoclonic

How to use

For generalized tonic-clonic, focal, or myoclonic seizures:

For children and adults, give 10 to 15 mg per kg of body weight by mouth in 1 to 3 doses per day for 1 week. Then increase this dose by 5 to 10 mg per kg per day each week as needed, up to 60 mg per kg per day.

For absence seizures:

For children and adults, give 15 mg per kg of body weight by mouth in 1 to 3 doses per day for 1 week. Then increase this dose by 5 to 10 mg per kg per day each week as needed, up to 60 mg per kg per day.

Important

Some people get painfully swollen and enlarged gums that may bleed. If this happens, medicine may need to be changed.

Side effects

Dizziness, feeling tired most of the time, diarrhea or upset stomach (reduced if taken after meal), blurred vision, skin rash, vitamin D deficiency especially in young children and teenagers, feeling sad and worried, memory and thinking problems. weight gain, hair loss, polycystic ovary syndrome (PCOS)

Warning Do not use during pregnancy or when trying to get pregnant. If pregnant, start replacing with another antiseizure medicine immediately.

Rescue medicines for status epilepticus

Status epilepticus is a medical emergency. It happens when a seizure lasts more than 5 minutes, or when many seizures follow one another without recovery in between. For focal seizures, this means continuous seizures for about 10 minutes, and for absence seizures, for 10 to 15 minutes. Anyone with status epilepticus needs urgent medical care. For more information on status epilepticus, see Chapter 3, page 57.

Medicines used to stop these seizures are called "rescue medicines." Some are only for status epilepticus, while others can treat different seizure types.

IMPORTANT Certain rescue medicines must be given directly into a vein (by IV), which requires special training and equipment found in hospitals. Only give IV medicines if you are trained to do so.

Diazepam *(Calmpose, Diastat, Paxum, Peptica, Valium)*

Diazepam is a benzodiazepine medicine. It is a rescue medicine for status epilepticus.

In what forms does this medicine come?

Tablet (5 mg, 10 mg)

Injection (10 mg in 2 ml)

Rectal gel (2 mg in 1 ml, 4 mg in 1 ml)

How to use

For status epilepticus:

For children younger than 1 month, give 1.25 to 2.5 mg in the rectum. Or slowly inject 0.3 mg per kg into a vein. If seizures do not stop 5 minutes after the first dose, give the same dose again. Do not give more than 2 doses total.

For children 1 month to 1 year, give 5 mg in the rectum. Or slowly inject 0.3 mg per kg into a vein. If seizures do not stop 5 minutes after the first dose, give the same dose again. Do not give more than 2 doses total.

For children 2 to 11 years, give 5 to 10 mg in the rectum. Or slowly inject 0.3 mg per kg into a vein. If seizures do not stop 5 minutes after the first dose, give the same dose again. Do not give more than 2 doses total.

For children 12 years and older and adults, give 10 to 20 mg in the rectum. Or slowly inject 10 mg into a vein. If seizures do not stop 5 minutes after the first dose, give the same dose again. Do not give more than 2 doses total.

Important

Diazepam does not work fast enough when injected into muscle (IM).

Side effects

Feeling tired and/or sleepy, muscle weakness, shallow and short breathing if dose is given very fast

Warning Giving too much diazepam can slow or stop breathing.

Giving diazepam for status epilepticus

Diazepam comes as tablets, a liquid, and a gel. All of these forms can be given in the rectum as rescue medicine for status epilepticus.

- **To use diazepam tablets,** crush them into fine powder and mix with clean, cool water. The powder will not dissolve completely. Then draw the mixture into a syringe without a needle.
- **To use diazepam liquid,** draw the liquid into a syringe and then remove the needle.
- **To use diazepam gel,** adjust the dose on the pre-loaded syringe by rotating the protective cap at the bottom of the syringe barrel. Push the circular lock ring upward. The dose will be locked in when you hear the click. Pull the protective cap off the syringe before using.

HOW TO Give diazepam in the rectum

- Put the person having seizures on their side in a place where they cannot fall. Rest their forehead on a pillow or something soft. Remove enough of their clothing to expose their buttocks. *For infants and toddlers:* Position on their stomach.
- Put petroleum jelly (*Vaseline*) on the tip of a syringe that has had the needle removed.
- Bend the person's upper leg forward and separate buttocks so the anus (opening of the rectum) is exposed. *For infants and toddlers:* Separate the cheeks of their buttocks with one hand and insert the syringe with the other.
- Gently insert the tip of the syringe into the rectum until the rim is snug against the opening of the anus.
- Slowly count "1, 2, 3" while pushing the plunger until it stops. Then hold the syringe in place for at least 5 minutes to keep the medicine from leaking out.
- Write down the time the medicine was given so that you will know when to give a second dose, if needed.

Levetiracetam *(Keppra)*

CAUTION

Levetiracetam treats tonic-clonic, focal, and absence seizures. It can also be used as a rescue medicine for status epilepticus.

In what forms does this medicine come?

Injection (500 mg in 5 ml)

How to use

For status epilepticus:

For children 1 month and older, slowly inject 40 mg per kg of body weight into a vein over 10 minutes. If seizures do not stop after the first dose, slowly inject an additional 20 mg per kg into a vein over 10 minutes. Do not give more than a total of 4500 mg.

For adults, slowly inject a single dose of 60 mg per kg of body weight into a vein over 15 minutes. Do not give more than 4500 mg in that single dose.

Important

How this drug affects a developing pregnancy and newborn babies is not clear. Use with caution during pregnancy and breastfeeding.

Side effects

Feeling tired, headache, dizziness, stomach upset or diarrhea, skin rash, feeling sad and worried, aggressive behavior

Warning Use with caution if you have heart or kidney problems such as acute kidney injury, chronic kidney disease, frequent urinary tract infections, or kidney stones.

Lorazepam *(Ativan, Novolorazem)*

CAUTION

Lorazepam is a benzodiazepine medicine.

In what forms does this medicine come?

Injection (2 mg in 1 ml, 4 mg in 1 ml)

How to use

For status epilepticus:

For children 1 month to 11 years, slowly inject 0.1 mg per kg of body weight into a vein. If seizures do not stop 10 minutes after the first dose, give the same dose again. Do not give more than 4 mg in each dose. Do not give more than 2 doses total.

For children 12 to 17 years and adults, slowly inject 4 mg into a vein. If seizures do not stop 10 minutes after the first dose, give the same dose again. Do not give more than 2 doses total.

Important

Use with caution during pregnancy and breastfeeding.

Side effects

Dizziness, feeling tired, diarrhea and stomach upset, difficulty with thinking and attention, soreness, redness or pain at injection site

Warning Do not drink alcohol while taking this medicine.

Midazolam *(Dormicum, Hypnovel, Midacum, Versed)*

CAUTION

Midazolam is a benzodiazepine medicine, the only one that can be injected into muscle (IM).

In what forms does this medicine come?

Liquid for injection, for administration between gum and cheek, or as nasal spray (1 mg in 1 ml, 5 mg in 1 ml)

How to use

For status epilepticus:

For children 1 month and older, inject 0.2 mg per kg of body weight into muscle 1 time. Or give 0.2 mg per kg between the gum and cheek. Or give 0.2 mg per kg as nasal spray. If seizures do not stop 10 minutes after the first dose, give the same dose again. Do not give more than 10 mg in a dose. Do not give more than 2 doses total.

For adults, inject 10 mg into muscle 1 time. Or give 10 mg between the gum and cheek. Or give 10 mg as nasal spray. If seizures do not stop 10 minutes after the first dose, give the same dose again. Do not give more than 2 doses total.

Important

To give midazolam between the gum and cheek, lay the person on their side. Fill a syringe with the dose of liquid midazolam and take the needle off the syringe. Put the tip of the syringe in the space between the gum and cheek on one side of the person's mouth. Give the medicine by slowly pushing the syringe plunger.

To give midazolam as nasal spray, lay the person in their side or back. Fill a syringe with the dose of liquid midazolam and add an additional 0.1 ml to the dose to account for liquid that will remain in the delivery device. Take the needle off the syringe and attach the device for giving medicine in the nose. Push the syringe plunger to spray the medicine into the person's nostril. You can spray some of the dose into each nostril or all into the same nostril.

Side effects

Dizziness, feeling tired, diarrhea and stomach upset, difficulty with thinking and attention, pain at site of injection (if injected), irritation of nostrils (if given in nose)

Warning Injecting this medicine very quickly can make a person choke. Giving too much medicine can slow or stop breathing.

Phenobarbital *CAUTION*

Phenobarbital and phenytoin are common daily medicines for treating tonic-clonic or focal seizures. They can also be used for status epilepticus but are not the first choice of rescue medicines because of their side effects.

In what forms does this medicine come?

Injection (200 mg in 1 ml)

How to use

For status epilepticus:

For children 1 month and older, give 20 mg per kg of body weight by IV infusion over 20 minutes. Do not give more than 1 g (1000 mg) in a dose. If seizures do not stop after this dose, give an additional 10 mg per kg by IV infusion over 20 minutes.

For adults, give 15 mg per kg of body weight by IV infusion over 15 minutes. Do not give more than 1 g (1000 mg) in a dose. Do not give more than 1 dose.

Important

Monitor breathing and blood pressure after treating with phenobarbital.

Side effects

Tiredness, slowed breathing, lowered blood pressure

Warning If possible, do not give to pregnant or breastfeeding people, or people trying to get pregnant. Can be used if no safer medicine is available.

Phenobarbital is habit-forming (addictive). It slows the functioning of several body systems and can make you sleepy. Be careful when driving or operating machinery while using this medicine.

Phenytoin *CAUTION*

In what forms does this medicine come?

Injection (50 mg in 1 ml)

How to use

For status epilepticus:

For children and adults, give 20 mg per kg of body weight by IV infusion. For people up to 50 kg, give infusion over 20 minutes. For people 50 to 75 kg, give infusion over 30 minutes. For people 75 to 100 kg, give infusion over 40 minutes. Do not give more than 2 g (2000 mg) in a dose.

Important

Closely watch the person's heart rate and blood pressure after giving phenytoin, as it can cause these to drop dangerously.

Use with caution in people using rifampin (rifampicin, taken for tuberculosis) or mefloquine (taken for malaria) as these medicines may make phenytoin less effective.

Side effects

Feeling tired, dizziness, stomach upset and diarrhea, heart problems

Warning If possible, do not give to pregnant or breastfeeding people, or people trying to get pregnant. Can be used if no safer medicine is available.

Do not give to people with heart problems, especially people with slow heart rates.

Medicines to lower fever

High fevers (temperatures over 38°C/100.4°F) can cause seizures in infants and toddlers. A fever seizure might stop quickly, but it might happen again if the fever continues or the child gets another fever. Finding and treating the infection causing a fever is important, but treating the fever seizure may also be necessary. Fever seizures usually stop by themselves and antiseizure medicines are rarely needed.

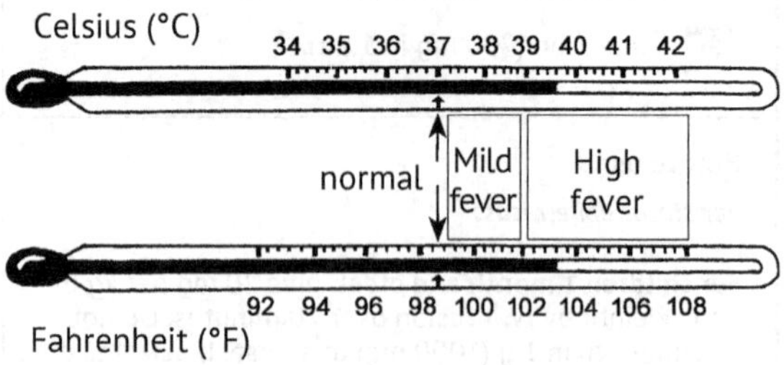

These temperatures are for temperatures taken by mouth.

If a fever seizure lasts longer than 5 minutes, it is an emergency. Give the child a rescue medicine like diazepam, lorazepam, midazolam, phenobarbital, or phenytoin. See pages 109 to 113.

If a child has fever seizures more than 3 times in 6 months, their parents or caregivers can keep rescue medicine on-hand and learn how to give it.

Use a thermometer after the fever seizure has passed to measure how much fever remains. If you don't have a thermometer, get a general sense of how hot the child is by touching their forehead or belly. Notice if the child is more drowsy or fussy than usual as these are common signs of high fevers.

How to lower a fever and help a child feel better

- Remove the child's clothes or wrappings.
- Give plenty of fluids to keep the child hydrated.
- Give a medicine to lower fever (see page 115).

Do not wrap a child in wet cloths or give a cool bath as these may cause discomfort and are not effective for lowering fever in most cases.

Most importantly, try to find and treat the cause of the fever. Could it be from an infection caused by a mosquito bite? Or from a virus like measles or HIV? Meningitis, a dangerous inflammation in the brain and spinal cord, can cause fever. Ask a health worker for help in discovering the cause and curing the fever.

Vaccinations, fever, and fever seizures. Sometimes a child may have a reaction to a vaccination that causes fever and, occasionally, a fever seizure. To lower the risk of fever, give ibuprofen or paracetamol, 1 hour before and 2 hours after the vaccination. See page 115 for further dosing information.

Ibuprofen *(Advil, Alivium, Brufen, Buprovil, Combiflam, Dolgit, Faspic, Fenbid, Gelofen, IBU, Paraped Plus)*

CAUTION

Ibuprofen is used to relieve pain and fever. Ibuprofen is not safe for very young babies. Use paracetamol instead.

In what forms does this medicine come?

Tablet (200 mg, 400 mg)

Oral liquid (100 mg in 5 ml, 200 mg in 5 ml)

How to use

For children, give by mouth 3 times a day and dose by age:

Age	Dose
3 to 11 months	50 mg
1 to 3 years	100 mg
4 to 6 years	150 mg
7 to 9 years	200 mg
10 to 11 years	300 mg
12 years and older	300 to 400 mg

For children under 12 years, do not give more than 30 mg per kg of body weight in 1 day. For children 12 years and older, do not give more than 1200 mg total in 1 day.

Important

To avoid stomach pain or indigestion, give ibuprofen with food or a large glass of water or milk.

Side effects

Stomach pain, indigestion

Warning Do not give to babies younger than 3 months old, and do not give to pregnant women in the last 3 months of pregnancy. Do not give for more than 10 days in a row.

Paracetamol, acetaminophen

(Tylenol, Calpol, Cetamol, Dexamol, Dolo, Dolex, Dolyc, Panadol)

Paracetamol is an effective, affordable medicine for fever and mild pain.

In what forms does this medicine come?

Tablet (100, 500 mg)

Oral liquid (120 mg in 5 ml or 125 mg in 5 ml, 250 mg in 5 ml)

How to use

For children, give by mouth every 4 to 6 hours and dose by age:

Age	Dose
under 1 year	62 mg (half of ¼ of 500 mg tablet)
1 to 2 years	125 mg (¼ of 500 mg tablet)
3 to 7 years	250 mg (½ of 500 mg tablet)
8 to 12 years	375 mg (¾ of 500 mg tablet)
over 12 years	500 to 1000 mg

Do not give more than 4000 mg a day.

Important

Cold medicines often contain paracetamol, so do not give them along with a separate dose of paracetamol or you may give too much and poison the liver.

Side effects

Stomach pain, indigestion

Warning Do not give for more than 10 days in a row.

Side effects of antiseizure medicines

Side effects are unintended changes a medicine causes in a person. Different people will feel the side effects of antiseizure medicines differently. Many side effects are uncomfortable or distressing but not dangerous. Some side effects lessen or go away completely as the body gets used to the medicine. Others can be severe and dangerous.

Get medical attention for these side effects

- Severe skin rash with blotchy, blistering skin
- Difficulty breathing or shortness of breath
- A sudden worsening of seizures
- Fast or irregular heartbeat, heart palpitations (a fluttering feeling in the chest or neck), chest discomfort or pressure
- Jaundice—causes whites of eyes and skin to turn yellow (less visible on darker skin), nausea, vomiting, or loss of appetite
- Sharp pain in the belly that may travel to the back
- Hallucinations (seeing things that are not there)
- Severe depression, thoughts of suicide
- Extreme sleepiness or confusion

Common side effects and what to do about them

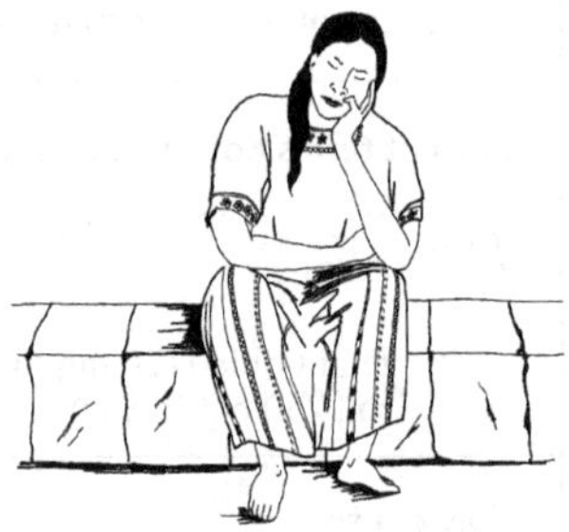

Side effect: Feeling tired

Antiseizure medicines that can cause tiredness: carbamazepine, diazepam, ethosuximide, levetiracetam, phenobarbital, phenytoin, topiramate, valproic acid

What to do: Tiredness is the body's signal that it needs rest, with or without antiseizure medicines. However, rest does not mean sleeping all day. A person taking antiseizure medicine must get up and move around during the day. Engaging in physical activity can help with tiredness and also can improve sleep.

If tiredness is so severe that a person cannot do daily activities like eating, bathing, or moving around, talk to a health worker. A different medicine or dose may be needed.

Side effect: Upset stomach or diarrhea

Antiseizure medicines that can cause upset stomach or diarrhea: carbamazepine, ethosuximide, diazepam, lorazepam, lamotrigine, midazolam, phenobarbital, phenytoin, topiramate, valproic acid

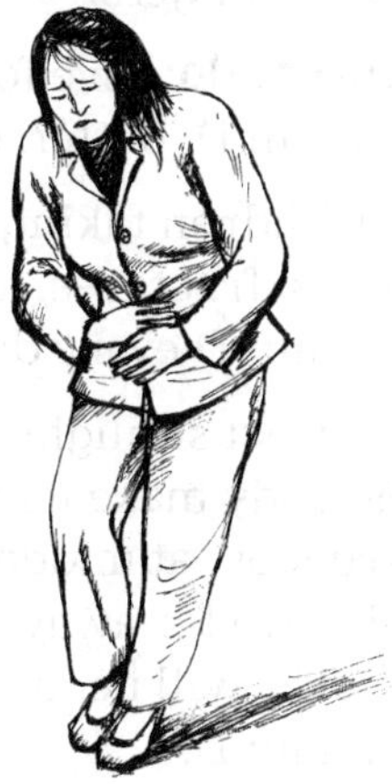

What to do: For diarrhea, drink plenty of water, herbal tea, or other liquids to ensure the lost liquid is replaced. Avoid spicy foods or animal milks if you have an upset stomach. Eat something light every 2 to 3 hours. Breastfeed young children with diarrhea more often. If diarrhea is so severe that it causes dehydration, use a rehydration drink (see recipe on page 183).

Get medical help if dehydration continues, there is blood in the stool, no desire to eat or drink, or the upset stomach or diarrhea continues for more than 2 days.

Side effect: Mild skin rash

Antiseizure medicines that can cause skin rash: carbamazepine, lamotrigine, phenytoin, valproic acid

What to do: Bathe a minor rash with cool water or water in which a handful of oats has soaked for an hour (less if the oats are ground into powder). Gently pat skin after bathing and leave skin open to the air to encourage drying. To calm itchiness, use calamine lotion. Neem tree oil also helps soothe inflamed skin.

A severe skin rash or a rash that spreads rapidly can be an emergency. See a health worker as soon as possible.

Side effect: Severe skin rash with blisters and peeling skin (Stevens-Johnson syndrome)

Antiseizure medicines that can cause severe skin rash: carbamazepine, lamotrigine, phenobarbital, phenytoin, valproic acid (rarely reported)

Some antiseizure medicines can cause a severe reaction of painful, blistering, and peeling skin, starting with the face and chest and spreading to arms, legs, and back. Flu symptoms like headache, cough, sore throat, and fever may begin before the rash.

IMPORTANT If the rashy area is larger than your hand, if there are red streaks, fever, or red and watery eyes, ***this is an emergency***. Quickly see a doctor or another health worker. Medicine may need to be stopped under supervision. Keep skin as clean and dry as possible.

Side effect: Vitamin D deficiency

Antiseizure medicines that can cause vitamin D deficiency: carbamazepine, phenobarbital, phenytoin, valproic acid (especially in young children and teenagers)

What to do: Give foods that are rich in vitamin D, including milk fortified with vitamin D, butter, egg yolks, animal fats, and liver, especially fish liver oil.

Children taking valproic acid risk developing weak bones, fractures, and rickets. Prevent this by giving them vitamin D every day (600 to 1200 IU of vitamin D2 or D3).

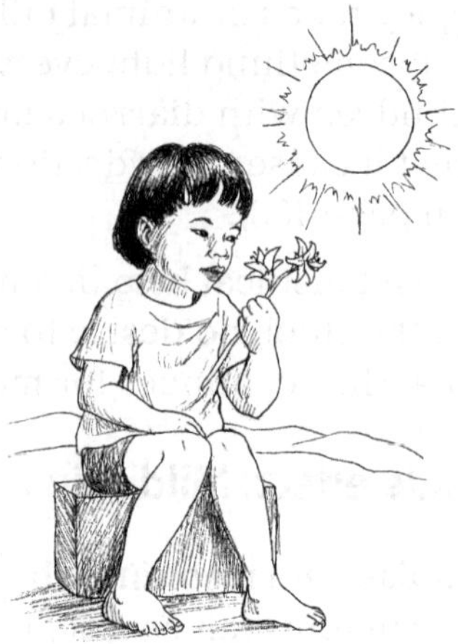

Direct sunlight on skin for 10 to 30 minutes can help the body make its own vitamin D. Sun exposure is strongest at midday. People with darker skin and people who live far away from the equator where the sun is weaker will need more time in the sun to get adequate vitamin D.

Side effect: Swollen and enlarged gums

Antiseizure medicines that can cause swollen gums: phenytoin and valproic acid

What to do: Clean teeth carefully every day. Brush with toothpaste, try to remove the tiny bits of food between the teeth, and gargle with a mouthwash of water, baking soda, and cloves or clove oil (see recipe below). Ask a health worker or epilepsy specialist about a change in medicine.

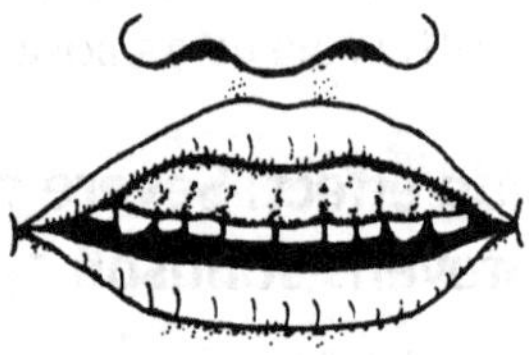

Mouthwash recipe:

- Filtered water (240 milliliters or 1 cup)
- Baking soda (6 grams or 1 teaspoon)
- If available, add 4 whole cloves or 4 drops of clove oil

Bring water to a boil and add whole cloves or clove oil. Remove pan from heat, let water cool, and remove whole cloves. Mix baking soda into mixture and store in a sealed jar. Shake before using as a mouthwash.

Side effect: Dizziness and loss of balance

Antiseizure medicines that can cause dizziness: carbamazepine, valproic acid, phenytoin, lamotrigine

What to do: Help a person sit or lie down and suggest they stay still until dizziness goes away. Closing their eyes may help. Give water to sip. If the medicine can be taken before bedtime, the dizziness may be less troubling.

Side effect: Blurred vision

Antiseizure medicines that can cause blurred vision: carbamazepine, levetiracetam, phenytoin, topiramate

What to do: Have the person's vision checked to see if they need eyeglasses. If vision remains blurry, change their epilepsy medicine. A variety of fresh fruits and vegetables contain vitamins and minerals that can help maintain vision: Vitamin A is found in sweet potato, carrot, pumpkin, and leafy greens. Vitamin C is found in peppers, avocados, mango, papaya, and orange. Vitamin E is found in nuts, seeds, whole grains, and avocados. The minerals lutein and zeaxanthin are in leafy greens and eggs. And oily fish are high in omega-3 fats.

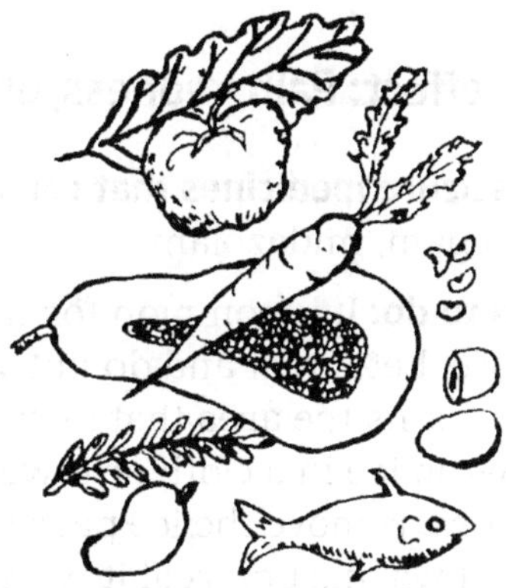

Side effect: Feeling sad, worried, depressed

Antiseizure medicines that can cause worry and sadness: carbamazepine, levetiracetam, phenytoin, phenobarbital, topiramate, valproic acid

What to do: Encouraging children and adults to talk about their feelings of sadness and worry can help improve the way they feel. If worry and sadness continue for a long time, see a health worker. Sadness that does not go away may be a sign of depression, and mental health support may be needed to help the person recover (see Hesperian's *Promoting Community Mental Health).*

Side effect: Difficulty thinking, remembering, and paying attention

Antiseizure medicines that can cause changes in the ability to think, memory, and attention span: carbamazepine, diazepam, levetiracetam, lorazepam, midazolam, phenobarbital, valproic acid

What to do: Sometimes a person taking antiseizure medicine may seem lost, forgetful, or take longer than usual to understand. These changes are not their fault, but may upset them. Reassurance and patience from friends and family can help a person understand these changes are caused by their medicine. Help people find ways to remind themselves about tasks and chores. If confusion or memory loss worsens, ask a health worker or epilepsy specialist if the antiseizure medicine can be changed.

Side effect: Pain, redness, or soreness at the site of injection

Antiseizure medicines that can cause pain, redness, or soreness at the injection site: lorazepam, midazolam

What to do: It is common for the skin at an injection site to swell and feel painful or sore. Let it rest and do not stress the muscles or joints near it. Avoid heavy work that strains the area that hurts. Cold often helps. Do not put ice directly on skin, but wrap ice in a cloth or towel and place it on the area that hurts. After 10 to 15 minutes, remove the ice pack and let the skin warm up. If the skin is still painful after it warms up, treat it with ice again.

Side effect: Unwanted hair on face or other body areas

Antiseizure medicine that can cause unwanted hair on face and other body areas: phenytoin

What to do: Remove unwanted hair by plucking with a tweezer, shaving with a razor, or using body wax or sugar wax.

HOW TO Remove hair with sugar wax

Ingredients:

- Sugar (250 grams or 1 cup)
- Juice from 1 small lemon
- Warm water (same amount as lemon juice)

To make wax:

- Mix all ingredients in a pot. Place on stove and stir continuously over medium-to-high heat so it does not burn.
- Lower heat when the mixture boils and continue to stir.
- Remove from heat when the mixture is golden-brown. It should be less thick than honey.
- Cool 15 to 20 minutes.

To use wax:

- Test temperature of wax by applying a small amount to the inside of your wrist. It should feel warm, not hurt or burn you.
- Apply wax with a flat wooden stick or small plastic spatula to a small section of skin where you want to remove hair.
- Spread wax in the direction the hair is growing.
- Place a cloth over the wax and press firmly. Use rectangular strips from an old shirt or piece of clothing. Leave the cloth on for 2 to 3 seconds.
- Hold the skin around the cloth tightly with one hand and then quickly pull cloth in the opposite direction of hair.
- Soothe skin by applying an ice pack.

When and how to stop antiseizure medicines

When to stop antiseizure medicines

Many people with epilepsy wonder: *If I have not been having seizures for some time, does this mean I can stop taking medicine?*

There is no answer to this question that is correct for everyone. Whether someone can stop medicine depends on their type of epilepsy, if they are taking one or more medicines, how easy or difficult it has been to control their seizures with medicine, and if seizures came back when they tried to stop using medicine before.

Certain epilepsy syndromes, such as Lennox-Gastaut syndrome, require a person to take medicine for their entire life. Some seizure types, such as myoclonic seizures in children, are likely to require ongoing treatment with medicine so that seizures are controlled. But for other epilepsies, medicine may not be needed forever, although in many cases, they are.

If you are thinking about stopping antiseizure medicine, it is very important to get help from a doctor or other health worker. Together, you can decide if the benefit (positive) of stopping the antiseizure medicine is greater than the harm (negative) that a seizure may happen again. A doctor or health worker's role is to share information, answer questions, and listen carefully to support you in the process of making a decision. The decision to stop or continue taking medicine is yours, but stopping medicine suddenly and without advice and guidance can be dangerous. Your seizures might restart immediately.

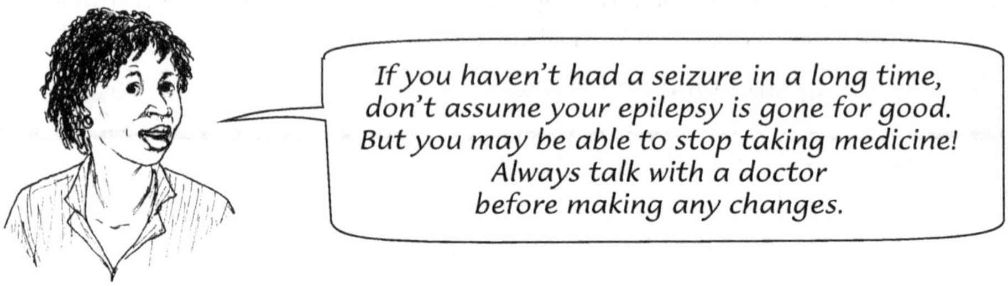

Another commonly-asked question is: *How long should I not have seizures before thinking about stopping epilepsy medicine?*

Research and medical practice around this topic (called "seizure freedom") have been changing. Some studies and doctors suggest that stopping medicine may be possible if a person has no seizures for 2 to 3 years while on medicine. However, other studies show that waiting at least 5 years without seizures while on medicine may be safer and may reduce the chances of seizures returning.

For any person with epilepsy taking daily antiseizure medicine, stopping medicine means freedom from side effects and an end to a dependency on medicine, which are concerns for many people. However, it also means living with uncertainty about having another seizure—taking antiseizure medicine offers emotional security as well as protection against seizures.

If seizures happen again after stopping medicine, it means that epilepsy is still present. The chances of seizures happening after stopping medicine are highest during the first year after stopping, especially the first 6 to 12 months. However, for some types of epilepsy, the risk that seizures may return can last several years. It can help to discuss your situation with a doctor or other health worker.

How to stop taking medicine

Just as the body gets used to taking antiseizure medicine every day, it will need some time to get used to not taking medicine. Ask your health worker about how much time you will need and what changes in the body you can expect as you slowly lower your dose of medicine.

Slow stopping of medicine is considered safest. Sudden withdrawal can increase the possibility, intensity, and frequency of seizures happening again. Stopping medicine suddenly is also associated with higher risk of death from seizures since it can cause rare cases of status epilepticus. It can also increase seizure frequency, a key risk factor for SUDEP (sudden unexpected death in epilepsy). For more about status epilepticus and SUDEP, see page 57.

To stop antiseizure medicine, slowly reduce the dose over 2 to 3 months, or even longer. The amount of time needed to stop taking medicine safely is different for each person, depending on their epilepsy and on what medicine they are taking. If a combination of medicines is being stopped, the process may take longer since each medicine will need to be slowly stopped, one at a time.

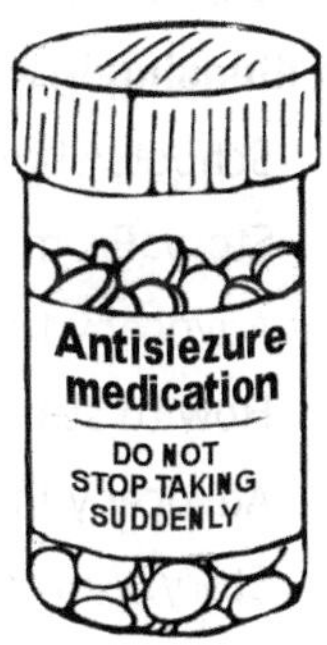

If seizures happen again after stopping medicine, the person probably needs to start taking medicine again to bring their seizures back under control.

Chapter 5

In this chapter

Understanding epilepsy stigma **125**
Story: Amani and her epilepsy 126
Three types of stigma 131
Identifying epilepsy stigma 132
Activity: Seeing epilepsy stigma in daily life 133
Women and girls face stronger stigma 135
Fighting stigma with support groups **136**
Starting an epilepsy support group 138
Encouraging participation in a group 139
Story: Making the internet a space for epilepsy support 142
Raising community awareness **145**
People with epilepsy can take the lead on education 145
Sharing information reduces stigma and harm 146
Activity: Epilepsy quiz: True or False? 146
Story: Concern for patients leads a faith healer to antiseizure medicine 150
Challenging institutional stigma **151**
Schools should not teach stigma 151
Story: From stigma to science: Teachers learn about epilepsy 151
Advocacy to improve laws and policies 152
How to start a policy advocacy campaign 153
Advocacy improves life for people with epilepsy 156
Story: Words matter: Changing the official word for epilepsy in Hong Kong 157
Appendix: Answer key to Epilepsy quiz: True or False? 158

Acting against epilepsy stigma

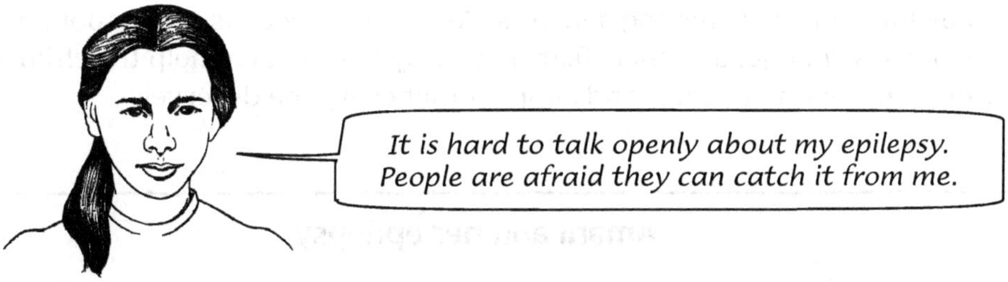

Understanding epilepsy stigma

When people do not understand what epilepsy is, they often feel afraid when someone has a seizure. The lack of clear, accurate information about epilepsy leads some to believe that seizures are contagious, or caused by evil spirits, curses, or as a punishment for wrongdoing. These negative beliefs are called stigma.

Epilepsy stigma leads to discrimination when someone is treated badly, unfairly, or as a less valuable person because they have epilepsy. People with epilepsy are often made fun of, denied support, kept hidden, or excluded from community life.

After my seizures started, my in-laws broke off relations with me. When my condition became known, my work mates said, "He has epilepsy, we don't want to get it from him." If my family and workplace won't accept me, how will I live?

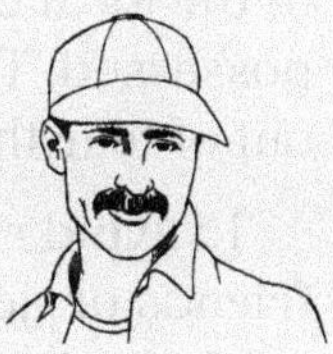

A person with epilepsy may be stopped from attending school, refused employment, or prevented from living in a certain place. Even health workers sometimes fear people with seizures or have harmful ideas about a seizure's effects. Stigma in health care settings prevents people with epilepsy from receiving the care they need and may lead them to avoid seeking care altogether.

My wife doesn't have epilepsy, I do. But at the village market, people won't let her stand in line with them. They move away and ask her to stand at a distance. Now she doesn't want to leave the house.

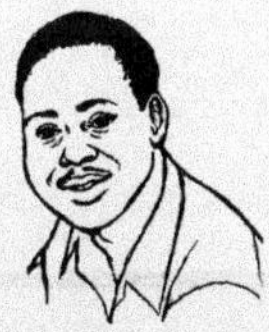

But when people come together to learn and share the truth about epilepsy, fear and harmful beliefs break down and are replaced with understanding. Families, health workers, teachers, and community members can create more inclusive environments to protect the rights of people with epilepsy.

Amani's story shows the range of reactions her family and community have when they find out she is having seizures. As everyone learns more about epilepsy, their responses change, and their fear gives way to efforts to help the child and her family get the treatment, care, and support that everyone deserves.

Amani and her epilepsy

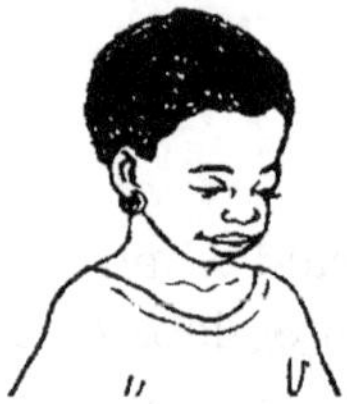

Amani and her family were sharing their evening meal when Amani suddenly toppled backward on her chair. Her 8-year-old body stiffened, and her arms and legs jerked. Then she lay still on the floor. After a few moments, she woke up, confused. Her family was shocked. No one really understood what had just happened. Amani's mother Jeane thought that maybe an evil spirit had entered her daughter's body, so she led her outside, lit a match, and told her to breathe in the smoke—that's how Jeane's own mother had taught her to drive spirits away.

Amani's seizures repeated several times over the next few months. The smoke from the matches didn't seem to help, but Jeane put off taking Amani to the local clinic because she believed that seizures meant a person was possessed. The grandmother convinced the family to keep the seizures secret out of fear that neighbors would stay away from the family if they found out.

To avoid rumors spreading, Amani was no longer allowed to play with her friends or go to school. Jeane worried it was her own fault that Amani was having seizures. As a young woman, Jeane had left her church and never went back. She now wondered if her daughter was paying the price.

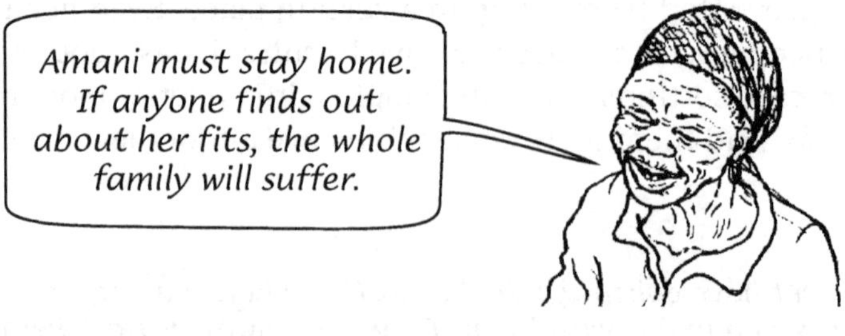
Amani must stay home. If anyone finds out about her fits, the whole family will suffer.

continues

Amani and her epilepsy *(continued)*

At first, Amani liked staying home and helping her grandma while her parents went to work. But when she listened to her brother talk about his friends in school, she was quiet and felt sad. She watched other children play and wished she could join them. No one answered her when she asked why she kept falling and then waking up on the ground, so she thought it was her fault.

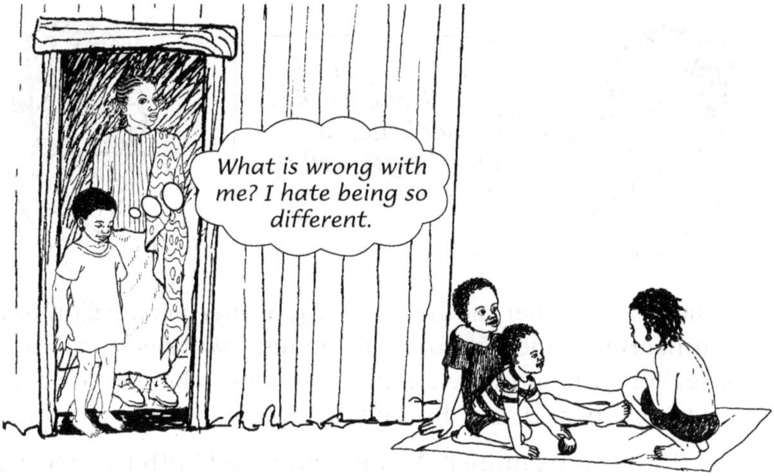

Self-stigma is when a person believes they are less worthwhile and less able. The person blames themself for their condition, feels shame, and believes their being different is a problem.

One day, while shopping in the town market, Jeane saw a shopkeeper's daughter have a seizure—just like Amani! The shopkeeper calmly moved a stack of pots and pans away from his daughter so she would not knock them over. After she woke up, he gently helped her sit and checked her for injuries. Jeane couldn't believe her eyes.

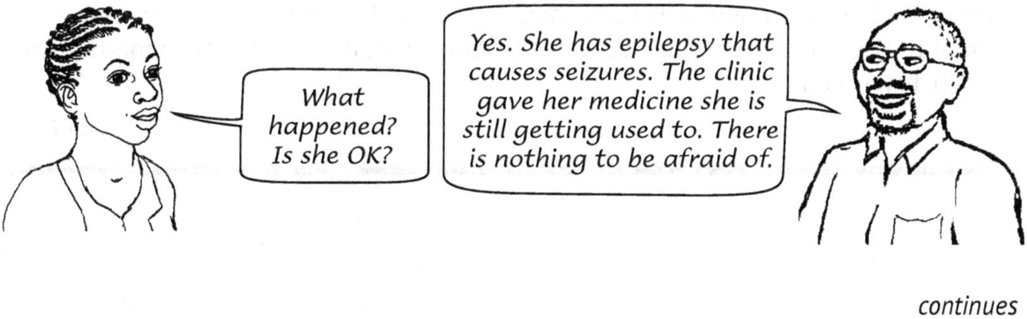

continues

Amani and her epilepsy *(continued)*

Jeane felt something she had not felt in a long time—hope. But she knew she would have to convince the rest of the family to let Amani try to get help. Her mother-in-law thought they should continue to hide Amani's condition. So Jeane reminded her how a doctor gave her medicine for her swollen feet, which she had long believed was caused by bad luck.

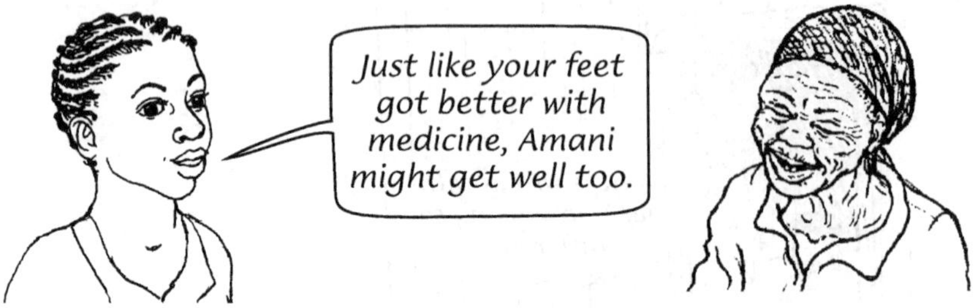

Jeane was relieved when her mother-in-law gave her permission to take Amani to the clinic. But Jeane's husband Emmanuel worried the clinic might be too expensive. When Jeane showed him the money she had put aside by not sending Amani to school and said it might be enough, Emmanuel agreed.

The doctor at the clinic examined Amani and asked both her and Jeane a lot of questions. Then he explained that he thought the seizures were caused by epilepsy—a brain condition that cannot be cured but most of the time can be managed with medicine, or the child "grows out of it." He gave Jeane a bottle of pills and told her to give one to Amani at the same time every day. He showed Jeane how to keep Amani safe during a seizure and told her to also explain this to the rest of the family. Then he asked Jeane to bring Amani back in one month to see how she was doing.

When Amani started taking the medicine, her seizures stopped, but the medicine made her so sleepy she just wanted to lie in bed all day. No one told them this would happen! Jeane stopped giving Amani the pills to get her energy back, but her seizures came back too. The doctor told Jeane to take Amani to the capital city for treatment because there were no other medicines at their town's clinic.

continues

Amani and her epilepsy *(continued)*

At the clinic in the city, Amani was given a different medicine with fewer side effects. Her seizures happened less often, and she began to smile and talk more. Eventually, Amani asked if she could go back to school, and Jeane and Emmanuel decided she was ready. But returning to class was not what Amani expected. On her second day, she had a seizure during lunch. The other children screamed, pointed at her, and ran away.

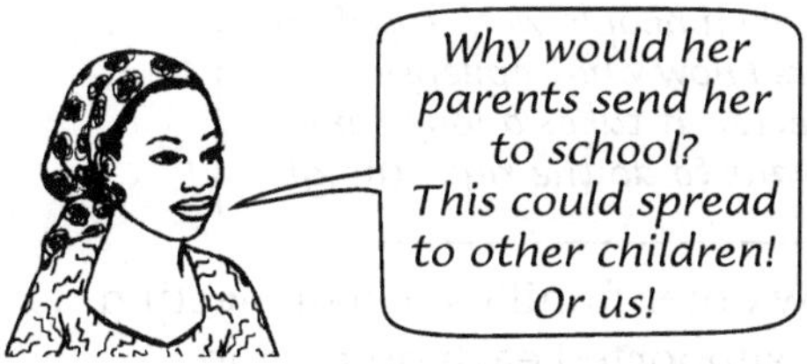
Why would her parents send her to school? This could spread to other children! Or us!

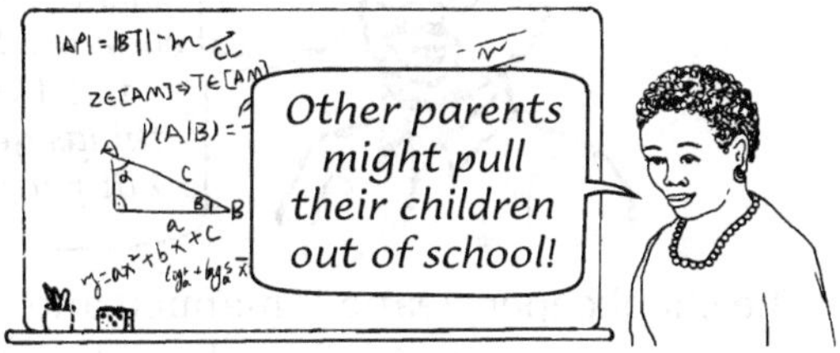
Other parents might pull their children out of school!

Interpersonal stigma is when others within families and communities react or behave negatively toward a person with epilepsy. Purposefully or unconsciously, they are telling the person with epilepsy that they are a problem.

Amani was so upset she ran home from school and cried herself to sleep. The next day, she did not want to go to school—she stayed home instead. Jeane went to talk to the principal. He listened uncomfortably to Jeane as she explained Amani's condition, but he insisted that Amani should be kept at home. The principal said the school's policy was not to accept students like Amani. Again, Amani was stuck at home. She felt lonely and helpless.

Emmanuel faced problems at work too. When a coworker heard him mention that Amani had epilepsy, the man looked frightened and refused to join Emmanual for their crew's regular noontime meal. Then, Emmanuel's boss called him into the office.

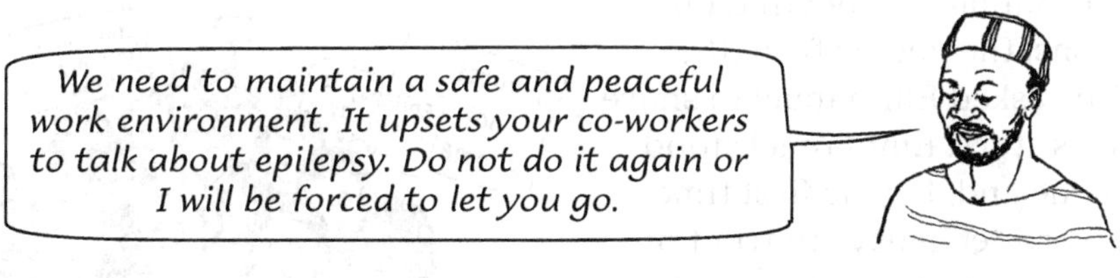

Institutional stigma is when organizations and governments have policies or rules that discriminate against people with epilepsy, unfairly limiting their rights and opportunities. They are telling communities and broader society that people with epilepsy are a problem.

continues

Amani and her epilepsy *(continued)*

Jeane and Emmanuel were hurt, angry, and unsure about what to do. They decided to ask for advice from the shopkeeper who had told Jeane about his daughter's epilepsy. Jeane and Emmanuel shared their experiences and frustrations. The shopkeeper offered them tea and related the problems his family had faced due to people's fear and lack of information about epilepsy.

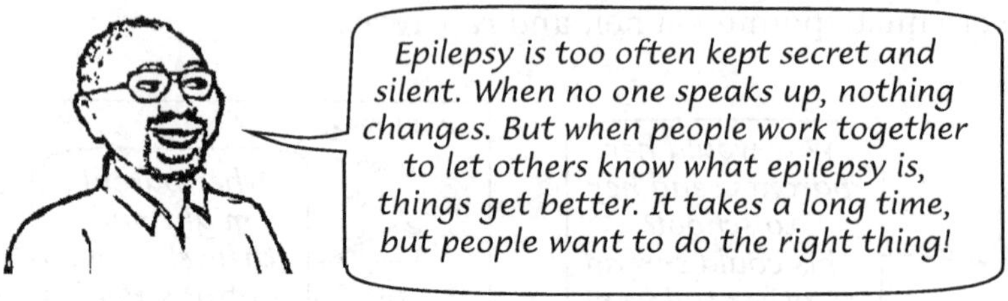

The shopkeeper, Jeane, Emanuel, and a few other families began meeting one evening each week. They shared stories, supported each other, and planned ways to help people in the community learn about epilepsy. A nurse from the town clinic began visiting schools and larger workplaces to explain basic information about epilepsy and to offer seizure first aid training and other first aid instruction. After some initial resistance, their group was able to meet with school officials and town leaders to propose ways to prevent epilepsy stigma and discrimination in education and employment, and to answer questions. Slowly, over many months, things began to change.

The next year, Amani returned to school. She was relieved to find that the teachers and staff had learned about epilepsy and seizure first aid. A small room was set aside for Amani or anyone else who needed to recover from a seizure or another health issue. Amani's schoolmates now understood that epilepsy is a health condition that affects a person's brain, not something to fear. Her old friends invited her to join their schoolyard games again.

After a community meeting on vaccinations, the doctor from the town clinic asked Emmanuel to share his family's story. Emmanuel stood beside Jeane and, for the first time, said the word "epilepsy" in front of a group of people. Everyone clapped when he finished speaking. Amani grinned in the front row, holding her grandma's hand. She felt nervous... and proud.

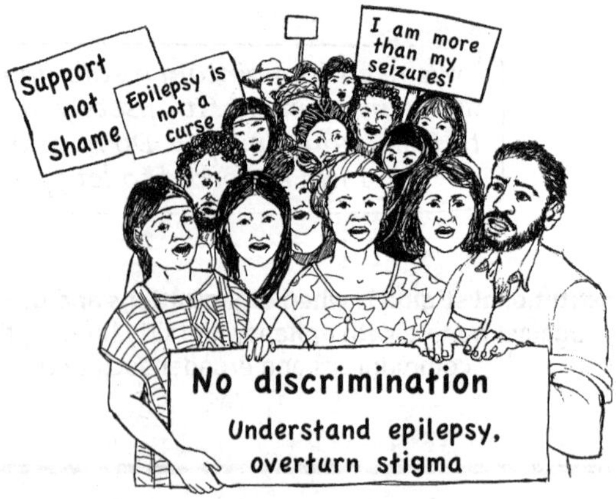
Support not Shame
Epilepsy is not a curse
I am more than my seizures!
No discrimination
Understand epilepsy, overturn stigma

Three types of stigma

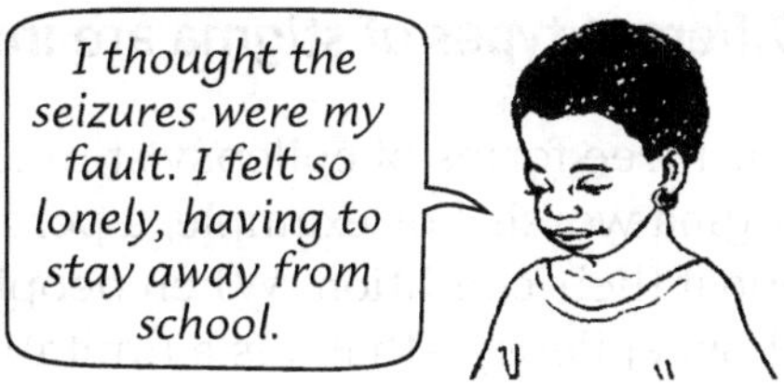
I thought the seizures were my fault. I felt so lonely, having to stay away from school.

Amani's story highlights three types of stigma.

Self-stigma can make a person with epilepsy:

- blame or shame themself for their condition.
- feel alone, anxious, worthless, depressed, hopeless.
- hide or lie about their epilepsy to others, including not getting medical care.
- limit what they do and not develop their abilities or friendships.

Amani's self-stigma made her hate feeling "different" from other children. She blamed herself for her seizures and felt ashamed for having them.

Interpersonal stigma can make others treat a person with epilepsy:

- as less capable or valuable than other people.
- like they should not participate in group activities, not develop social relationships, and not be recognized as community members.
- as if they should not and cannot lead a full and rewarding life.

Despite their love for her, Amani's family showed interpersonal stigma by stopping her from playing with her friends, attending school, and getting medical help, and by worrying about how epilepsy would reflect on the family's community acceptance. Amani's teachers showed interpersonal stigma by sharing their fears of epilepsy with each other. Emmanuel's coworkers showed interpersonal stigma when they refused to eat lunch with him.

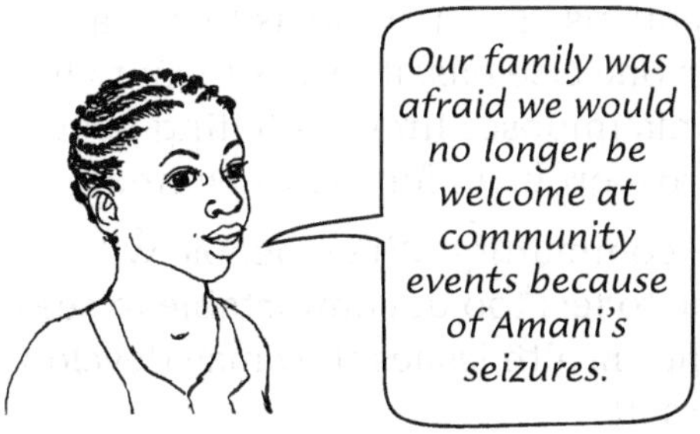
Our family was afraid we would no longer be welcome at community events because of Amani's seizures.

Institutional stigma harms people with epilepsy when:

- education, employment, marriage, and housing policies and laws discriminate against people with epilepsy and their families.
- health workers are not trained on how to support and treat people with epilepsy and seizures.
- medical systems do not provide access to trained health professionals and safe and affordable antiseizure medicines.

Amani and her family faced institutional stigma when the school principal enforced a policy banning children with epilepsy from attending school, and when Emmanuel's boss threatened to fire him for talking about epilepsy at work.

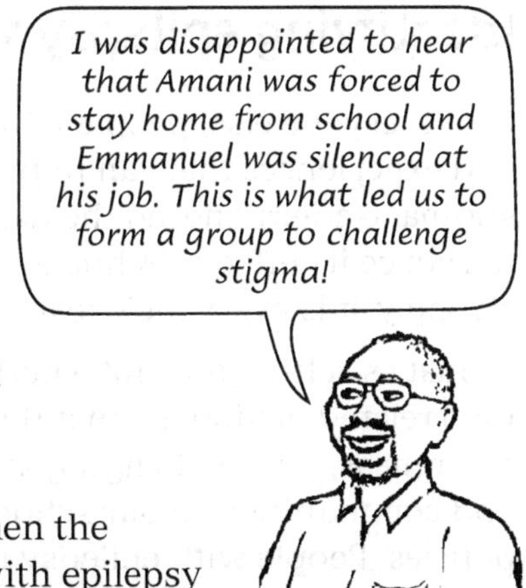
I was disappointed to hear that Amani was forced to stay home from school and Emmanuel was silenced at his job. This is what led us to form a group to challenge stigma!

Different types of stigma are interrelated

The three forms of epilepsy stigma are connected and often interact to make stigma worse. For example, a person with epilepsy may feel **self-stigma** as shame about their condition. When people around them share and spread harmful beliefs about epilepsy—that it is a limitation on what a person can achieve or a curse—this **interpersonal stigma** increases the self-stigma the person already feels. When neighbors, teachers, or employers discriminate against the person with epilepsy by creating policies or rules that prohibit them from attending school or working, this is **institutional stigma**. Where institutional stigma is in place, community members feel justified in their mistreatment of people with epilepsy, and the person with epilepsy feels worse about themself.

Stigma takes on a life of its own

Epilepsy stigma is not always intentional. A lack of information or understanding can cause people to treat someone with epilepsy poorly just because that is the way they have learned to behave. This is why education about epilepsy can make such a difference. When people learn their fears of epilepsy are unfounded, they are often willing, even eager, to make changes. Most people do not want to cause harm.

When laws or traditions prevent people with epilepsy from living as they want to, with the same rights and opportunities that everyone else has, it forces them to hide their epilepsy. A community where epilepsy stigma imposes limits is telling people with epilepsy they are less deserving and they are a problem for their neighbors.

Stigma also threatens the overall health of the community. When people with epilepsy are denied access to health care or made to feel too uncomfortable to seek it, they are less likely to get care for whatever other health issues they may develop, including ones that could spread and make others ill.

Identifying epilepsy stigma

Like everyone else, people with epilepsy can develop a broad range of talents, skills, and experiences that can improve a community—if they do not live behind a wall of stigma. Understanding the different types of stigma can help you think about how to reduce its effects. While a person with epilepsy feels the effects of stigma most strongly, it is everyone's responsibility to oppose the harm it causes.

Just as self-stigma, interpersonal stigma, and institutional stigma are interrelated, acting against them is interrelated too. Increasing support, raising awareness, and challenging stigma happen in our hearts and minds, in our families and communities, in our schools and workplaces, and in our laws and national policies. People with epilepsy have a right to live free of stigma and discrimination, and the more people we can involve, the closer we will be to achieving this.

ACTIVITY Seeing epilepsy stigma in daily life

Recognizing ways in which the three types of stigma cause harm is an important step in acting to stop it. Making and looking at simple drawings can point out epilepsy stigma in daily life that we might not otherwise see.

1 Form small groups

Divide people into groups of 2 or 3, and give each group paper and markers. If the group prefers not to draw, ask them to act out their scenes.

2 Read the descriptions and draw (or act)

Ask for volunteers to take taking turns reading the sample descriptions out loud (see below), then ask each group to choose 1 or 2 descriptions to draw or act out. They can also draw or act scenes from their own experiences. Allow the groups time to draw or practice acting out scenes like these:

Three friends are sitting on a bench in a park. One is whispering to another. Third friend has epilepsy and is on the corner of the bench looking uncomfortable.

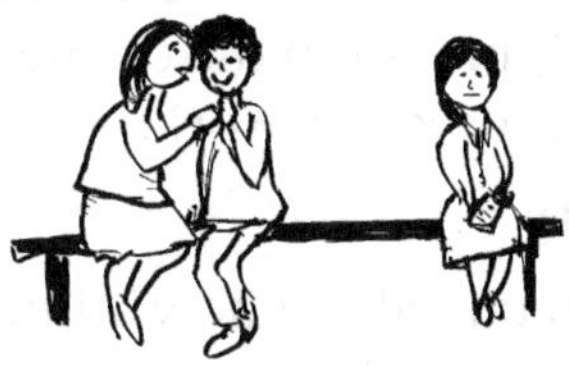

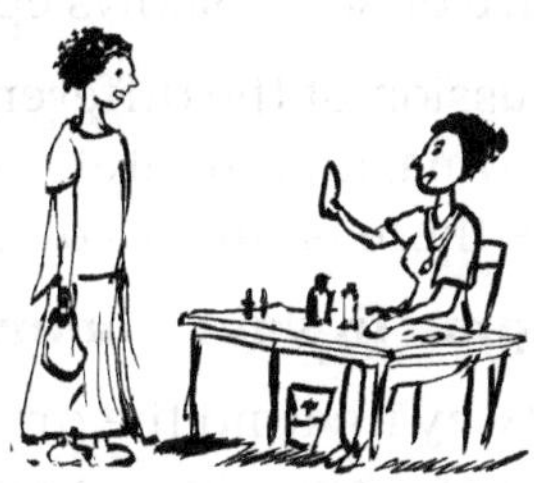

A health worker will not touch the person with epilepsy because she believes epilepsy can spread that way.

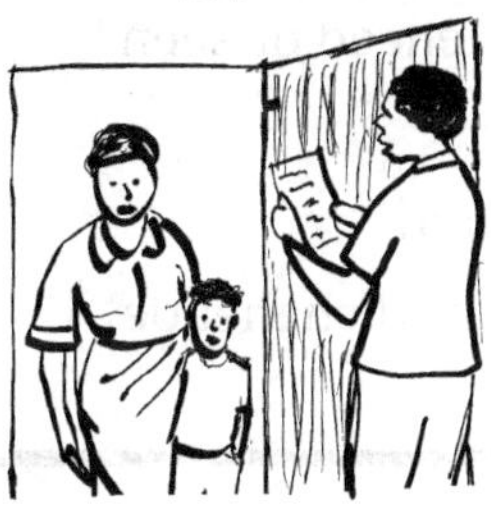

A landlord says it is his right to ask a family to leave their rented home because a family member has epilepsy.

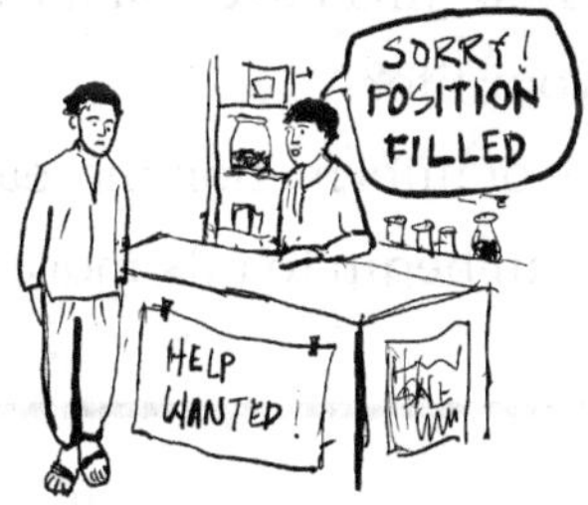

A person is not hired for a job because the employer will not hire someone with epilepsy.

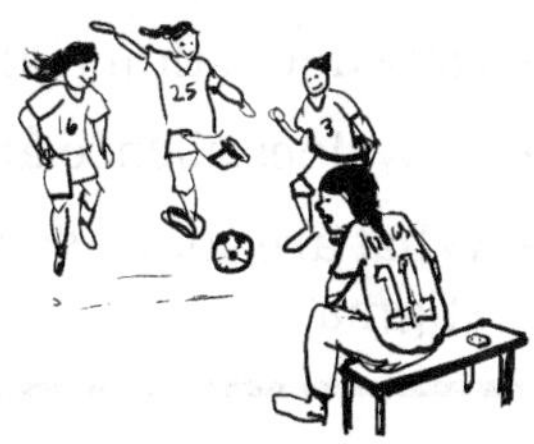

A young woman is not allowed to play football even though her epilepsy is well-controlled with medicine.

continues

ACTIVITY Seeing epilepsy stigma in daily life *(continued)*

Neighbors will not allow a woman in the line for the communal water tap because she has epilepsy.

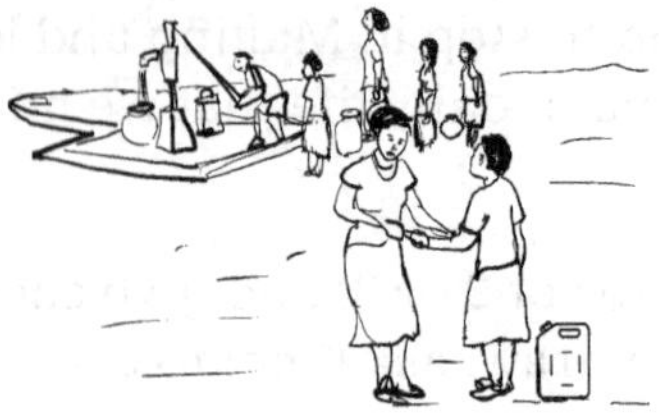

3 Share and discuss

When all the small groups are finished, have them show their pictures or act out their scenes to the entire group. Ask them to describe:

- what is happening in the picture or scene.
- how the picture or scene shows epilepsy stigma.

Promote discussion of the different kinds of stigma—self-stigma, interpersonal stigma, and institutional stigma—and the connections among them. Make sure there is time to discuss everyone's work.

4 Talk about stigma in your community

Close the activity by inviting the group to talk about how stigma happens in their community and how they can challenge it. Here are some questions that can help get the conversation going:

- What examples of epilepsy stigma have you have experienced or seen?
- How does stigma affect your life?
- How does silence and lack of information increase stigma?
- What are some ways we can begin to talk more openly and challenge stigma?

Women and girls face stronger stigma

In all communities, girls and women with epilepsy face different and stronger stigma than men. The stigma of having a feared or overlooked health condition becomes more intense as it interacts with gender discrimination. Where women are treated as second-class citizens, epilepsy stigma can further lower their self-esteem and confidence. These challenges are even worse for women with disabilities and those from minority groups.

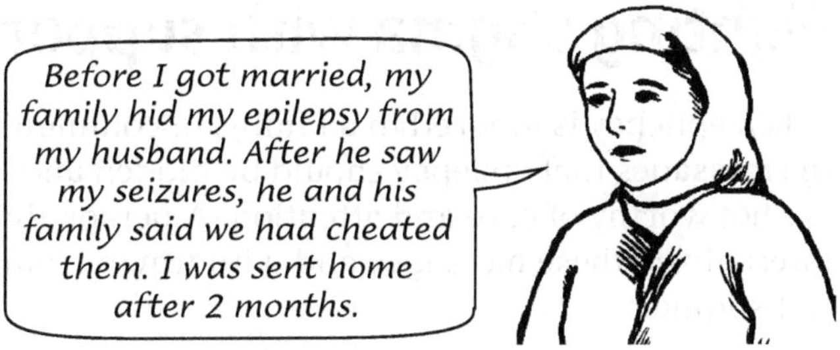
Before I got married, my family hid my epilepsy from my husband. After he saw my seizures, he and his family said we had cheated them. I was sent home after 2 months.

Marriage and family life. On top of facing discrimination and exclusion in education or work due to their gender, women with epilepsy are often considered unfit to be wives and mothers. Some women are forced to use contraception out of fear their condition will be passed on, so they are denied the right to have children. Families may try to hide a daughter's epilepsy, especially during marriage arrangements. If she does marry, her husband and in-laws may see her as a "burden," "cursed," or "dishonest" for concealing her illness, often leading to rejection or divorce. If her marriage ends, a woman with epilepsy is more likely to lose custody of her children.

Abuse and assault. A woman with epilepsy is at higher risk for neglect and abuse by family members. Women and girls have also reported finding themselves being groped or sexually assaulted by strangers or health providers as they recover from seizures.

Dignity and respect. Self-stigma among women with epilepsy can be especially harmful. Just as women are taught to devalue themselves due to their gender, a woman may believe incorrect information she has been told about epilepsy, for example, that she should not have children or breastfeed because seizures are contagious, or that her epilepsy prevents her from caring for others. This may make her feel unworthy of respect and likely to accept unjust treatment from her family and the community.

Community life and support. Gender inequality may allow a husband or other family member to restrict a woman's movements and prevent her from attending public events. This can make it harder for women with epilepsy to work or to participate in support groups or other activities that challenge stigma, either in the community or online.

It is usually easier for men to access epilepsy information and support groups online because they generally work outside the home and are more likely able to afford devices and data. Many women do not have paying jobs and must rely on the men in their families for mobile phones and internet connections.

Gender discrimination makes it more difficult for women and girls to talk openly about their epilepsy, find support, and become involved in community actions against stigma, but many people face additional barriers in lessening the effects of stigma on their lives. Poverty, racism, religious bigotry, homophobia, and other beliefs that divide our communities can make seeking support sometimes feel impossible. Make a conscious effort to overcome those divisions so your outreach and programs include everyone in the community.

Fighting stigma with support groups

When epilepsy is ignored in a family, in communities, or in larger society, it sends the messages that epilepsy should be hidden and that people who have epilepsy are not worthy of care and attention. A person living with epilepsy may have internalized these messages and withdrawn from family and community, due to self-stigma.

Epilepsy support groups provide a space for people with epilepsy to learn more about their own epilepsy, grow more comfortable talking about it, and form meaningful and supportive friendships with others who have it. Support groups can become a base from which people with epilepsy and their families can spread awareness throughout a community. They play a central role in reducing stigma.

When someone speaks about their experiences with epilepsy and stigma, it can help others think about their own situation. For example, when a person with epilepsy—or the parent of a young child who has severe epilepsy—describes what it feels like to be left out of community life and how they have handled it, others who face the same challenges may feel less alone and find some new ideas that help them. For the person sharing, talking openly about epilepsy can bring relief and validation, and help them become more confident in managing and living with the condition.

As you and others share your experiences of challenges, you can identify possible solutions together.

Support groups help people with epilepsy:

Recognize and allow feelings. We often hide our feelings or do not even admit we have them because we may think feelings are bad, shameful, or a sign of weakness. In some families or cultures, people tend to ignore feelings rather than talk about them. Hearing others talk about their feelings can help us recognize and become comfortable with our own.

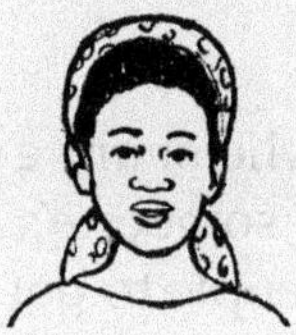

I felt so much shame and inner pain, I could never find the words for it. My epilepsy group showed me I was not alone and helped me see that the seizures are not my fault.

Get support. Feeling bad about your epilepsy, or that of a family member, can leave you drained and discouraged. Meeting as a group can spark energy and ideas, helping everyone cope with daily problems and mental health challenges. Group members can also check in with each other between meetings.

Understand the causes of problems. Talking together helps people realize that we share problems that need a common solution. Identifying causes of epilepsy stigma stops us from blaming ourselves.

Share good information. A support group can help find and share resources about epilepsy. This can reduce stigma that people may be facing. Guest speakers from health organizations or epilepsy support networks can visit to share useful and accurate medical information.

I look forward to hearing the university doctor who talks every other month about new research in epilepsy. It might not help me now, but it does give me hope.

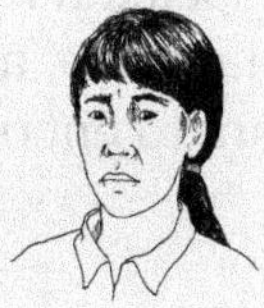

Recognize strengths. Support groups provide spaces where we can celebrate each other's strengths and remind each other that we have successfully overcome challenges before. Ask the group: "What did you do well that helped you oppose stigma?"

Build power together. Acting together is always more powerful than acting alone. When a group identifies ways to reduce stigma in the community, knowing that some or all of the group members can work together makes fixing it feel more possible.

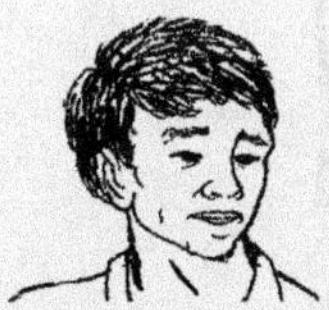

At first, I felt nervous talking about my seizures in the group. But I realized no one was judging me. That made me feel lighter, as if the weight of stigma was lifted off my shoulders.

Starting an epilepsy support group

Anyone can start an epilepsy support group. It just takes a few people who share a common goal to arrange to meet regularly. Support groups can meet in someone's home or in a shared community space. Find a location that is easy for people to get to and offers privacy.

The warmth of human connection that comes with an in-person gathering offers the greatest benefit. But you can also meet online (see "Making the internet a space for epilepsy support," page 143).

Here are some ways to help make a support group a positive experience:

Plan in advance. Try to set the dates for your meetings in advance to make sure people can plan to attend. Consider planning and letting people know of the agenda too. Knowing what to expect may help group members come ready to participate with thoughts, questions, or information related to what will be discussed.

Set group agreements. Decide on basic rules before you begin meeting so everyone feels comfortable participating and sharing. To create a space where people can speak openly, one basic rule might be to keep group discussions private. Other agreements might cover taking turns running meetings, giving everyone a chance to speak, listening and not interrupting, avoiding judging people or telling them what to do, and a commitment to starting meetings on time. The group may also want to encourage honest communication, humility, kindness, and respect.

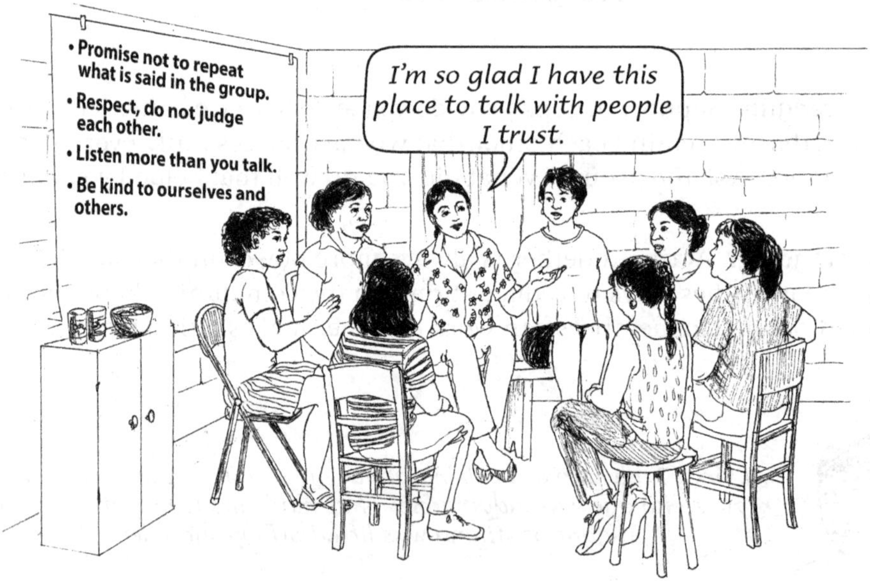
• Promise not to repeat what is said in the group.
• Respect, do not judge each other.
• Listen more than you talk.
• Be kind to ourselves and others.
I'm so glad I have this place to talk with people I trust.

The group can develop a list of agreements and refer to it when needed. Check in occasionally to see if any adjustments or additions are needed.

Beginning a meeting. Beginning each meeting in the same way can help people shift from their previous activities to join in common purpose. Try different ways to start the meeting so the group can decide what they like best. Some groups start with an "ice breaker" exercise or have each person respond to a prompt—for example, "Say something you are grateful for." Other groups start with a prayer or song, or by spending a few quiet moments to "reset" by writing or drawing their thoughts on "How I feel right now." If meetings begin with each person checking in about how they are feeling, it may become clear that someone needs special attention that day.

Decide what you hope to do. Choose your main topics. Give everyone a chance to express what they would like to get from the group: a chance to talk about feelings, share ideas about facing stigma, learn techniques to manage epilepsy and seizures, and other things. Try to keep expectations realistic. Support groups can be helpful in many ways, but they will not fix everything for everyone all the time.

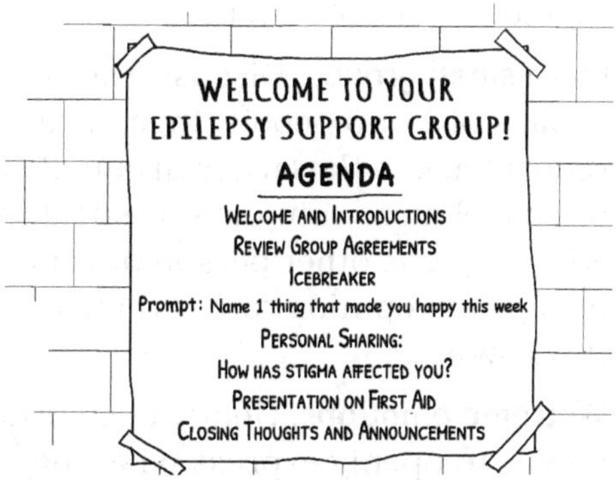

Encouraging participation in a group

Group discussions work best when everyone participates fully and equally, even if this does not come naturally. Try to draw people out and help everyone feel their ideas are valuable and worth sharing. This is especially important when people have been made to feel shame about their epilepsy. Here are some ways to make your group a place where people want to spend time.

Be a good listener. Show interest in what people say. It may help both individuals and the group if you briefly echo the main point of what a person said so they know they have been understood. Then invite the next person to speak.

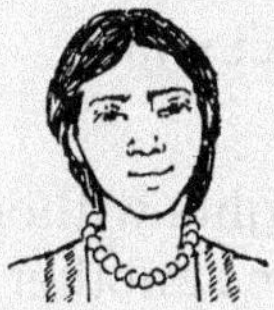

When I'm leading the group and someone says something that does not make sense to me, instead of correcting them, I ask: "Can you say more about why you believe that?" or "Can you explain more about those feelings?" I think this helps all of us understand them better.

Use a "talking stick" to take turns. Use a seashell, stone, feather, or other object that has meaning for your group. When someone holds the object, everyone else listens and does not interrupt them. If the object comes to a person who does not wish to speak, they pass it to the next person.

Give people a moment to prepare their thoughts before starting a discussion. This helps people prepare and feel more confident to speak. Do not be afraid of silence during a group. It can be a sign of group members taking time to feel what they are feeling rather than nervously filling the silence.

Be aware of people who are quiet or shy. Some people need more time to feel comfortable sharing. You can make participation easier, for example, by going around the circle and giving everyone a turn to speak. Or you might ask people to write questions or comments anonymously and then read them out loud without saying who wrote what.

Make small groups. Discuss issues in groups of 2 or 3 people, then have them report back to the larger group. People often feel more comfortable speaking with only one other person or reporting on a group opinion rather than stating their own.

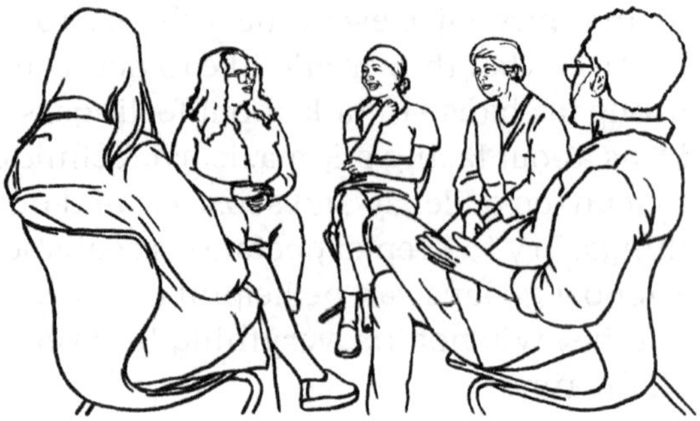

In a support group, unlearning and new learning can happen, and action can follow!

Welcome emotions. Gently encourage people to openly express what they are feeling, recognizing that not all members of the group may feel comfortable opening up. Assure the group that strong feelings and tears are not a problem. Have tissues available and be ready to offer support if needed (see "How to support a person in distress," page 141).

Aim for a balance of voices. Consider using terms like "step up" to encourage people who usually speak less and "step back" for those who tend to talk more, to help make participation equal. Find kind but direct ways to ask people to step up or step back such as: "Thanks for adding that. Would someone we haven't heard from like to go next?"

Keep the conversation on topic. If someone strays from the topic, first acknowledge their input (for example: "That's a good point.") and then invite them to relate what they were saying to the topic at hand (for example: "How does that affect your anxiety about your epilepsy at work?").

Address conflict. If conflict arises, encourage people to share their thoughts without interrupting, and remind the group that everyone is there to support one another. Use simple, clear language, and try to find shared understandings to guide the discussion so it stays focused and respectful. If needed, take a break and return to the discussion later. Solving conflict together can help a group grow stronger and more united.

HOW TO Support a person in distress

Support group discussions can stir deep feelings, whatever the topic. When a person with epilepsy speaks about experiences of stigma, they may get very emotional. The group can help the person acknowledge, accept, and manage their feelings. Here are some ways a facilitator and group members can offer support:

- If a person is overcome with emotion and unable to continue speaking, say something like, "It's OK, please take the time you need. We're here for you."
- Ask the person if they would like you to sit close to them and if they are comfortable with you gently placing your hand on their back. Follow their lead on physical contact. For some people, it can be grounding and reassuring. For others, if may feel uncomfortable.
- When a person begins to cry, remind everyone that tears are not a problem or something to be embarrassed about. Have tissues or soft cloths on-hand. Allow them some time and then offer a glass of water.
- If they are unable to recover in the group, invite the person to take a "time out" and talk privately with them to find out what might help. They may want to hear supportive thoughts from others, receive hugs, or sit quietly for a while on their own.
- For those remaining in the group, ask for a volunteer to continue leading the discussion and suggest that everyone move to a new place in the circle. This will literally change their point of view and can "reset" the group.

When the person in distress feels ready to rejoin the group, let everyone know what they said would be supportive and ask that people limit their responses to that. Ask if someone is willing to lead a breathing exercise or a song to unify the group. Then, allow the meeting to move on naturally, discussing the topic at hand.

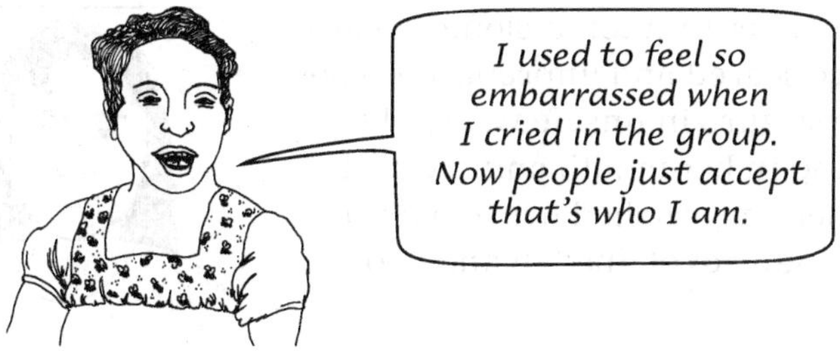
I used to feel so embarrassed when I cried in the group. Now people just accept that's who I am.

Know yourself as a facilitator

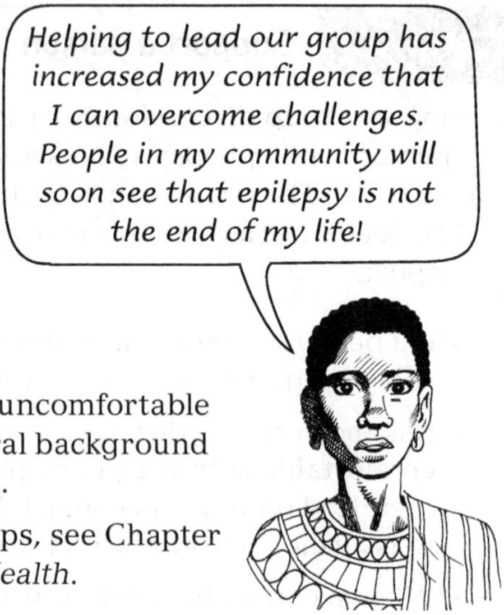
Helping to lead our group has increased my confidence that I can overcome challenges. People in my community will soon see that epilepsy is not the end of my life!

When starting a support group or leading an educational activity, it helps to be aware of how your comfort talking about epilepsy developed. Ask yourself: "What made me feel shame about my epilepsy and what did I want to keep secret? How can I encourage others to speak about their feelings?" Also, be aware of how people in the group may see you. Perhaps some women will have a hard time trusting men, or it will feel uncomfortable to have a person of one racial, religious, or cultural background being guided by someone of another background.

For more information on leading support groups, see Chapter 8 of Hesperian's *Promoting Community Mental Health.*

Making the internet a space for epilepsy support

Ivana began having absence seizures when she was 13. Her parents noticed she would "zone out" and briefly stop responding, but none of her doctors could explain it. They gave Ivana a medicine that reduced the episodes, and her mother made sure she took it every day, but no one explained why she needed it.

Not understanding what was happening made life confusing for Ivana. One summer when Ivana was away at a school camp, her mother called the organizers to remind them to give her the medicine. They made an announcement over the loudspeaker, which embarrassed Ivana in front of everyone. Her friends asked why she needed medicine and if she was sick. Ivana had no answers.

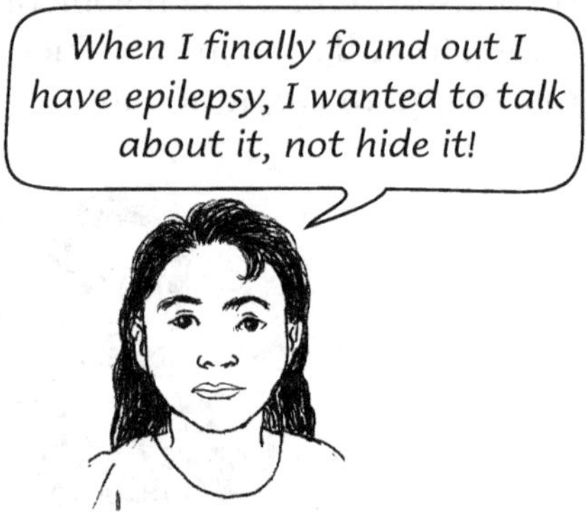

At 21, Ivana had her first tonic-clonic seizure. Her parents were scared and unprepared. They tried to stop the seizure in unsafe ways, like putting something in her mouth and trying to hold her still. Then they rushed her to a clinic where a doctor finally explained: Ivana had epilepsy.

continues

Making the internet a space for epilepsy support *(continued)*

Knowing she had epilepsy changed everything for Ivana. The uncertainty, mystery, and fear all fell away. The stigma that had prevented Ivana, her family, and her health providers from learning or speaking about epilepsy could now be replaced with understanding, care, and support.

Ivana began volunteering at epilepsy awareness events and meeting others who lived with epilepsy and stigma. One day, she met an unhappy teenage girl with epilepsy whose family helped her with medicine and checkups but refused to talk to her about her condition.

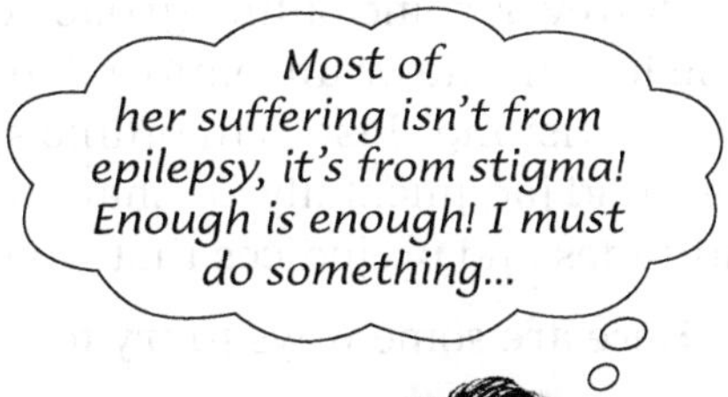

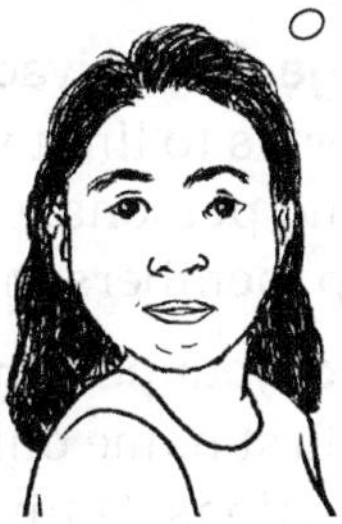

Ivana started a Facebook group called Espacio Epilepsia—a space for Spanish-speaking people with epilepsy to find support, information, and community. She began by inviting family and friends to join. As members encouraged others to participate, people with epilepsy from all over the world found the group.

Ivana posts interviews with health workers and people with epilepsy on Espacio Epilepsia. Her short, clear messages, images, and memes make learning about epilepsy easier, and sometimes even funny.

As the group grew, Ivana listened to members. Parents wanted to know about medicines. Students wanted advice and complained about school. Now, Ivana goes everywhere people with epilepsy gather online—Facebook, Instagram, and newer platforms. She asks what topics they want to discuss and makes space for new conversations to begin and go wherever they will.

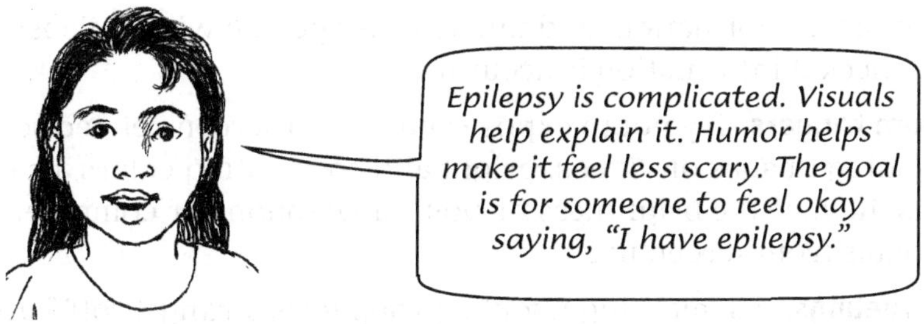

Safety and privacy online

Online spaces can make it easier for people with epilepsy to talk openly about their lives and feelings. These communities can offer support and health information. For people with access to the internet, online networks provide a way to connect and create friendships with others who share similar experiences.

However, some online groups can feel bad instead of helpful. If a group makes you feel unsafe or uncomfortable, it is not your fault and it is probably not a place worth visiting. Just as in offline spaces, people online can say unkind things, respond judgmentally, or share misinformation. They can express the same attitudes and prejudices that would make you avoid them in person.

Here are some ways to try to maintain online and digital safety and privacy:

Manage your privacy. Adjust the privacy settings on social media and online platforms to limit who can see your posts and personal information. Go slow about sharing personal details online. After joining a group, spend some time seeing how group members interact before you begin to participate.

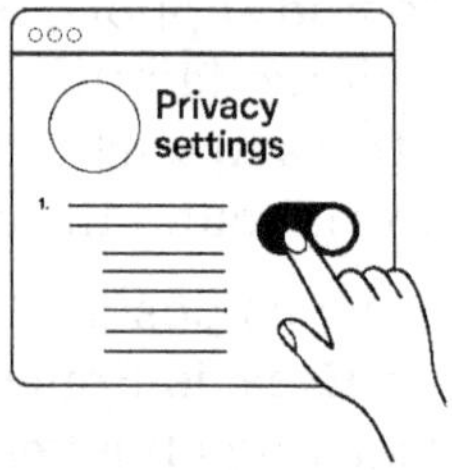

Protect your personal information. Decide if you want to use your first name only or a different name for your online interactions. Online communities often feel more anonymous than they really are. Think carefully before you share photos or information about where you live, work, go to school, etc.

Join moderated groups. Check if the online group has safety rules about connecting with other members and has group moderators or support teams. These can reduce the risk for abuse and bullying by providing ways to report harmful behavior. If someone online is abusive, report them, to protect both yourself and others.

Fact-check health information. Do not immediately believe information you find online. Be curious and ask questions. Look elsewhere online to see if other sources provide the same information, and talk to other people with epilepsy or a health worker, to check if information is accurate.

Avoid seizure triggers. Try not to expose yourself to screen-related seizure triggers, such as flashing images or videos, bright and contrasting colors, or fast-moving animations. Reduce the brightness on your smartphone or computer and take regular breaks from screen use.

Trust your feelings. If something about a group feels strange, "off," unsafe, or just somehow not good or not able to meet your needs, you can leave or take some time away from it. Try looking for support in a different online group or locally in your community rather than online.

Raising community awareness

Silence allows harmful ideas to spread and prevents useful information from being shared. Activities that raise awareness about epilepsy help break the silence and undo stigma.

Helping neighbors and community members understand epilepsy and seizures is key to reducing stigma and the harm it causes. Because stigma prevents people from talking about epilepsy, one way to act against stigma is to do the opposite—support a broader discussion of epilepsy.

People with epilepsy can take the lead on education

Public sharing by a person with epilepsy or a family member can show that epilepsy is both manageable and nothing to be ashamed of. They are more likely not to just share information but to speak from the heart. Stories and explanations from people with epilepsy carry the strength of their experiences of fear, courage, and resilience and can have a huge impact. People listen to them more closely, ask more questions, and often recognize how their own ideas and actions reflect stigma and discrimination. This encourages change in the community.

When people with epilepsy do not want to speak, or have a severe form of epilepsy that prevents them from speaking, a family member or caregiver can share what it means for someone with epilepsy to live the best life they can. Family members and caregivers can also talk about how epilepsy stigma affects the entire family and community.

Interacting personally with people affected by epilepsy is a powerful antidote to misinformation and stigma. It breaks down fear and builds empathy and understanding, all of which are necessary for people to act against stigma.

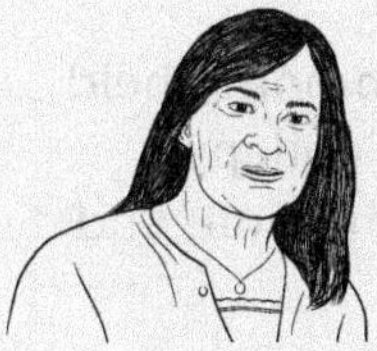

It felt good to be asked to share my story as part of a training on the harms of epilepsy stigma. For years, I would not have felt comfortable doing it. But this time, I was ready. Everyone really listened, and lots of people said that hearing from me made them "get it" in a new way.

Sharing information reduces stigma and harm

No matter what beliefs exist about epilepsy in a community, sharing correct information about what does and does not cause epilepsy and seizures, and how people with epilepsy can be helped, is one way to begin educating your community.

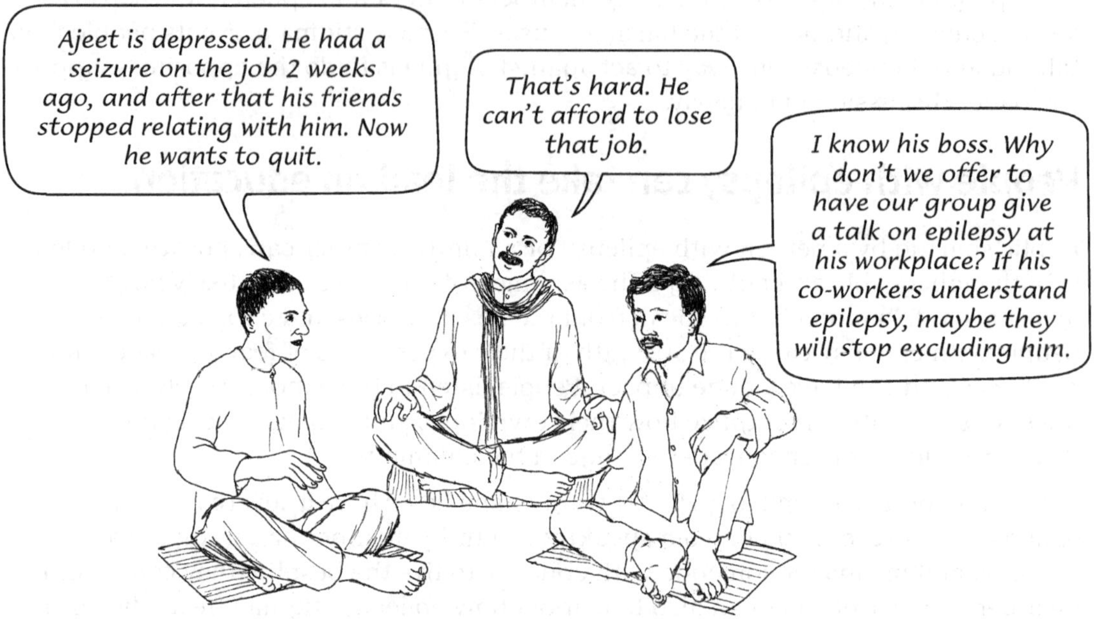
Ajeet is depressed. He had a seizure on the job 2 weeks ago, and after that his friends stopped relating with him. Now he wants to quit.
That's hard. He can't afford to lose that job.
I know his boss. Why don't we offer to have our group give a talk on epilepsy at his workplace? If his co-workers understand epilepsy, maybe they will stop excluding him.

ACTIVITY Epilepsy quiz: True or False?

When people do not talk openly about something, all sorts of ideas and explanations can develop that may or may not be true. This is certainly the case with epilepsy.

This activity can help a group raise and talk about the many commonly-held beliefs about epilepsy. The purpose of the activity is to learn about epilepsy and oppose beliefs that are wrong and can lead to stigma, discrimination, and harm. It can work with any number of people.

To prepare, create a deck of cards where each card has one of the statements provided on it (see next page). On the back of each card, write "True" if it is a true statement, and "False" if it is incorrect. For correct answers, brief explanations, and references to places in the book with more information, see pages 158 to 159.

continues

ACTIVITY

Epilepsy quiz: True or False? *(continued)*

Statements:

- Epilepsy can be caused by a head injury.
- You can get epilepsy by touching someone who had a seizure.
- Seizures are a punishment from a past life.
- A woman who has seizures should not get married or have children.
- Epilepsy is a medical condition that can be treated with daily medicine.
- Rubbing animal blood on a person with epilepsy will help them heal.
- Taking daily medicine can help control seizures.
- Hammer nails into a person's head to release the spirit causing seizures.
- People with epilepsy should not play sports.
- A baby can develop epilepsy if the brain is injured during birth.
- Sharing food or dishes with a person who has epilepsy is dangerous.
- Anyone can get epilepsy.
- A person having a seizure can swallow their own tongue.
- Stress or trauma can sometimes lead to seizures.
- Smoke from burning herbs will stop a seizure.
- Rest, exercise, and healthy food can help control seizures.
- Epilepsy can be caused by a curse.
- Rare forms of epilepsy can cause lifelong problems with speech, learning, and movement.
- Put a stick in the mouth of a person having a seizure, to stop them from biting their tongue.
- Sudden unexpected death in epilepsy (SUDEP) is a myth.
- Sometimes people get seizures, and no one knows why.
- A baby can get seizures from a high fever.
- Some children "grow out of" having seizures.
- If a mother has epilepsy, her children will also.
- You can get epilepsy by kissing.
- Some people can tell when they are going to have a seizure.

Create more statements based on common beliefs in your community.

continues

ACTIVITY

Epilepsy quiz: True or False? *(continued)*

1 Introduction

Start the activity by pointing out that people have heard many different things about what causes seizures or how to treat epilepsy. Some of the ideas are true and helpful, and others are false, based on myths, rumors, or fear, and often contribute to stigma.

2 Play the cards

People form a line and one at a time pick a card, read it aloud, and say whether they think it is true or false. Ask people in the group who agree with the answer to raise their hand. Then ask the person with the card to turn it over and share the correct answer. Give clear instructions that a card should not be turned over until it has been read aloud and they have shared whether they think it is true or false. Briefly discuss the answer if necessary. As the next person steps up, the other goes to the back of the line.

3 Group reflection

After all the cards have been read and discussed, ask questions like these and others that flow from your discussion:

- What was it like to share your statement and hear people's responses?
- What surprised you?
- How do these beliefs affect people with epilepsy in our community?
- How do some of the beliefs promote epilepsy stigma, including self-stigma, interpersonal stigma, and institutional stigma?
- What can we do to share helpful information that will reduce stigma?

As you lead the group discussion, ask people to share examples of what happens when falsehoods are believed to be true. While we may not always be able to change a person's beliefs, we can try to keep wrong information and harmful beliefs from hurting people with epilepsy.

End the discussion by emphasizing that correct information protects people with epilepsy from injury, shame, isolation, and harm. Sharing correct information also promotes dignity, inclusion, and belonging.

Traditional healers can help end stigma

Traditional and faith healers help people stay healthy in all parts of the world. They offer hope and comfort, lead prayers and rituals, promote a sense of community, and, increasingly, encourage people to seek other forms of care when health problems are beyond what they can address.

Health workers may be distrustful of faith healers if they are unfamiliar with the herbs they use or traditions they carry on. They may worry about illnesses getting worse when medical treatment is postponed, and the cost of those treatments. In return, their distrust or opposition makes traditional healers even less likely to put any trust in modern medicine.

But when health workers begin to accept healers as trusted leaders in their communities, faith healers can be enlisted to get people with epilepsy help that can stop their seizures. By training traditional healers to recognize different types of seizures, learn seizure first aid, and bring people to medical settings where seizures can be treated, support for people with epilepsy grows. Traditional healers can be encouraged to use their influence by speaking out against the mistreatment of people with epilepsy, challenging stigma and discrimination.

Some religious leaders believe epilepsy comes from possession by evil spirits, curses, or sin which can be cured by prayer, and that if a person continues to have seizures, it is because they are not praying hard enough. This kind of blaming can cause stigma, fear, and isolation. While praying for healing may comfort the person, their seizures can be stopped by using antiseizure medicine. Even if you do not share the same religious beliefs, it is important to help religious leaders learn that epilepsy is a brain condition, not a spiritual problem.

Traditional healers and religious leaders depend on their communities for support, income, and respect. They may worry that sending people to clinics for treatment will undermine their role and the importance of spirituality in the community. But when collaboration is built slowly, with mutual recognition of the services that both health workers and spiritual guides provide to a community, it can be possible to find common ground and work for the benefit of all.

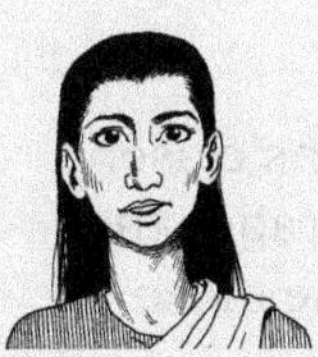

Recently, one of our temple priests began to refer patients with seizures to hospitals after learning about epilepsy. This helped shift community beliefs away from seeing epilepsy as a curse, and it encouraged people with other problems to seek medical care too.

Health workers can invite pastors and healers to trainings and make health visits to their homes or places of worship. As religious and traditional leaders understand that epilepsy is best treated medically, they can assert their leadership by making clinic referrals that lead to healing.

Concern for patients leads a faith healer to antiseizure medicine

Mtambo, a traditional healer in Malawi, uses herbs, prayer, and rituals to help people communicate with their ancestors and restore harmony in their lives. When people with seizures consulted him, he tried to help them expel the evil spirits or curses he believed caused their seizures. Some people improved, but others returned again and again with the same or worse problems, and that bothered him.

After visiting many different healers, a young man named Joseph sought out and prayed with Mtambo for help with his seizures. When his seizures continued, Joseph told Mtambo how he once used a daily medicine that stopped his seizures, but it was expensive and he could no longer afford to take it.

Mtambo became curious. He visited a clinic where a nurse explained how epilepsy works and how medicine can prevent seizures. After speaking with a patient about his experience with antiseizure medicine, Mtambo realized that medicine can help in situations where prayer cannot.

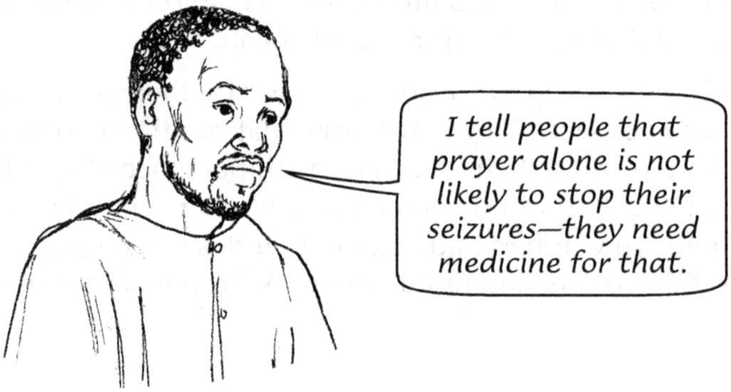
I tell people that prayer alone is not likely to stop their seizures—they need medicine for that.

Now, when people reveal they are having seizures, Mtambo listens closely, prays with them, then urges them to go to the clinic. He also encourages the clinic to travel to villages to hold epilepsy camps and make medicine more available.

Challenging institutional stigma

Many of the problems faced by people with epilepsy are resolved by accepting and learning to deal with the condition, and by educating families, neighbors, and friends about the realities of epilepsy. However, overcoming self-stigma and interpersonal stigma is often not enough to break through the barriers preventing people with epilepsy from getting the medical care they need, accessing education, finding fulfilling employment, and participating in many aspects of community life. For society to recognize that people with epilepsy have the same rights as people without epilepsy, we all have to challenge the harms caused by institutional stigma and discrimination.

Schools should not teach stigma

Engaging educational and community leaders in epilepsy education projects is a good way to ensure programs and policies that benefit children with epilepsy will continue. When school teachers, principals, administrators, and local politicians have some direct exposure to projects, they can speak up within school or government bodies about the importance of making schools work for children with epilepsy (see "Build trust and allies," page 154). Invite them to visit or participate in your efforts so they will support and make permanent programs that challenge stigma and discrimination in the education system.

From stigma to science: Teachers learn about epilepsy

For many years, schoolchildren with epilepsy in the Indian city of Mumbai did not have their teachers' support. Many teachers believed that a child with epilepsy was cursed or controlled by an evil spirit, or that seizures were a sign of laziness or lack of focus.

The epilepsy advocacy group Samman Association decided it was time to change these harmful ideas, fight stigma in the classroom, and bring epilepsy education to classrooms in their city. They launched a pilot epilepsy education program with middle school and high school teachers. It included a talk about epilepsy from a neurology (brain health and medicine) specialist, followed by a person with epilepsy sharing their experiences, and ending with a question-and-answer session.

continues

From stigma to science: Teachers learn about epilepsy *(continued)*

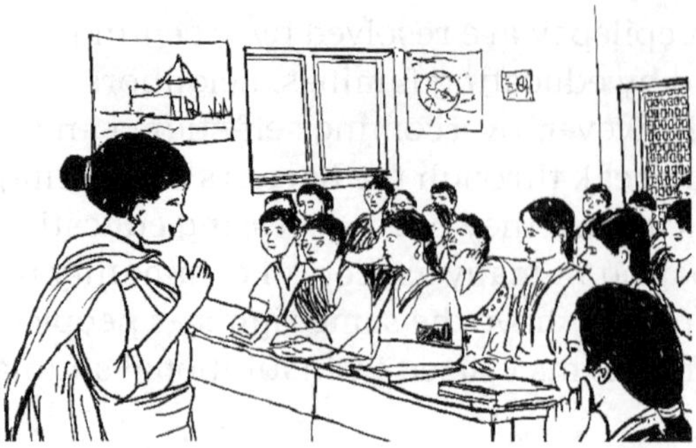

Encouraged by the positive response, Samman expanded the program to reach 250 teachers in 12 schools within a few months. Then they approached the city leaders with a proposal to train teachers at every public school to recognize, support, and advocate for children with epilepsy.

Their project was approved just as the global COVID-19 pandemic forced schools to close. So Samman adapted their program to an online format with Zoom talks and WhatsApp groups where epilepsy information was shared, questions were answered, and harmful ideas were challenged.

The program reached 7,000 teachers in a year and a half, helping them to identify seizures (including an understanding that absence seizures are not the same as daydreaming), provide safe first aid (no spoons in mouths during a seizure!), and speak out against bullying of children with epilepsy. Through follow-up surveys, Samman found the program had succeeded in reducing stigma and improving education for children with epilepsy.

Advocacy to improve laws and policies

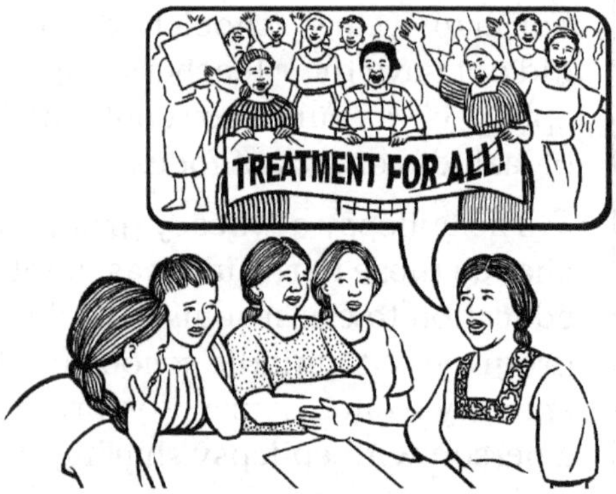

When people get their governments and health institutions to make laws and policies that recognize epilepsy as a disability, provide access to affordable medicines, and recognize everyone's right to housing and employment, people with epilepsy are more likely to be treated with dignity, equality, and respect. If enforced, laws protecting people with epilepsy can hold people and institutions accountable for discrimination and prevent further mistreatment.

When you compare these goals to current conditions, they may seem like wishful thinking, but taking steps to get there over time is very realistic. By speaking up, organizing, and working together as a community, you can begin to advocate for changes in laws and policies, so they better support human rights.

HOW TO Start a policy advocacy campaign

Identify a problem to work on. Talk to people with epilepsy, their families, health workers, parents of children with epilepsy, teachers, and others in the community to understand how institutional stigma and discrimination affect people.

Work together to clearly identify the issue you want to change. For example:

- Are people with epilepsy denied the right to marry?
- Do mothers with epilepsy lose custody of their children after divorce?
- Are children with epilepsy kept out of school?
- Is epilepsy left out of disability rights laws?
- Are antiseizure medicines not covered by national health insurance?
- Are people with epilepsy not allowed to work?

Then, find out exactly what the laws say about these issues in your country. This information may be found on government websites, in libraries and public databases, or with help from lawyers, government officials, or advocacy organizations. Look for specific laws related to epilepsy, disabilities, education, employment, and discrimination.

Discuss what you find with the people you have spoken with already. As you narrow your focus to the issues that interest most people, organize them to take the next steps in the campaign you are getting off the ground!

Decide exactly what you want to change. Write down your goal. Be clear and specific. For example:

- Change existing marriage laws so epilepsy cannot be used as a reason for preventing or ending a marriage.
- Ban housing and employment discrimination against people with epilepsy.
- Enact a policy that requires training teachers to safely respond to seizures and support children with epilepsy in schools.
- Get the health ministry to include antiseizure medications in a list of essential medicines that should be included on the national health insurance list.
- Change disability laws to recognize epilepsy as a disability.

continues

HOW TO **Start a policy advocacy campaign** *(continued)*

Gather stories and evidence. Collect information and stories that have to do with your chosen issue. Here are some ideas about what to gather. They are from a group working on adding antiseizure medicines to the approved list of medicines provided by their country's national health system.

- Stories and personal experiences of how people with epilepsy have faced institutional stigma and discrimination at the hands of health organizations.
- Examples of how that stigma and discrimination have harmed their health.
- Examples of and information about how access to medicines or health care is inadequate or unaffordable. (Are medicines available? Are there clinics that can treat epilepsy?)
- Examples of how lack of access to antiseizure medicines has stopped people with epilepsy from working, participating in community life, or enjoying their lives.

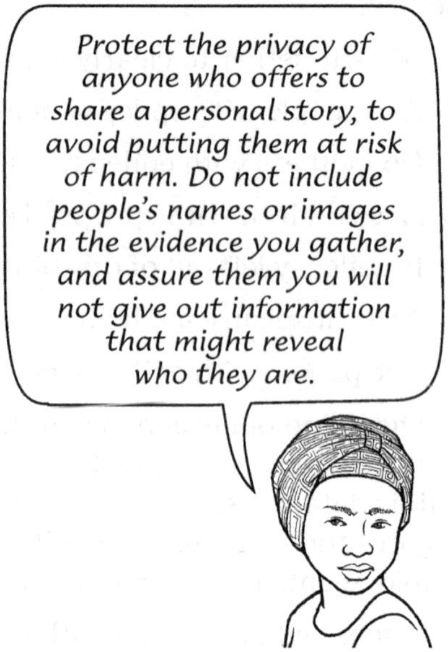
Protect the privacy of anyone who offers to share a personal story, to avoid putting them at risk of harm. Do not include people's names or images in the evidence you gather, and assure them you will not give out information that might reveal who they are.

Build trust and allies. The stories and evidence you gather will help your group convince others that a law or policy needs to be created or changed. People willing to support and stand with your cause can become your allies. They can help raise awareness, open doors to officials, and work to advance your goal. Their support makes it more likely that the government will pay attention to your cause.

Make a plan to connect, engage, and build trust with:

- epilepsy support groups.
- disability rights groups.
- health professionals.
- teachers and parents.
- religious and community leaders.
- women's groups and labor unions.
- media workers.
- concerned community members.

continues

HOW TO Start a policy advocacy campaign *(continued)*

Develop your message. Create clear messages that explain:

- the problem.
- why it matters.
- what you want to change.

You may want to prepare messages of different lengths: short, simple slogans that fit on a sign or leaflet, and longer messages that better explain why the change is needed. Find ways to share your message through community meetings, street theater, posters, leaflets, radio, or social media—whatever works in your area. When more people know and care, it will be easier to build support for change.

Talk to decision-makers. Find out who has the power to influence or change the law or policy you wish to work on, such as local health or education leaders, town council members or other government officials, or elected representatives at the local, regional, or national level. Request meetings to promote your cause, try to get them to commit their support, and follow up after the meeting to provide more information and remind them of your request.

Be patient and keep going. Policy change can take a long time. You may face challenges or delays from community members who do not fully understand the need for protections against stigma and discrimination, from institutions reluctant make changes in their policies and practices, and from government officials who do not want to provide resources or have conflicting interests. But by building support among allies and by being persistent, your struggle will keep moving forward. Support each other—the members of your group and your allies—and celebrate and share your achievements along the way. Tell the community about your progress, thank your supporters, and encourage others to act too. Every positive change can open the road for many more.

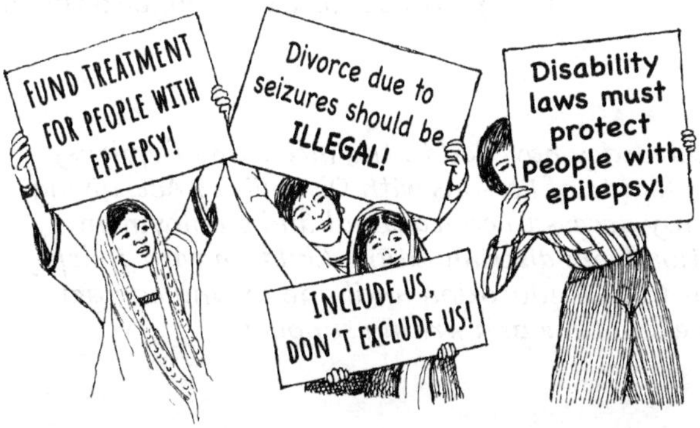
FUND TREATMENT FOR PEOPLE WITH EPILEPSY!
Divorce due to seizures should be ILLEGAL!
Disability laws must protect people with epilepsy!
INCLUDE US, DON'T EXCLUDE US!

Advocacy improves life for people with epilepsy

Advocacy is about changing laws and policies to build a more just and supportive world. When people with epilepsy experience improvements in their lives and communities through policy changes, the message shifts from "you are a problem" to "you have the same rights as everyone else." This message is a counterweight to all kinds of stigma. Here are just a few of many examples of advocacy efforts underway or already successful, from around the world.

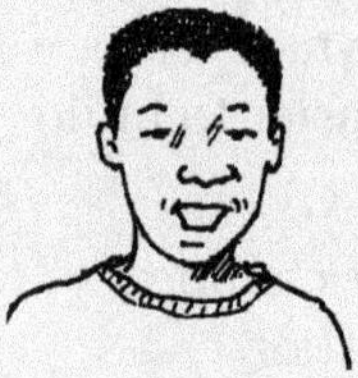

In Kenya, the Kenya Association for the Welfare of People with Epilepsy is working with the government and the National Council for Persons with Disabilities to make sure people with epilepsy receive support through the legal recognition of epilepsy as a disability. We are also pushing for epilepsy care and antiseizure medicines to be included in the country's National Health Insurance Fund, so more people can get treatment.

In Poland, our group of epilepsy advocates has successfully changed the law that says who is allowed to provide emergency care for people with epilepsy and other health conditions. Teachers and other bystanders are now legally allowed to give prescription medication—such as emergency medicine for seizures—if the person has it with them. This important change also requires training for teachers on how to respond in medical emergencies.

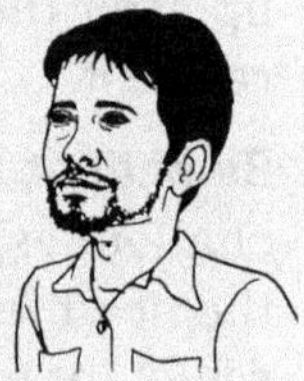

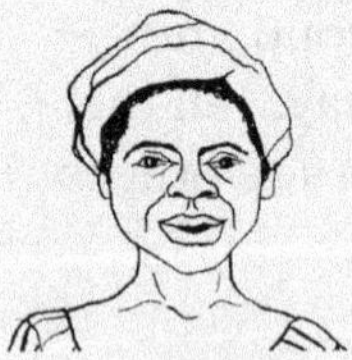

In Tanzania, we are challenging a law that allows a marriage to be annulled if one partner has repeated seizures. This law reinforces stigma and denies people with epilepsy the right to love and have a family. Through our Mothers On A Mission (MOM) Forum, people with epilepsy come together in support groups to share experiences, build confidence, and speak out for this change to the law.

In India, years of advocacy have led to the inclusion of epilepsy as a disability in the Rights of Persons with Disabilities Act, giving people with epilepsy access to educational and employment support, and protection from discrimination. Children with epilepsy now have the right to free education until age 18 and can get extra exam time and writing support.

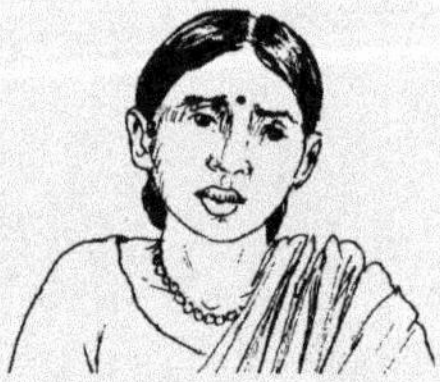

Words matter: Changing the official word for epilepsy in Hong Kong

One of the three characters in the written word for epilepsy in Chinese translates to "crazy" or "mad" (癲癇症). In Hong Kong, this has led to people with epilepsy being viewed and labeled incorrectly, making their lives very difficult. Stigma carried in the word for epilepsy makes people fear they will be isolated or mistreated when they talk about their condition. It even prevents some people from getting medical help!

To change this, epilepsy support groups and health workers began to organize with civic groups and social impact organizations in Hong Kong. They advocated for changing the word used for epilepsy to a more appropriate term that is both simple and clearly explains the condition. They campaigned at local and international conferences and through social media to make sure people understood the reasons behind the desired name change and would agree to use a new name.

They finally convinced Hong Kong's health authorities, who introduced a new Chinese name to be used, one that highlights epilepsy as a brain health condition. The new name—腦癇症—translates to "brain seizure disorder."

If the word for epilepsy in your language is harmful and you want to change it, here are some lessons from Hong Kong:

- Work with people with epilepsy, their friends and caregivers, health workers, and people in the government.
- Think of terms and names for epilepsy that are based on science and make it clear that it is a brain health condition.
- Collect possible new names from community members.
- Test your proposed name with people inside and out of the epilepsy community to find out if the new name and the reason for the name change make sense to them.

Having a new name for epilepsy will only make a difference if people learn it and start using it once a name is approved. Plan public education and awareness activities to make sure that the new name is adopted.

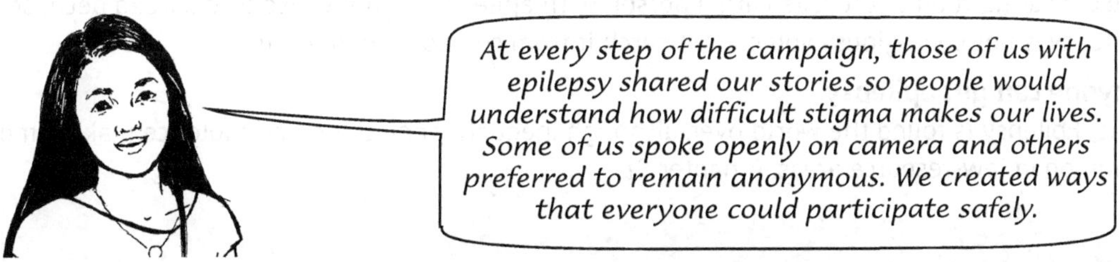

Answer key to Epilepsy quiz: True or False?

These are the answers to the true or false quiz on page 146.

Epilepsy can be caused by a head injury.
True. Head injuries are one of the many causes of epilepsy and seizures, but sometimes no cause can be identified. (Chapter 3)

You can get epilepsy by touching someone who had a seizure.
False. Epilepsy is not contagious. It does not spread by touching or being near a person who has epilepsy.

Seizures are a punishment from a past life.
False. A seizure is a temporary disturbance in the brain's electrical activity. It can be triggered by a variety of causes.

A woman who has seizures should not get married or have children.
False. Women with epilepsy can get married, become pregnant, and raise children just like anyone else. (Chapter 7)

Epilepsy is a medical condition that can be treated with daily medicine.
True. There are many effective antiseizure medicines that control seizures in people with epilepsy. (Chapter 4)

Rubbing animal blood on a person with epilepsy will help them heal.
False. Rubbing any blood on a person with epilepsy does not help and can cause infection or illness, especially if there are any cuts, scrapes, or open wounds.

Hammer nails into a person's head to release the spirit causing seizures.
False. Epilepsy is not caused by spirits or demonic possession. Hammering nails into a person's head is very harmful. It can cause bleeding, serious and permanent brain injury, or death.

People with epilepsy should not play sports.
False. People with epilepsy can play sports. Focus on avoiding seizure triggers, taking safety measures, and training coaches and communities in seizure first aid. (Chapter 6)

A baby can develop epilepsy if the brain is injured during birth.
True. A baby who does not get enough oxygen or whose head is injured during birth may develop epilepsy or another brain condition.

Sharing food or dishes with a person who has epilepsy is dangerous.
False. Sharing food or utensils with a person with epilepsy cannot cause it to spread because epilepsy is not contagious—you cannot catch it from someone who has it.

Anyone can get epilepsy.
True. Epilepsy is found the world over, although inequality and structural violence make it more common in low-resource areas. (Chapter 9)

A person having a seizure can swallow their own tongue.
False. It is not possible to swallow the tongue because it is connected to the bottom of the mouth. A person's tongue may fall back towards the throat during a seizure, as it does during snoring or sleep apnea, to temporarily block the airway.

Stress or trauma can sometimes lead to seizures.
True. Seizures can have psychological causes. Not all seizures are caused by epilepsy. (Chapter 3)

Smoke from burnt herbs will stop a seizure.
False. Breathing any kind of smoke will not help, but it can cause breathing problems or burns.

Rest, exercise, and healthy food can help control seizures.
True. Staying physically active, eating nutritious food, and getting enough sleep can help control seizures, especially when combined with the use of antiseizure medicine. (Chapter 6)

Epilepsy can be caused by a curse.
False. Epilepsy is not caused by a curse, witchcraft, evil spirit, or spiritual illness. Epilepsy is a brain condition that causes repeated seizures.

Rare forms of epilepsy can cause lifelong problems with speech, learning, and movement.
True. Several rare epilepsy syndromes can cause serious disabilities in young children. (Chapter 3)

Put a stick in the mouth of a person having a seizure to stop them from biting their tongue.
False. Putting a stick in the mouth of a person having a seizure does not help and can cause serious injury. (Chapters 3 and 4)

Sudden unexpected death in epilepsy (SUDEP) is a myth.

False. SUDEP is when a person with epilepsy dies without warning signs and no cause of death can be found. (Chapter 3)

A baby can get seizures from a high fever.
True. A high temperature can cause a child to have a fever seizure (a "febrile" seizure) which is not epilepsy. Help the child by using fever-reducing medicines. (Chapter 3)

Some children "grow out of" having seizures.
True. When seizures start at a young age, they sometimes stop happening as children get older.

If a mother has epilepsy, her children will also.
False. Epilepsy has many causes and only rarely is it passed from parent to child. (Chapter 3)

You can get epilepsy by kissing.
False. Epilepsy is not contagious and does not spread from person to person.

Some people can tell when they are going to have a seizure.
True. An "aura" warns some people with epilepsy that a seizure is starting. When noticed, it can prompt the person to get to a safe place and sit down. (Chapter 3)

Chapter 6

In this chapter

Physical activity and exercise help our bodies **161**
- Make it about movement 162
- Making physical activity and exercise safer 163
- Supporting physical activity for children with epilepsy 166
- Growing older and physical activity 167
- Contact sports 167
- Climbing, swimming 168
- Story: Kwame fights his fear of swimming—by swimming! 169
- Yoga for epilepsy 170
- Social and cultural barriers to staying physically active 175
- Story: Bicycling to beat stigma, fear, and sadness 177
- Physical activity for women with epilepsy 178
- Story: I will travel everywhere with my epilepsy 178

Eating well with epilepsy **180**
- Eating and food-related seizure triggers 181
- Fasting and epilepsy 184
- Food and antiseizure medicines 185
- Cooking safely 186
- Story: Cooking to feel bright in low moments 187
- Special food plans to control seizures 187
- Story: Managing Keilah's seizures with a keto diet 189
- Food security: Healthy eating for all 191

Sleeping well with epilepsy **192**
- Managing disturbed sleep 192
- Seizures during sleep 194
- Story: Manta's sleep seizures 195
- Preventing injuries from sleep seizures 196
- Effects of antiseizure medicines on sleep 196

Appendix: Recipes for a ketogenic diet 197

Living well with epilepsy

Nutritious food, dignified housing, clean air and water, sufficient physical activity, rest, and love—these things help everyone lead a healthy life, including people with epilepsy.

Physical activity and exercise help our bodies

Our bodies work better when we are physically active. When you exercise, you can feel your heart beat faster, your blood circulate more strongly, your muscles stretch and contract, and your lungs breathe deeply.

Exercising helps oxygen from the air we breathe and nutrients from the food we eat reach our lungs, brain, heart, bones, muscles, and skin. Regular activity reduces the body's risk of infection and illness and helps prevent pain. When you exercise regularly, your body produces chemicals that balance your mood and improve sleep.

Exercise is just as important for people with epilepsy as it is for people without epilepsy. Exercise hardly ever makes seizures worse, and it helps people who take daily antiseizure medicine reduce side effects like tiredness, sleepiness, and increased body weight.

Everyone benefits from having accessible, safe, and attractive places where they can exercise and stay physically active. Encouraging physical activity can also include educating and sharing information about the importance and safety of physical activity.

Regular physical activity makes the body stronger. This strength can decrease seizures triggered by strains on the body. For example, physical activity can strengthen the body of a person with epilepsy to handle tasks like lifting heavy things or keeping up with an active child. When exercise is done safely, it can build self-confidence, and triggers can be avoided and managed.

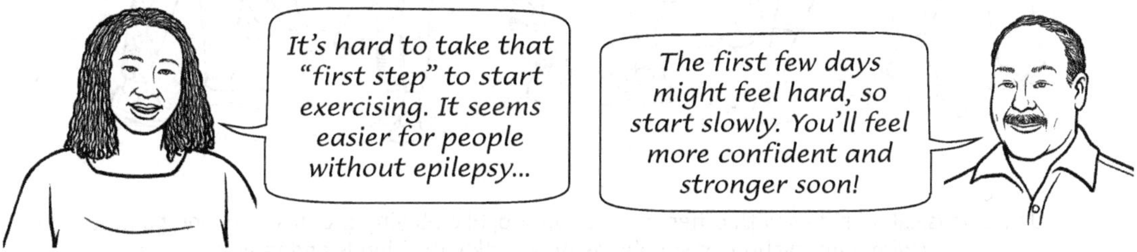

Make it about movement

Walking around your neighborhood, cycling or walking to work, gardening, and doing household chores are all things we do in our daily lives that keep us physically active. You can build upon daily life activities to get the exercise you need.

Household chores: Cleaning your home, fetching water, firewood, and groceries, washing and hanging clothes to dry, preparing meals, gardening...

Childcare: Lifting, carrying, bathing, and playing with children, tidying spaces and toys, walking children to and from school...

Farming: Clearing fields, digging and planting, weeding, harvesting your produce, cleaning and processing maize (corn), wheat, rice, and other crops...

Sports and social activities: Football, volleyball, ping pong, cricket, track and field events, jogging, jumping rope, dancing...

Spending less time on screens and moving your body more will help you feel happier and have more energy for your day. Even small amounts of movement can make daily life easier.

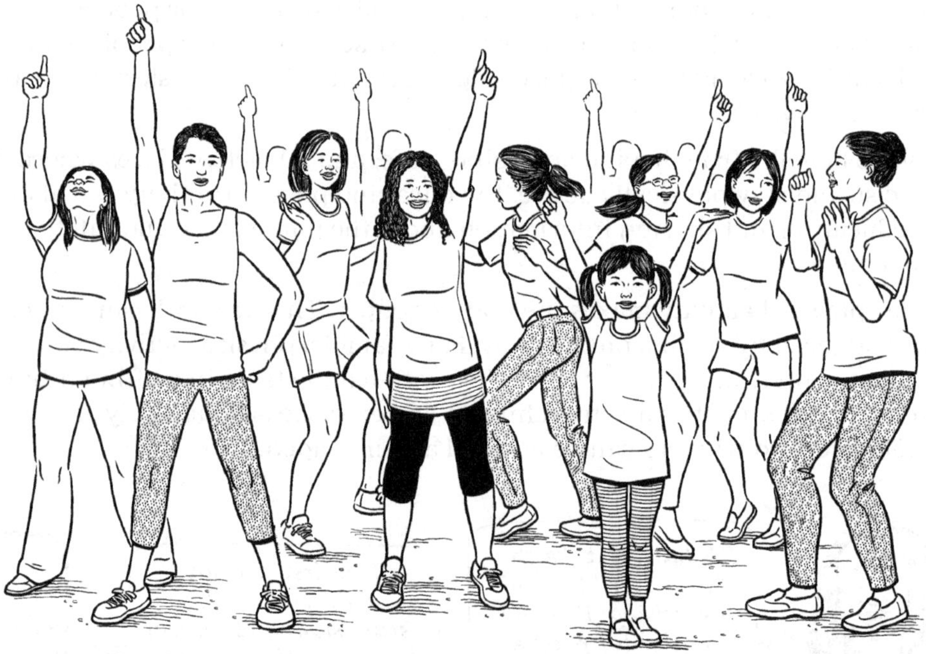

Doing physical activities with others can be fun too, like playing group sports and games, swimming, cycling, or simply taking a walk with friends and family.

Making physical activity and exercise safer

A seizure during or after physical activity might be triggered by different conditions. Tiredness, hot temperatures, dehydration, hunger, low blood sugar, and not taking medicines on time can all cause seizures for some people.

Pay attention to conditions or activities that seem to trigger seizures. Seizures can be prevented or avoided by modifying those activities or conditions.

Keep track of your seizures by noting the situation and your activities before the seizure. This can help you identify your seizure patterns so you can make changes to avoid seizure triggers.

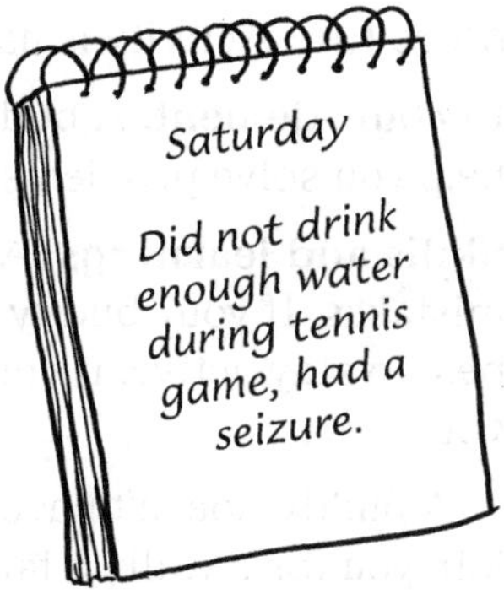
Saturday
Did not drink enough water during tennis game, had a seizure.

To prevent seizures during physical activity:

- Take medicines as directed.
- Drink water before, during (every 15 to 20 minutes), and after exercise.
- Eat a light snack about 1 hour before beginning. Nutritious snacks include bananas, apples, oranges and other fruits, and yogurt or milk. Nuts and seeds are also great because they release energy slowly.

If a specific physical activity triggers your seizures:

- Decrease the intensity of the activity and the length of time you do the activity.
- Try a different physical activity that is gentler on your body.

When a seizure happens during or soon after a physical activity you enjoy, it can be disappointing and difficult to resume the activity. Ask for support from a friend or family member to help you try again or choose a different activity.

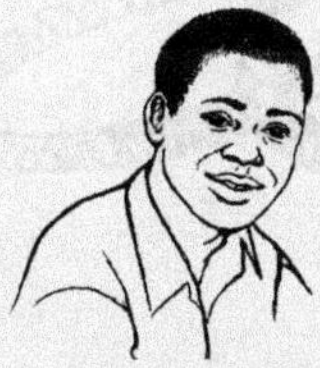

When my brother has a seizure during exercise, I remind him to slow down and help him get his confidence back. I also remind him that it is OK to take breaks when he needs them—his safety is important!

Get a buddy for safety, support, and encouragement

A buddy can be a friend, family member, or anyone willing to pair up with you for support, assistance, and encouragement during physical activity. A buddy can help provide:

Physical safety: A buddy can make sure you are physically safe and protected from injury, especially if you have a seizure. For information about seizure first aid, see Chapter 2.

More fun: Activity is usually more fun when shared with others.

Encouragement: A buddy can encourage and remind you to stay active. They can help you solve problems that get in the way of your activity.

Skills and learnings: An experienced buddy can help you develop skills and avoid mistakes. If your buddy also has epilepsy, they can share their experience about how best to stay active. If your buddy does not have epilepsy, they can learn about it from you.

A buddy doesn't have to be the same person all the time. Sometimes a friend can join you for a walk, a family member can check in on you, or a neighbor can look out for you. Different people help in different ways. Some give emotional support, some help you feel safe, and others can stand up for you if anyone tries to limit your participation in physical activities.

By letting someone know where you're going and when you'll be back, a buddy can check on you if needed. A buddy is there for support, however you choose.

Let people know you have epilepsy

Stigma sometimes prevents people from letting others know they have epilepsy and might have a seizure. Especially for times when you are not with a buddy or someone who knows and understands your epilepsy, it is good to wear an identification tag or have information visible on your phone.

Epilepsy ID bracelet, necklace, card, or tag. Make an ID necklace or a bracelet to wear on your wrist or ankle. Or hang a card on your bag or keychain, or keep one in your pocket. Whatever you choose, make sure the ID clearly says Epilepsy, or "I have epilepsy," and includes the name of an emergency contact and, if you use one, an emergency medicine. This will help others help you.

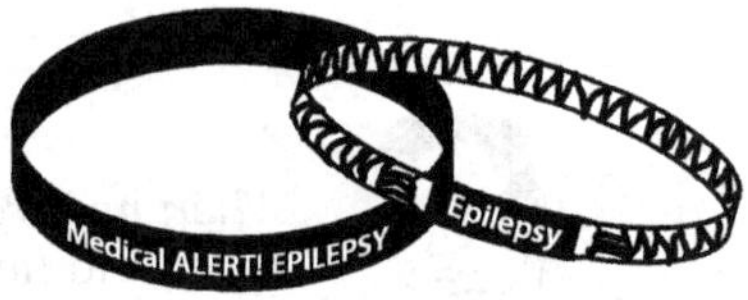

Epilepsy information on your phone. If your phone has a GPS locator, keep it turned on so people can find you in case you lose consciousness or do not return home when expected. Put a message like "I have epilepsy" on your phone screen. Keep your phone unlocked during physical activity. Save emergency information of people to contact and identify them as sister, partner, father, etc. so they are easy for someone else to find.

HOW TO Make it easy and fun to stay active

- **Keep it simple.** Find activities with low or no requirements for special equipment that can be done easily wherever you are, like walking or propelling yourself in your wheelchair. Stretching can be done almost anywhere while standing, sitting, or lying down. For examples of basic yoga poses, see page 170.
- **Set goals and commit to meeting them.** Think about the kinds of physical activity you want to do and can do. Make a plan for when, where, and how long. Commit to start slowly and work towards your goals, despite difficulties that may arise.
- **Track your progress.** Honest tracking of activity helps you stay motivated.
- **Do not get discouraged.** Even if all your goals are not met, the important thing is to be active in some way, every day. It is OK to miss a day. Just keep moving forward.
- **Pay attention to your body.** Pause and rest when you are hot, thirsty, or tired. You may need a break or to eat or drink before you start again.
- **Get help to remove barriers.** Talk to someone you trust or get a buddy for support, safety, and encouragement.

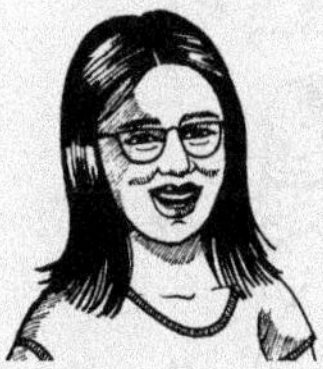

I've been going to dance classes with my best friend. We encourage each other, and it's a great chance for us to connect a couple of times a week.

For health workers

Daily physical activity is something most people with epilepsy can do safely without medical support.

Worry and safety concerns about a person with epilepsy are understandable. Family members and friends often find themselves balancing the desire to encourage physical activity with feelings of protectiveness. But overprotection can limit a person's independence and lower their self-confidence. Health workers can help familly members find the right balance between protection and encouragement.

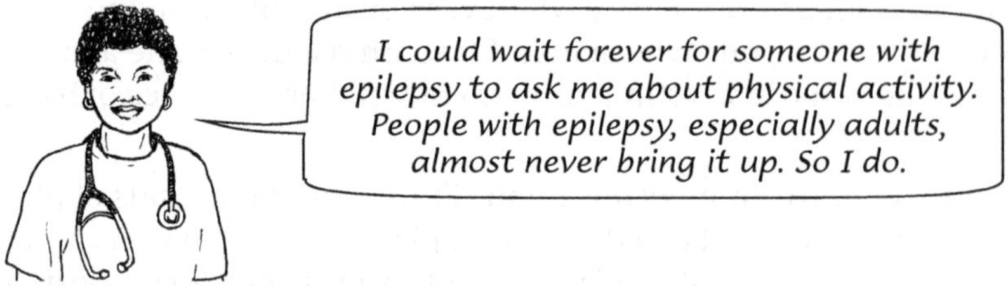

Supporting physical activity for children with epilepsy

Physical activity and playing with other children are important for growth. Playing with others helps children learn, develop, and make friends. Movement and play give pleasure and confidence, let children support each other, and offer a break from difficulties.

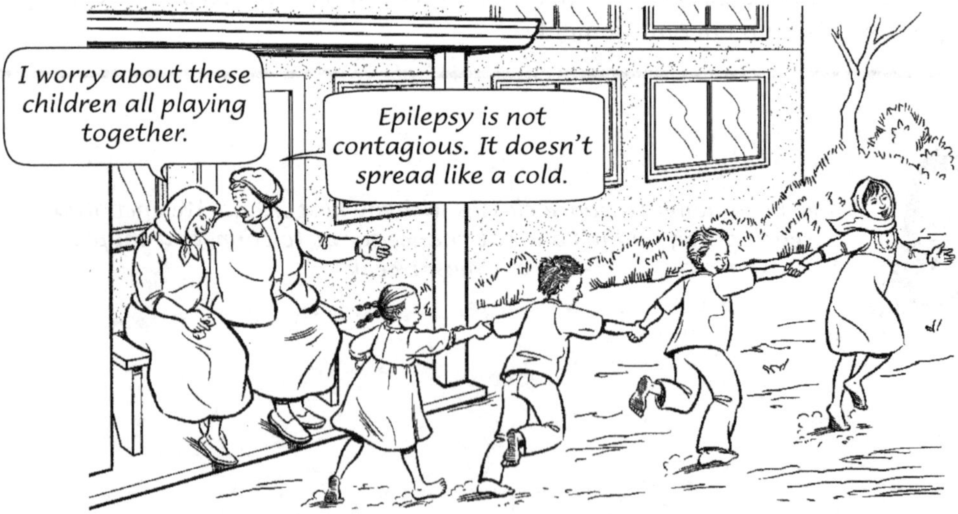
I worry about these children all playing together.
Epilepsy is not contagious. It doesn't spread like a cold.

Children with epilepsy need the same opportunities to move their bodies and play as other children and should not be excluded or treated differently during physical activities. Encourage exercise in ways that match each child's abilities. Parents, teachers, and other children and adults can teach and learn about epilepsy and seizures at schools, playgrounds, churches, child care centers, and other places where children spend time and play.

Growing older and physical activity

Seizures and epilepsy can begin at any age, including later in life. No matter when they start, staying active is key to good health. As we grow older, we might need to adjust how we move, but regular physical activity still brings big benefits. Older adults can:

- walk 15 to 20 minutes a day to keep up stamina.
- do arm exercises to build upper body strength.
- stretch or do yoga to stay flexible and improve balance.

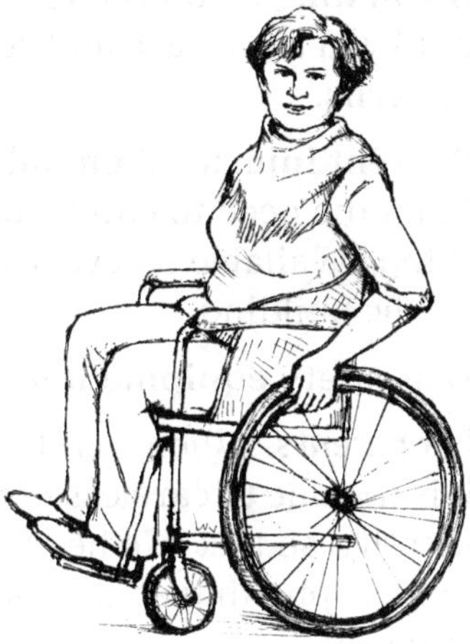

If an older adult with epilepsy joins an exercise group, others can learn seizure first aid to help keep everyone safe. It is important to adapt activities as the body and its needs change. You can move your wheelchair with your arms if you cannot walk, and do chair yoga rather than floor yoga. Make adjustments so you can stay active.

Contact sports

Hitting, tackling, or pushing are all features of contact sports like football, basketball, rugby, hockey, and wrestling, among others. Many people, including those with epilepsy, think the enjoyment from playing contact sports outweighs the chances of getting hurt.

Having epilepsy does not make you more likely to get hurt in these sports. But if you are hit on the head, it could trigger a seizure. You might want to limit or adapt your participation in contact sports if your seizures are not controlled by medicine.

To prevent head injury during contact sports and support participation from people with epilepsy:

Let people know you have seizures so those who you play with are aware and can offer seizure first aid if a seizure happens. Everyone—players, coaches, and others—can learn simple steps to prevent injury during a seizure (see Chapter 2).

Wear a safety helmet during games and practice.

Climbing with epilepsy

Climbing happens in various settings—on stairs or ladders, during sports, while picking fruit or trimming trees, and during play, especially among children.

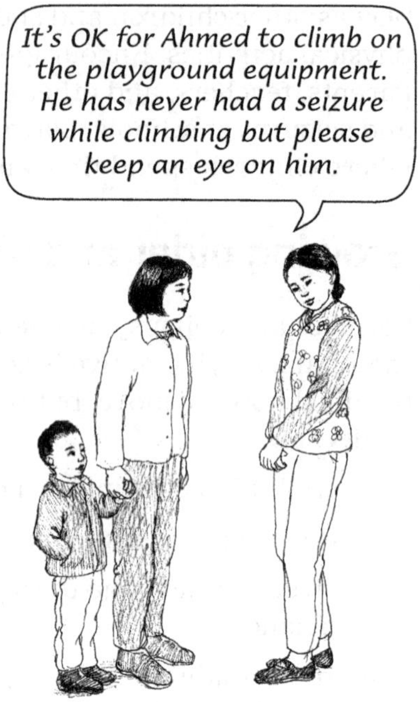
It's OK for Ahmed to climb on the playground equipment. He has never had a seizure while climbing but please keep an eye on him.

Safety tips for climbing with epilepsy

If seizures are not controlled with medicine: Avoid climbing ladders or stairs, or being on ledges or balconies with no railings, especially when alone.

If you take medicine for epilepsy: Avoid climbing until you are aware and confident of your seizure patterns.

Prevent injuries from falls: Use handrails on stairs. Limit the need to climb stairs by making often-used things available on every floor of a home, school, or public building.

Use safety equipment for climbing: Wear a helmet, harness, etc.

For parents. When a child with epilepsy is climbing and falls because of a seizure, it is not due to carelessness or clumsiness. Childhood seizures can be difficult to identify, so talk to a health worker about what medicines might prevent a seizure from happening again and finding a support group for parents of children with epilepsy.

Swimming with epilepsy

A buddy can make swimming safe for someone with epilepsy. In fact, it is a good idea for anyone swimming to have another person nearby. People with epilepsy are often told they must not swim because of fear of drowning during a seizure. This is not true.

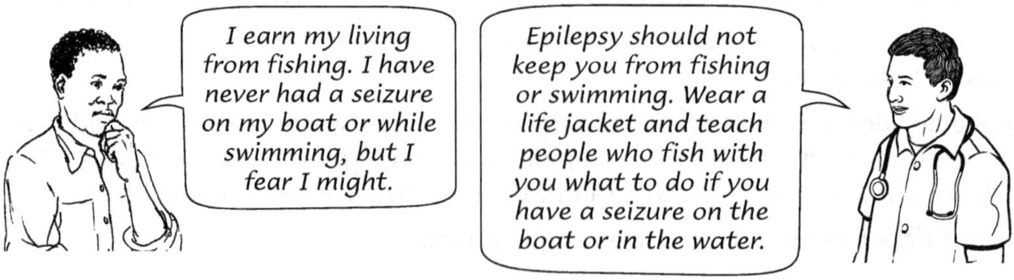

Safety tips for swimming with epilepsy

Swim with a buddy who knows seizure first aid and can help if a seizure happens.

Choose safe swimming locations, like a public pool, or a lake, river, or ocean with a designated swim area. Stay in shallow water to make swimming safer.

Inform others about your epilepsy. If you swim someplace regularly, teach people who work there or visit often what to do if you have a seizure.

For information about what to do when a person has a seizure in water, see Chapter 2, page 20.

For parents. Children who have seizures need constant supervision while swimming. A person watching them nearby can help prevent serious injury or drowning if a child has a seizure in water.

Kwame fights his fear of swimming—by swimming!

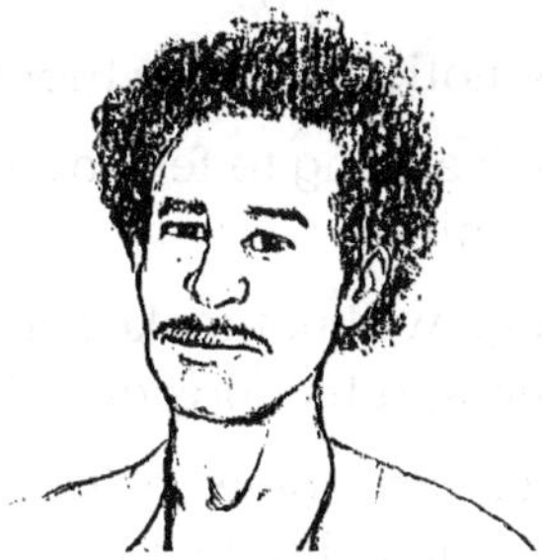

Last year, I had a seizure in the changing room at the swimming pool. Thankfully, it was after my swim and I was out of the water. But it made me nervous. What if my next seizure happened in the water?

I'm not sure if this fear will ever go away completely, but each time I swim, I work to conquer it. I've tried other sports, but I enjoy swimming so much that I do it every day.

I told the people managing the pool that I have epilepsy and they could help me when needed by learning simple seizure first aid. They agreed.

At some other pools, the managers refuse to let me swim because they think I am dangerous. The truth is, I have a disability, and it is simple to learn what to do if I ever need help. What is dangerous is not knowing what to do when someone needs help!

When more people are open to learning how to help people having seizures, more people with epilepsy will feel safe and confident to swim. When more people understand what epilepsy is, people who have it will face fewer restrictions and will live happier, freer lives!

Yoga for epilepsy

Yoga benefits our bodies and our minds. It is one of the pillars of traditional Indian medicine. It has been around for thousands of years, long before antiseizure medicines were invented.

Yoga views the body, breath, and mind as connected. Practicing yoga and this feeling of connectedness every day helps keep stress levels low, making it easier to manage daily life and reduce stress-triggered seizures. A regular yoga practice can build self-reliance and strength.

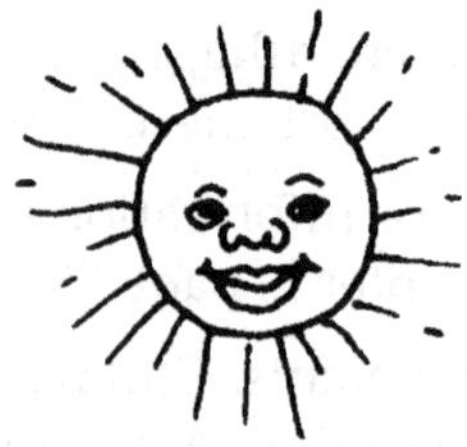

A person doing yoga is working on several things at once. Yoga involves:

- movement and poses that stretch the body, build strength, and improve balance. Yoga is a great addition to activities like walking, swimming, or cycling.
- breathing with a specific purpose or objective in mind.
- noticing all the thoughts that come up during movement.
- learning to feel joy, confidence, and energy despite challenges in the body and mind.

Yoga will not make seizures go away, but it can reduce stress, panic, sadness, anger, and feelings of "why me?"

Here are some basic and gentle yoga postures and breathing techniques that relax and calm the mind, and improve oxygen flow to the brain, where seizures start. Follow the step-by-step instructions at home every day or as often as you can.

Getting started with yoga

To do yoga, you don't have to go anywhere or do anything special. Just decide you want to do it and do it every day or a few days each week. Soon you will feel a shift in your body, mind, and spirit.

If it makes you feel more secure, ask someone who knows seizure first aid to be near you when you are doing yoga. Invite them to join you in the movements and breathing. If there is someone in your community who does yoga, ask for their support. Let them know you have epilepsy.

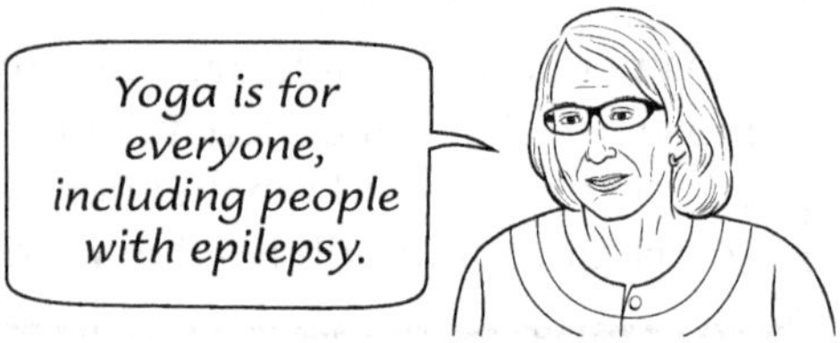

If you experience an aura or a feeling that a seizure is about to happen while you are practicing yoga, sit down and stop moving. Connect with your breath.

Make sure the space where you are doing yoga is clear of sharp or dangerous objects that might hurt you or cause injury if you have a seizure. Yoga poses involve standing, sitting, and lying down. Cushion hard surfaces with a mat or blanket to make yourself comfortable. Practice breathing and moving in and out of poses slowly.

Alternate nostril breathing (*Anulom Viloma Pranayama*)

1. Find a quiet place and sit with your shoulders relaxed and back straight, either cross-legged on the floor or on a chair with your feet flat on the ground. Rest your hand on your knees and close your eyes and relax.
2. Use your right thumb to gently close your right nostril. Hold your ring finger near your left nostril. Do not block the left nostril.
3. Breathe in slowly and deeply through your left nostril. Hold your breath.
4. Now close your left nostril with your ring finger, release your right nostril, and breathe out slowly through your right nostril.
5. Breathe in through your right nostril.
6. Switch and exhale left.

This completes one round. Repeat for 5 to 10 rounds, breathing slowly and gently to relax. If you feel uncomfortable, stop and breathe normally.

Benefits of alternate nostril breathing

- Helps calm mind and relax body
- Releases stress

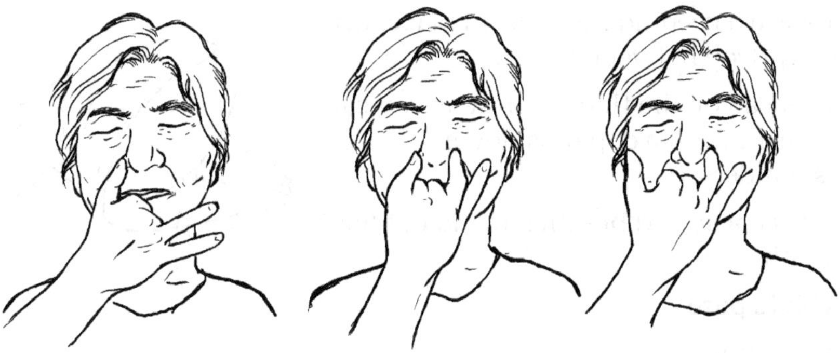

Hissing breath (*Sheetkari Pranayama*)

1. Sit with relaxed shoulders and straight back, as described for alternate nostril breathing.
2. Gently bring your upper and lower teeth together. Part your lips slightly and gently so your teeth can be seen.
3. Roll your tongue up to touch the roof of your mouth, if comfortable. Breathe in slowly through the gaps between your teeth, making a soft sound. Focus on the cool sensation of the air.
4. If comfortable, close your mouth and hold your breath for a few seconds, letting the coolness spread.
5. Close your mouth and breathe out slowly and completely through your nose.

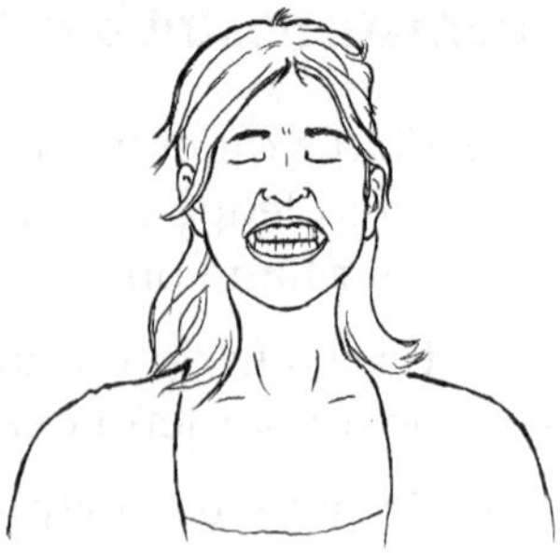

Try this for 5 to 10 rounds, staying relaxed and focused on your cooling, calming feeling.

Benefits of hissing breath

- Cools body and lowers body temperature (great during hot weather after exercise)
- Releases stress and tension
- Relaxing can help lower heart rate

Child's pose (*Balasana*)

1. Sit with buttocks resting on or slightly above heels, knees apart.
2. Lean forward keeping buttocks in place. Let your belly drop between knees.
3. Rest forehead on the floor as best as you can. Stretch arms forward, palms down. Relax shoulders.
4. Stay in this pose and breathe in and out for 7 to 8 breaths.

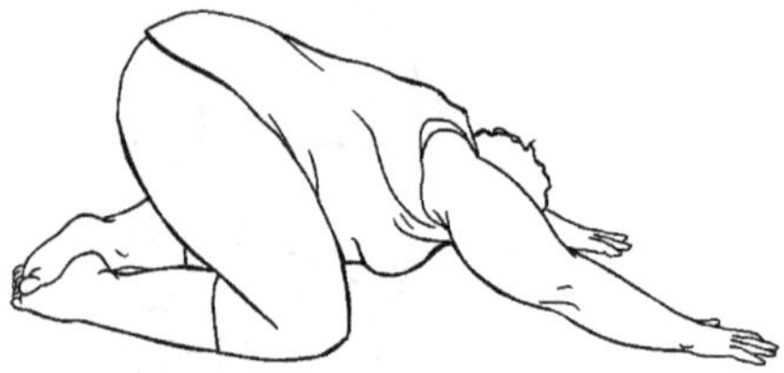

Benefits of child's pose

- Releases stress
- Improves blood and oxygen flow to the brain
- Stretches back, thighs, hips, arms, and shoulders
- For a person recovering from a seizure, this pose relaxes aching muscles and bones

Tree pose (*Vrikshasana*)

1. Stand up straight with feet shoulder distance apart, arms at your sides.
2. Shift body weight onto one foot.
3. Slowly lift other foot off the ground. Focus on balance and stability—use wall or a chairback for balance, if necessary. Bend raised knee and bring bottom of raised foot to rest against inner thigh. If this is challenging, bring foot to lower part of leg, but avoid the knee. If you lose balance or are shaky, do not be disappointed—just try again.
4. Bring hands together in front of chest, folded as in prayer. Or raise arms overhead, palms facing each other.
5. Keep your gaze fixed on a point on the floor or wall to help keep your balance.
6. Stay in this pose and breathe in and out for 7 or 8 breaths.
7. Slowly lower arms and the raised foot to return to a standing position.
8. Repeat the same steps on the other side.

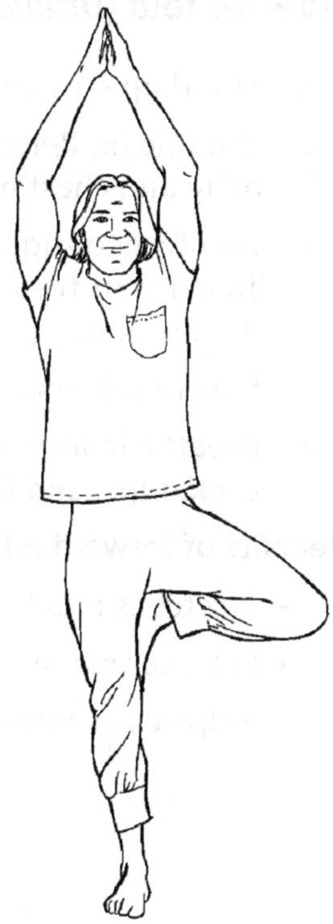

Tree pose to inner thigh

Benefits of tree pose

- Improves balance and stability, which can reduce risk of falls or injuries during seizures
- Releases stress
- Over time, as balance improves, builds sense of achievement, self-esteem, and increases self-confidence

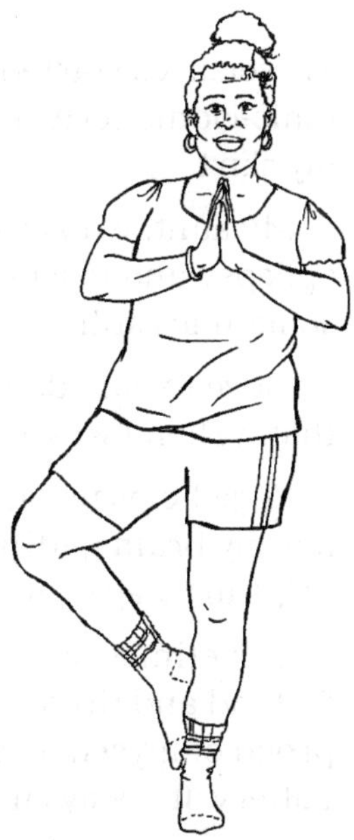

Tree pose to lower leg

Forward fold (*Uttanasana*)

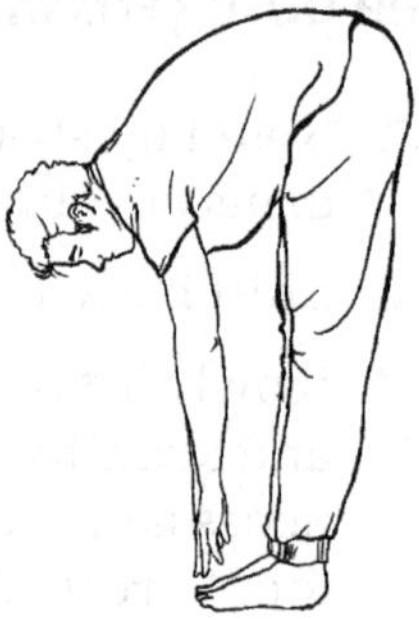

1. Stand up straight with your feet shoulder distance apart.
2. Breathe in. Release breath and bend forward from hips so belly and chest move closer to thighs.
3. Feel free to slightly bend knees as torso moves downward. Touch your toes, hold your ankles, or place your hands on the ground.
4. Stay in this pose and breathe in and out for 7 or 8 breaths.
5. Breathe in as you roll up slowly. Feel the stretch in your back, hips, and legs.

Benefits of forward fold pose

- Stretches and lengthens the spinal column
- Releases stress, feelings of panic, and tiredness
- Helps clear mind

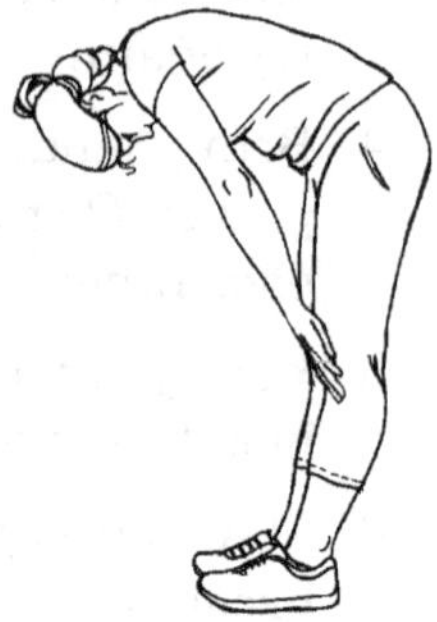

Roll up slowly

Biban says yoga helps her epilepsy

My seizures started when I was 5 years old. When I was 10, I had a generalized tonic-clonic seizure at school. I fainted. When I woke up, I had passed urine in my skirt.

My aunt, who is a nurse, took me to a hospital where they told me that I have epilepsy and must take medicine every day. But even with the medicines, I sometimes still have seizures.

I love to run, dance, and go for long walks and didn't want to stop any of that. When I was 15, my aunt suggested I try yoga.

Yoga helps me deal with my epilepsy in a positive way. Before a seizure, I can feel my brain getting excited, but doing yoga helps me stay calm and relaxed.

Sometimes having epilepsy makes me feel sad and tired, but when I do yoga, I feel proud of myself. It is like charging my body's battery. It always makes me feel better.

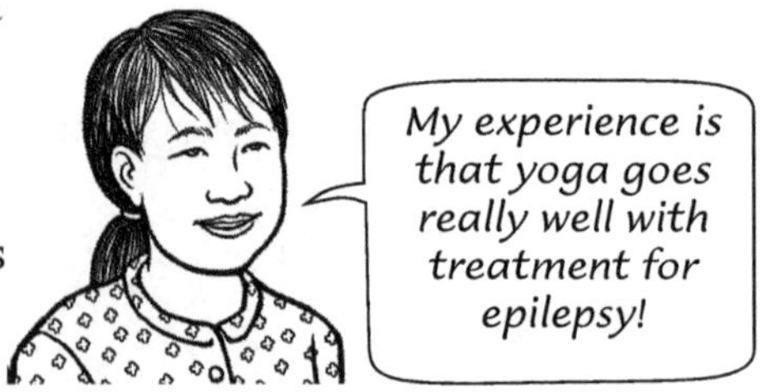
My experience is that yoga goes really well with treatment for epilepsy!

Social and cultural barriers to staying physically active

Stigma and lack of information about epilepsy can make people believe too much physical activity causes seizures or makes epilepsy worse, or that people with epilepsy are dangerous to be around.

This can make people with epilepsy feel bad about their bodies and believe something is wrong with them. They may withdraw from group activities, exercise, games, and sports. See Chapter 5: Acting against epilepsy stigma, for ideas about how to challenge these beliefs and reactions.

The barriers that prevent people without epilepsy from being active in their daily life, such as time, cost, and access, also harm people with epilepsy. Added to these challenges are stigma and safety concerns. But people can work together to remove these barriers for everyone.

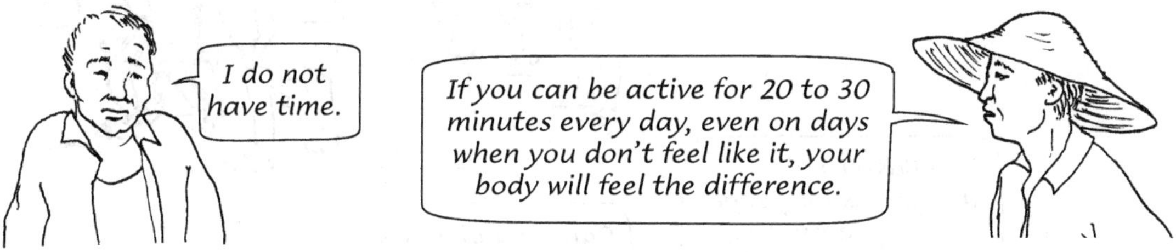

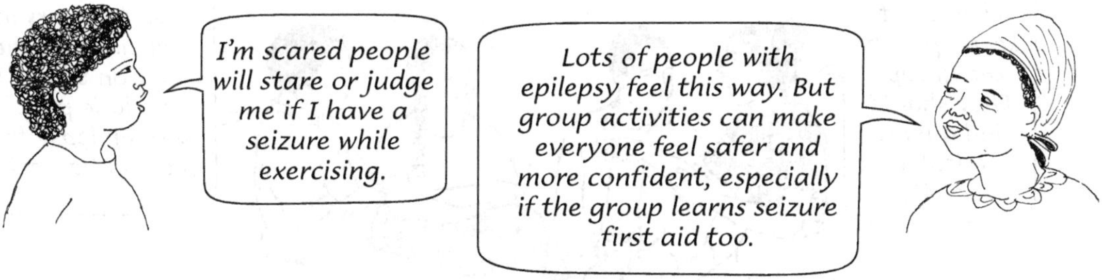

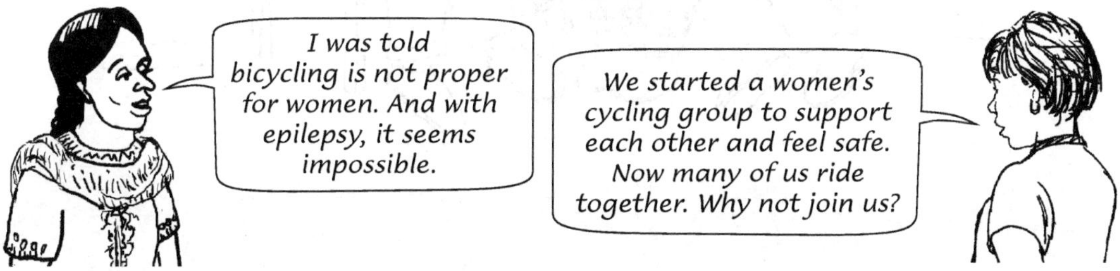

Team sports

People are often fearful of what they do not understand. Talking openly about epilepsy and seizures can help change wrong ideas and beliefs. It also allows people who might be great players onto your team so you can win together! Accepting each other, with all our strengths and weaknesses, helps everyone improve and appreciate life in all its richness.

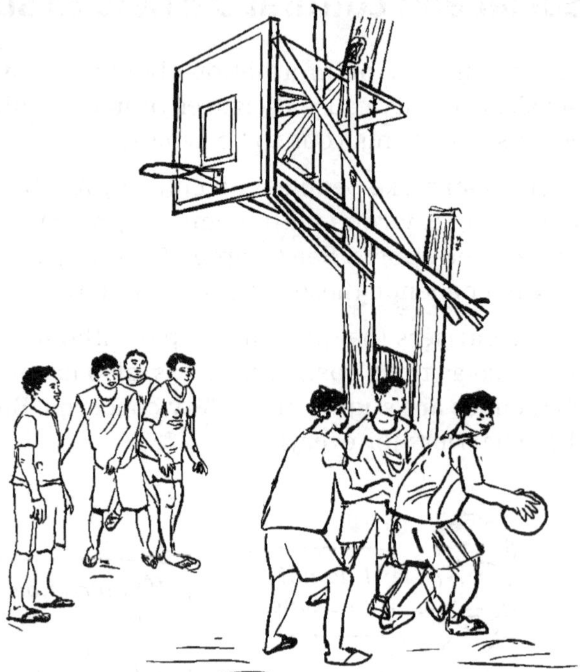

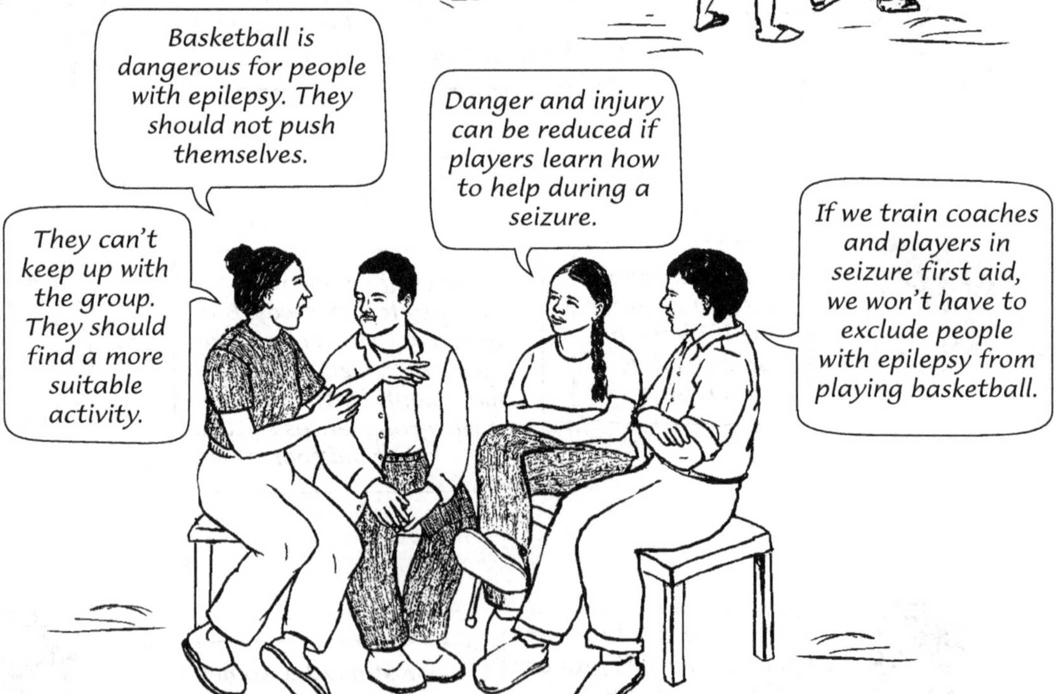
Basketball is dangerous for people with epilepsy. They should not push themselves.
They can't keep up with the group. They should find a more suitable activity.
Danger and injury can be reduced if players learn how to help during a seizure.
If we train coaches and players in seizure first aid, we won't have to exclude people with epilepsy from playing basketball.

Bicycling to beat stigma, fear, and sadness

I am Vinay Jani. At 21, I started having focal seizures. No one in my family knew about seizures or epilepsy. So, for 3 years, I did not use medicines. I tried doing things suggested by traditional healers, homeopathy, and ayurveda (Indian medicine). Nothing worked.

I felt extremely sad and lost the will to do anything. One day, I had an intense seizure and lost consciousness. After that, I was diagnosed with epilepsy. My seizures could be controlled with medicine, but the doctor said I had to take a very high dose because I weighed close to 135 kilos, and high doses can be dangerous. All this caused me more sadness and worry.

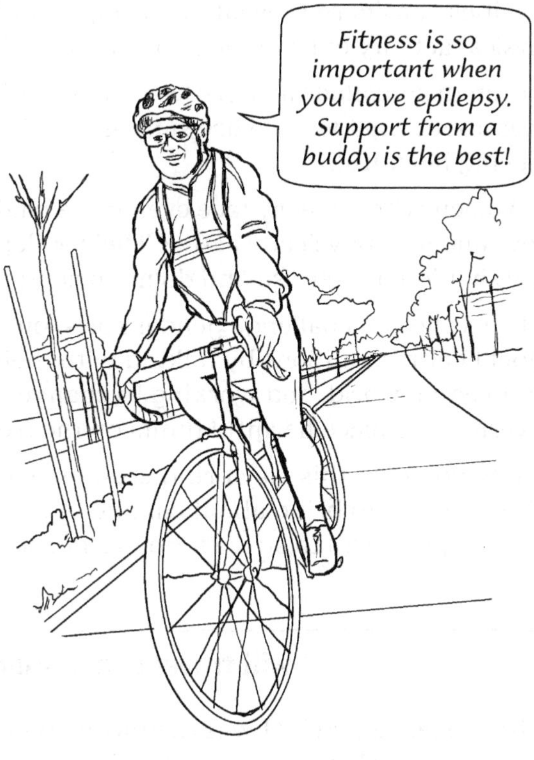
Fitness is so important when you have epilepsy. Support from a buddy is the best!

I decided to break through my sadness and worry with physical activity. I started taking the medicine and exercising at the same time. With medicine, I felt confident I would not have seizures.

I signed up for an indoor cycling class at the gym. I suggested that a friend go with me to the gym, and I told the staff about my epilepsy and my physical activity goals. They asked me how they could offer support. The more I opened up about my epilepsy, the better I felt.

One day, the trainer asked me, "Why don't you join an outdoor cycling ride?"

I was hesitant, afraid of having a seizure outdoors where people could see. I was honest about my fears with the trainer. To my surprise, she said, "Don't worry, I will learn seizure first aid and train some others in our group too." So I got a new bicycle and opened a new chapter in my life!

Physical activity for women with epilepsy

Many cultures still consider physical activity a taboo for women.

Traditional gender roles assign women to care for the household and family, not for themselves or their bodies. Some cultural and religious traditions claim to preserve a woman's honor and reputation by not allowing her to do physical activities considered revealing or improper for women. When women engage in physical activity outside the home, they challenge these beliefs.

Even in so-called "modern" societies, body image and beauty standards influence ideas about what women are supposed to look like and often link physical weakness to being beautiful.

Women with epilepsy face even more challenges in meeting their body's need to move and stay physically active. Their epilepsy makes them more likely to be told they should not exercise and do not belong in gyms or on playing fields.

Everyone can challenge gender roles, outdated traditions, and mistaken ideas about health conditions by talking with their partners and families, raising children for an equal world, and working to change how schools, religious institutions, and governments place harmful limits on the freedom of women with epilepsy.

Talking about this may bring up shame or fears about what others think, but it is necessary to bring about change. A person who stands up and speaks out encourages others to strive for more fairness and equality.

I will travel everywhere with my epilepsy

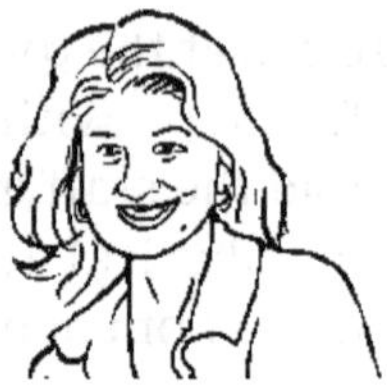

Namaste. I am Priti. I was diagnosed with epilepsy at a very young age. My parents faced ridicule in our small Indian community, where sons are considered blessings but daughters bring shame. My parents protected my sister and me from those harmful opinions and encouraged us to dream big.

My dream was to travel the world. I did not know of any women with epilepsy who did that. Even my close friends refused to travel with me. I could tell they were afraid I would have a seizure and they would not be able to help me. But their fear did not make me give up my dream.

At 23, I took my first trek up a mountain to a hill town. That gave me confidence that I could do more. Along the way, I met other women who told me how they often do not feel safe while traveling and trekking alone, because of crime and violence against women.

continues

I will travel everywhere with my epilepsy *(continued)*

This experience made me realize: A woman does not have to have epilepsy to feel unsafe while traveling! I felt a need to challenge these barriers so women, especially women with epilepsy, can travel independently in groups with other women, without partners or parents. So I started an all-women travel program.

It was tough to convince parents to send their daughters on trips. When I told them, "We will not be in danger because we will travel as a group," they had other concerns: A female tour guide with epilepsy? How can she be a leader?

When I hear that, I say, "The more women travel together, on their own and with friends, the more they develop life skills and grow confidence, and the more they show the world what is possible."

When people have doubts about me because of my epilepsy, I also share that thousands of people across the world, including myself, manage their epilepsy with medicine. People who have seizures and epilepsy are encouraged to carry emergency medicine, in addition to their daily medicine, on trips. Many people have been very curious and also very accepting.

Fear usually forces women with epilepsy to sit at home and wait for their next seizure. But like everyone else, we have the right to live our lives as we want, on our terms. Today, I can proudly say my epilepsy has led me to strengthen my community and society by encouraging people to break barriers together!

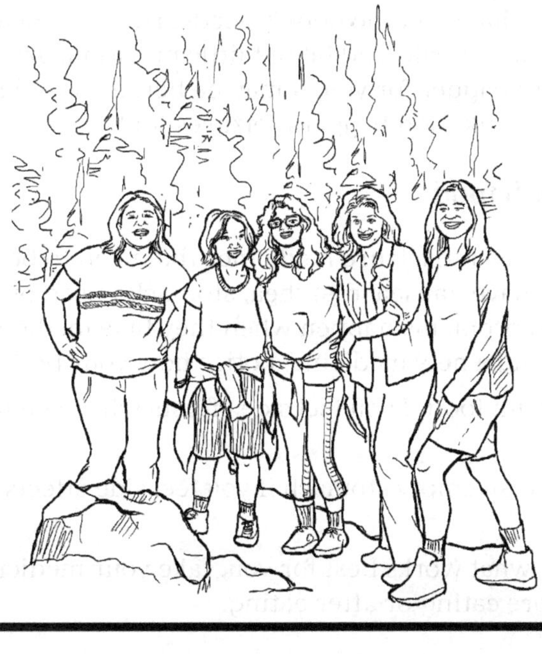

Physical activity during pregnancy

Many traditional beliefs try to limit a person's activities during pregnancy. Continue physical activity during pregnancy, though you may need to adjust what you do as your balance changes and to avoid injury. Being active during pregnancy supports better energy, mood, and health for both you and your growing baby.

It can be hard to stay physically active during pregnancy, especially if you are feeling tired or worried about having a seizure. But safety concerns and challenges like changes in medication or sleep are not reasons to stop exercising. Making group and outdoor spaces welcoming and safe for pregnant people, both with or without epilepsy, will help make pregnancy healthier for everyone.

Eating well with epilepsy

Good nutrition is important for everyone. It supports physical growth, provides the energy needed for daily physical activities, and protects against illness and stress. Good nutrition is especially important for people with epilepsy since poor nutrition and its resulting tiredness, illness, and stress can trigger seizures.

Good nutrition → Energy for physical activity → Regular physical activity → Less stress → Fewer seizures caused by stress

In much of the world, people eat one main low-cost food and add other foods to make nutritious meals that meet the body's needs. Highly processed "junk" foods, which contain lots of sugar, salt, and fat but little nutrition, are best to avoid. But if low energy is a seizure trigger for you, it may be better to eat junk food than to eat too little food—unless junk food triggers seizures too!

Timing medicine with food

Medicines, including the antiseizure medicines that need to be taken every day, cause some people to have nausea, diarrhea, stomach upset, or pain when taken with food. For others, problems happen when they take medicines on an empty stomach. When starting a new medicine, notice how your body responds.

- Take medicine with food if you feel side effects when you take it without eating, or
- take medicine on an empty stomach if you feel side effects when you take it with food.

Once you discover what works best for you, take your medicine the same way every day, either before eating or after eating.

Eating and food-related seizure triggers

Food does not cause epilepsy. But for some people with epilepsy, certain foods may trigger a seizure. For example, food and drink that contain caffeine and sugar, such as coffee, chocolate, tea, and cola drinks, can cause problems if they make it harder to sleep well, because poor sleep is a common seizure trigger. Alcoholic drinks may also trigger seizures. Alcohol interacts with some epilepsy medicines, making them less effective or increasing their side effects.

Because triggers are different for everyone, it can be difficult to identify if a certain food or drink is a seizure trigger for you. And, not everyone with epilepsy has food or drink triggers. Talk with a health worker before making big changes to your diet.

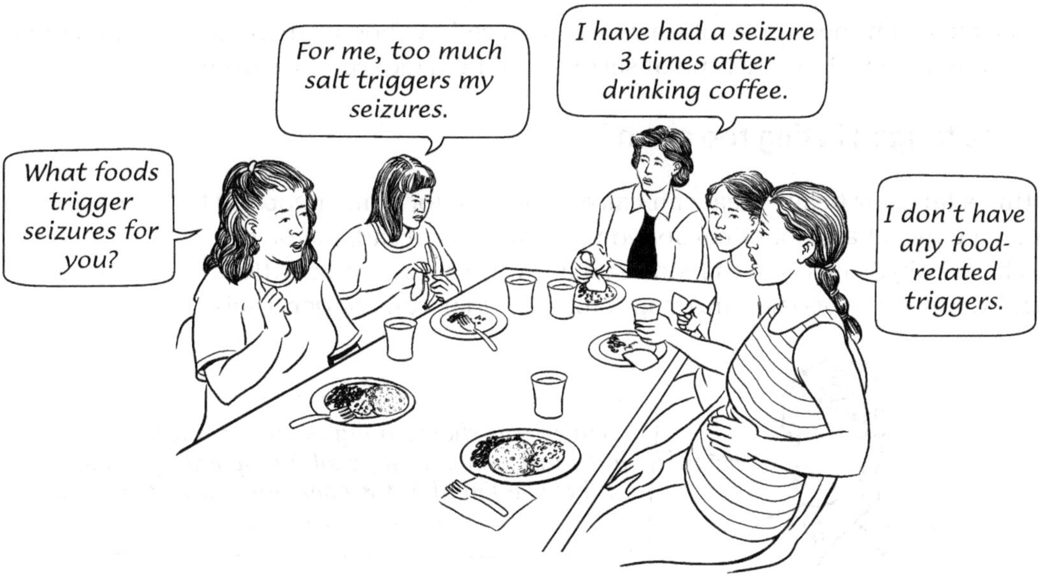
What foods trigger seizures for you?
For me, too much salt triggers my seizures.
I have had a seizure 3 times after drinking coffee.
I don't have any food-related triggers.

To find out whether a seizure was triggered by eating or drinking—or by not eating or drinking—ask yourself these questions:

- What foods were you eating before the seizure? Or had you not eaten for a while?
- Did the foods (or lack of food) also make you feel different in any other way?
- Was there another time you remember having a seizure after eating the same food or not eating anything for several hours?

Finding seizure triggers can take time. Noting and sharing details about a few seizures can help you and your health worker understand your eating patterns and food-related triggers.

Keep track of:

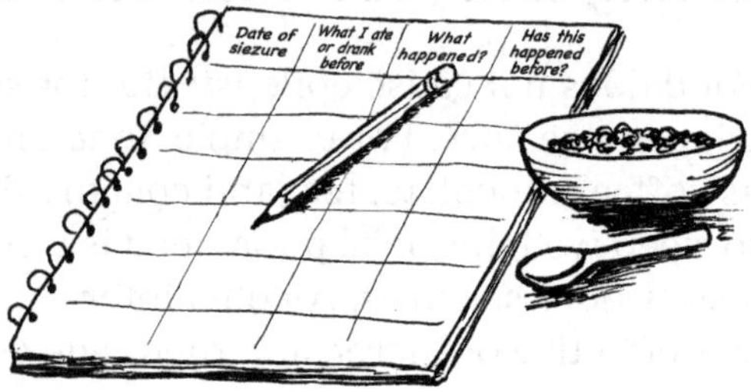

- Date of seizure
- What you ate or drank before
- What happened
- Has this food/seizure combination happened before?
- Did any other condition (heat, stress, tiredness, etc.) also happen before the seizure?

When you think certain foods or activities trigger your seizures, try to avoid them. Share what you are learning about your seizures with your health worker.

The most common types of seizures triggered by food or drink are focal seizures with convulsions, but any type of seizure can be triggered by eating.

Seizure trigger: Eating too much

Eating a large or heavy meal can cause a seizure for some people. This is most likely when the meal has a lot of carbohydrates, such as bread, pasta, or rice. Eating too much carbohydrates causes blood sugar levels to rise, and a little later, to decrease rapidly. For some people, the drop in blood sugar can trigger a seizure.

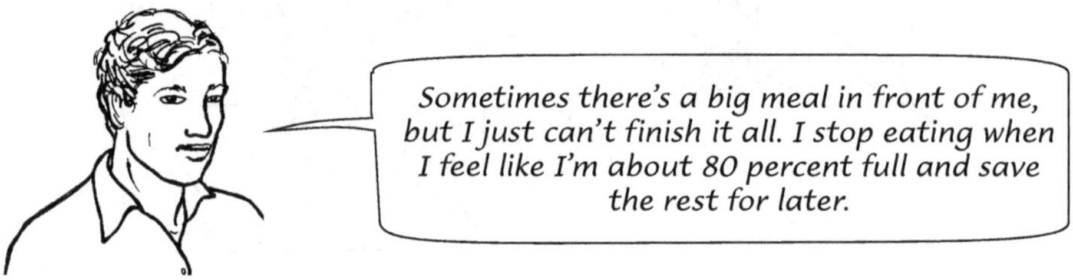

The right amount of food is different for everyone. It is affected by age, amount of daily physical activity, how quickly the body converts food into energy, and other things. But a simple way to know the right amount for you is to notice when your stomach feels full. Then stop eating.

Here are some ways to avoid eating too much:

- **Eat slowly.** Chew each bite thoroughly. Some people count and chew each mouthful 32 times before swallowing to help themselves eat more slowly.
- **Use smaller plates and bowls.** This can help limit the amount of food you eat in one serving.
- **Avoid skipping meals.** When you skip a meal, it is likely you will be hungrier at the next meal, leading you to eat more, and more quickly.

Seizure trigger: Not drinking enough liquid

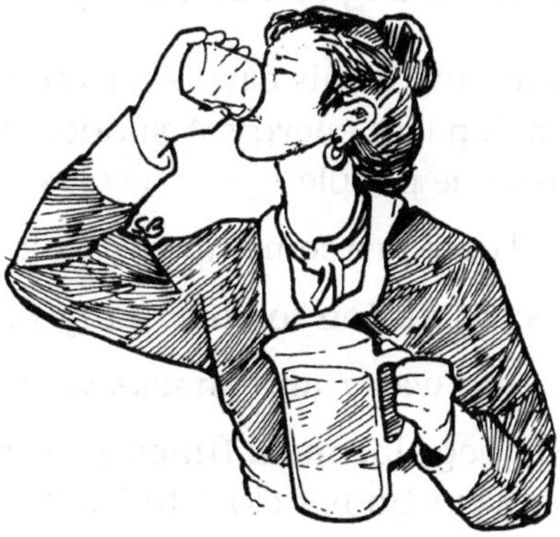

Drinking enough water can prevent seizures.

Our bodies need water to function. Not having enough water in the body is called dehydration and is a common seizure trigger.

Because drinking water helps maintain body temperature, not drinking enough water can cause the body to overheat. This can also be a seizure trigger.

Prevent dehydration and seizures triggered by dehydration by drinking about 8 glasses of water throughout the day. Some people need more water than others, especially in hot weather.

SIGNS Dehydration

Diarrhea, even if there are no other signs of dehydration.

Thirst. Remember that children and older people do not always say when they are thirsty.

Dry mouth and tongue. The inside of a person's cheek is dry.

Urinating less often. Urine may be dark-colored. Older people, to avoid getting up or leaking urine at night, often drink too little in the evening.

Treatment for dehydration

A rehydration drink will help replace liquid the body has lost through dehydration. With diarrhea, food passes through the body too quickly and nutrients are lost. This recipe for rehydration drink also replaces some of those nutrients.

Recipe for rehydration drink

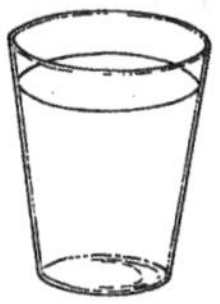

Water

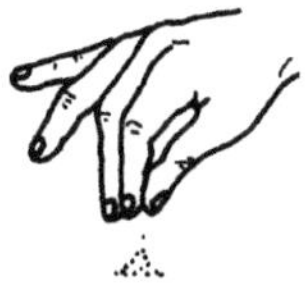

+ a little salt

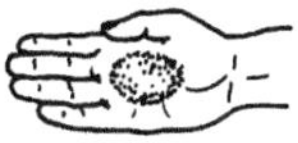

+ some energy food (sugar or rice or corn meal)

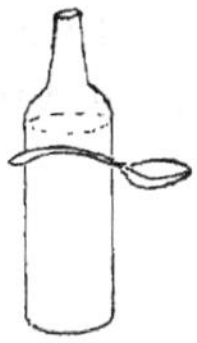

= rehydration drink

Seizure trigger: Skipping meals

Skipping meals can lower the amount of sugar in the blood, which can lead to having less energy. A sudden drop in blood sugar and energy levels causes seizures in some people.

These are some tips to avoid skipping meals:

Pay attention to your body's signals that it is hungry. Eat when you feel hungry.

Carry water and snacks with you when you leave home.

Set regular meal times and try to eat around the same times every day. This can set your body's clock to feel hunger at the same time every day.

Meal routines can be easier to keep when everyone is involved. Family members, friends, or caregivers can help by reminding each other about eating regularly, making it a group effort rather than one person's job. Letting people know about your need to stick to a meal routine will make it easier to stay on track—others can gently remind you if you forget, without it feeling like pressure.

Fasting and epilepsy

Fasting means going without food for a period of time. Some people do not drink water while fasting, but others do. People fast for different reasons, including religious and spiritual ones, or for health reasons.

Tips for fasting with epilepsy:

Do what is best for your body. If you know that fasting without food and water is not good for your epilepsy, do not force it on your body. Find ways to adjust your fast so it does not harm your health. Talk with a health worker about how to make your beliefs work with, not against, your body.

Do not stop taking your antiseizure medicine. Taking antiseizure medicine every day is important during fasting. If you use meals or tea- or coffee-time as a reminder to take medicine, link taking medicine with a non-food daily activity instead.

Rest, sleep, and drink water. Try to get enough rest and sleep, at least 8 hours every day. If you choose not to drink water during a fast, drink lots of water before and after the fast.

Can I safely fast with epilepsy?

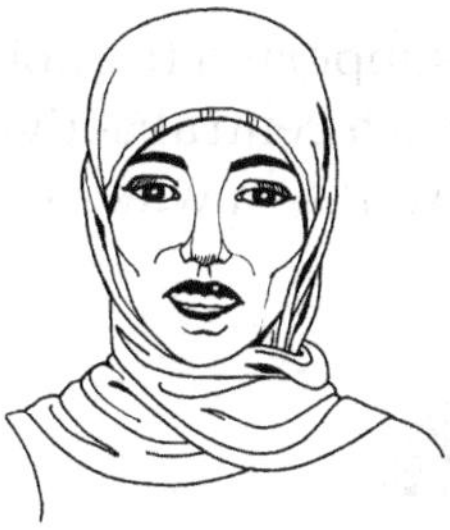

Salaam alaykum. My name is Rehab Magdy. I treat people with epilepsy and seizures. A concern for people with epilepsy in the Muslim community is how to fast safely. This is because during the holy month of Ramadan, we fast from before sunrise to sunset every day—no food, no drink.

Going without food or drink for almost 16 hours is a concern for people with epilepsy because it can affect sleep and cause dehydration, weakness, and tiredness, all of which are seizure triggers for some people.

After talking to many people with epilepsy before, during, and after Ramadan, I found that people who have focal, myoclonic, and absence seizures actually have fewer seizures when they are fasting during Ramadan. But this is not true for people with generalized tonic-clonic seizures.

Like many links between food, epilepsy, and seizures, fasting affects different people differently. Talk to a health worker who will support you to fast in the way that works best for you.

Food and antiseizure medicines

People using antiseizure medicines to manage their epilepsy need the same nutrition as a person without epilepsy. But the side effects of using some antiseizure medicines make it harder to get enough of these important vitamins and minerals:

Vitamin D: Some antiseizure medicines can cause low vitamin D levels, especially in young children and teenagers. Vitamin D helps the body use calcium better to strengthen bones.

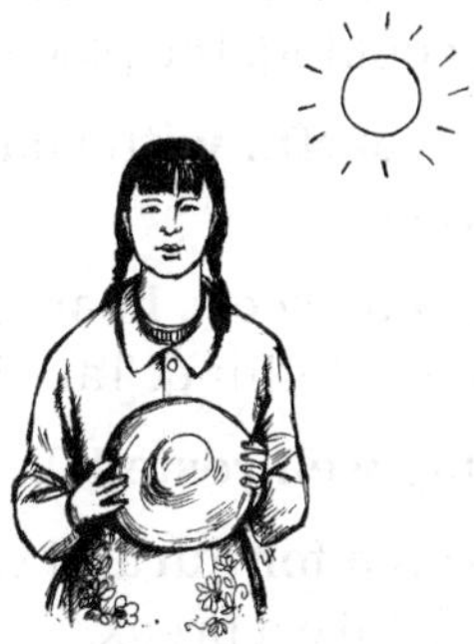

Our body makes its own vitamin D when sunlight shines on skin, but the amount it makes depends on where a person lives and the time of year. For people with lighter skin, being outside in the sun for 15 minutes every day helps the body make enough vitamin D. Those with darker skin may need up to 30 or 40 minutes each day.

Foods with vitamin D include: milk, butter, egg yolks, animal fats, oily fish, and liver.

Calcium: The antiseizure medicine carbamazepine can lower calcium levels. Bones and teeth need calcium to be strong. It is also needed to make breast milk.

Foods with calcium include: milk, curd, yogurt, cheese, ground sesame, almonds, beans (especially soy), and shellfish.

Cooking safely

People with epilepsy who enjoy cooking can be encouraged and supported to cook—not kept out of the kitchen! Making and sharing food with others is a central activity of many people's lives—a necessary task to keep away hunger as well as a way to build community and express love and creativity.

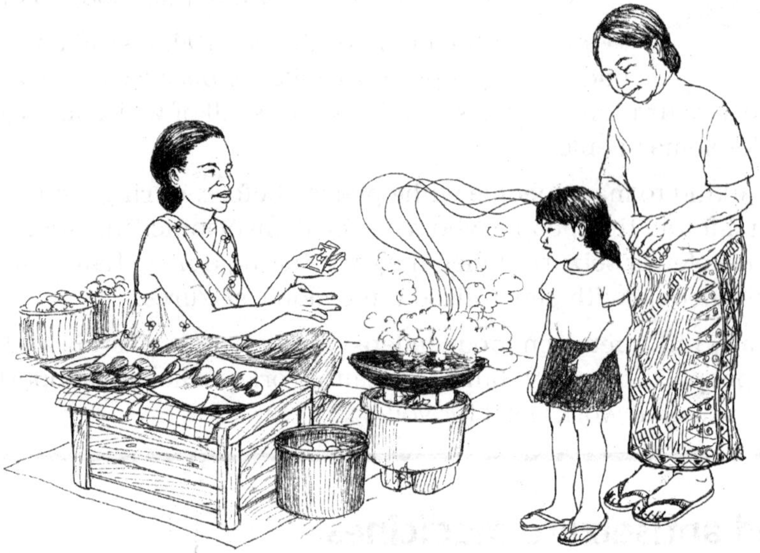

Prevent injuries while cooking

To protect against injury and prevent accidents if a seizure happens while a person is cooking, the place where food is prepared and cooked can be made safer.

Be careful with sharp tools. Keep knives and scissors in a box with a lid or inside a drawer.

Avoid excess heat. Open windows or use a fan while preparing food. Wear light, loose clothing. Take breaks away from a hot stove.

Stay well rested. Don't cook while tired, when seizures are more likely.

Watch for aura. If you sense a seizure is coming (aura), turn off the stove, sit down, and take a break.

Pay attention to fire and burn safety. Avoid cooking on open fires. On a hot stove, turn handles of pots and pans to the side when you are not using them. This can prevent injury if you fall or spill hot food during a seizure.

Find a kitchen buddy. Have someone with you when you cook on a stove or open fire. Cooking together can be more fun.

Cooking to feel bright in low moments

My name is Bright Bwalya and I have epilepsy. People ask, "How do you manage to live with epilepsy and still wear a smile on your face every day?" Well, a lot of positive practices help me when things get difficult. One of them is cooking. I love to cook. It relaxes me. When I cook, I go all out and try new and different things. Give me a stove, good ingredients (greens are a must!), a knife, and a nice chopping board, and I'm good to go. Dear friends with epilepsy: if cooking is your passion, try it out when those low moments hit. But be careful: If high temperature is a seizure trigger for you, you might specialize in making salads or cooler foods.

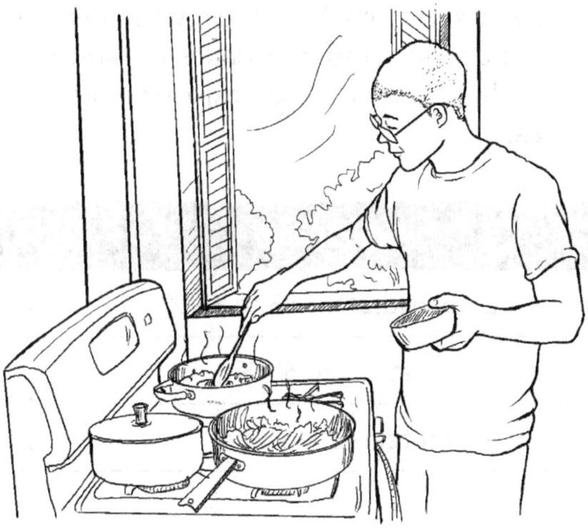

Special food plans to control seizures

For some people with epilepsy, especially children whose seizures are not well-controlled by medicines, special diets can lessen their seizures. One special daily food plan is called the "keto" or ketogenic diet (similar to the Atkins diet). This diet guides people to:

- Eat food rich in healthy fats (oil, meat, milk, butter, cheese, avocado, nuts, seeds).
- Eat higher protein foods (eggs, cheese, fish, other seafood, and meats such as chicken, beef, pork, and lamb). They have very low or no carbohydrates and fit well into a keto meal plan.
- Avoid foods with sugar and carbohydrates (bread, cassava, potatoes, pasta, sweets).
- Eat fruits and vegetables with less sugar and carbohydrates (melons, berries, avocado, greens, lettuce, and cauliflower).
- Avoid foods high in both protein and carbohydrates, such as legumes (beans, lentils, chickpeas) and grains (rice, wheat, corn). These are not part of a keto diet because they contain a lot of carbohydrates.

How low sugar, low carbohydrates, and more fats help epilepsy

A low carbohydrate and high fat diet helps manage epilepsy by getting the body used to a new main source of energy called ketones. The body produces ketones from fats. They are a different energy source than glucose, a form of sugar produced from carbohydrates, which is what our bodies are most used to. Because sudden increases and decreases in blood sugar levels are a common seizure trigger, keeping these levels steady by lowering sugar from carbohydrates helps to manage seizures.

Typical diet	Keto diet
Carbohydrates—45 to 65 %	Carbohydrates—5 to 10 %
Fat—20 to 35 %	Fat—70 to 80 %
Protein—10 to 35 %	Protein—15 to 25 %

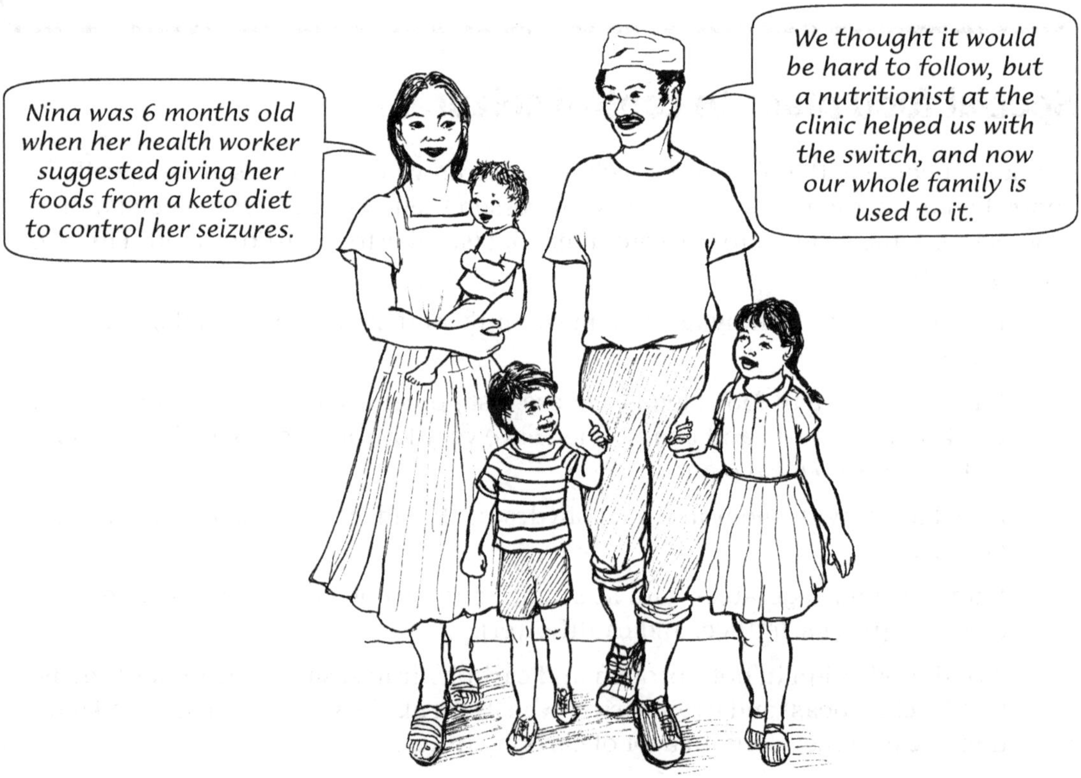
Nina was 6 months old when her health worker suggested giving her foods from a keto diet to control her seizures.
We thought it would be hard to follow, but a nutritionist at the clinic helped us with the switch, and now our whole family is used to it.

Starting a ketogenic diet

A keto diet requires changing what you eat. It can take some time for your body to get used to the diet. Some people may switch all at once, while others may find it easier to reduce foods with carbohydrates over a few weeks.

It usually takes about 2 to 4 weeks for children and adults to get used to the new mix of foods and for the body to start using fat for energy instead of sugars. As the body adjusts, you might notice changes in energy, mood, or appetite. It is important to stick to the plan. Being on a special diet is similar to taking medicine—you need to follow the instructions every day for it to work properly.

See some easy-to-prepare and delicious keto recipes at the end of this chapter.

Talk about keto or other special food plans with a health worker who has experience with the care and treatment of people with epilepsy. Discuss these issues:

- Will it be possible for you to follow a food plan different from what you and your family are used to?
- Are the foods you will need available and affordable?
- Does the health worker know others who have tried this? What was it like for the person with seizures and their family?
- Can the health worker advise you on how to adapt the dishes you commonly cook to make them high in fats and low in sugars and carbohydrates?

Special diets are often designed in a health clinic or hospital. They include carefully measured amounts of particular foods. Sometimes, medicines may need to be adjusted when changing your diet. If you are interested in a ketogenic plan for yourself or your child, talk to a health worker with knowledge of epilepsy, nutrition, and local food, to make sure a change is safe.

IMPORTANT People with Type 1 diabetes, liver, kidney or pancreatic diseases, or other metabolic disorders often cannot tolerate a ketogenic diet. Talk with a knowledgeable health worker.

Managing Keilah's seizures with a keto diet

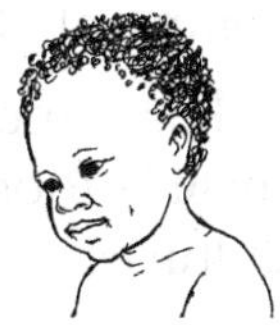

Keilah's seizures started when she was 14 months old. Her first seizure was a generalized tonic-clonic seizure that lasted for 10 minutes. After the seizure, Keilah closed her eyes and went limp. Her mother was terrified that Keilah was dying and rushed her to the hospital.

continues

Managing Keilah's seizures with a keto diet *(continued)*

Health workers thought Keilah's seizure was from fever and gave her medicine for that. They also tried to find the cause of the fever but could not.

The next week, Keilah began seizing again. This time, she had multiple atonic seizures: her body went limp and her head dropped forward. Back at the hospital, health workers counted 3 head drops, and a few days later, Keilah was having over 100 head drops each day.

The health workers gave Keilah antiseizure medicine, but it only made her seizures worse. So they asked her mother if she would agree to switch Keilah to the ketogenic diet instead.

At first, her mother was unsure. But she decided to try the keto diet. It took a few weeks to get Keilah used to the new foods and then to find the right dose of a different antiseizure medicine. With the new diet and medicine, Keilah had fewer seizures and they did not last as long.

After a few months, it became clear that the combination of diet and medicine was controlling Keilah's seizures. They became less frequent until they seemed to stop completely!

In 2013, Keilah's doctors held a workshop in Cape Town to discuss the importance of diet plans in epilepsy care. Almost 120 community health workers attended from all over South Africa. A network grew and organized trainings and community education in different cities. Two more clinics were opened to support children with epilepsy who could benefit from a keto diet.

When a nurse from an orphanage in Uganda heard about the keto diet, she started using it with a child whose seizures were not stopped by medicines. She got advice by phone on how to adapt food available in her orphanage to a ketogenic plan for the child. She stayed in touch with the clinic in South Africa to track the child's progress—and to celebrate when the seizures stopped!

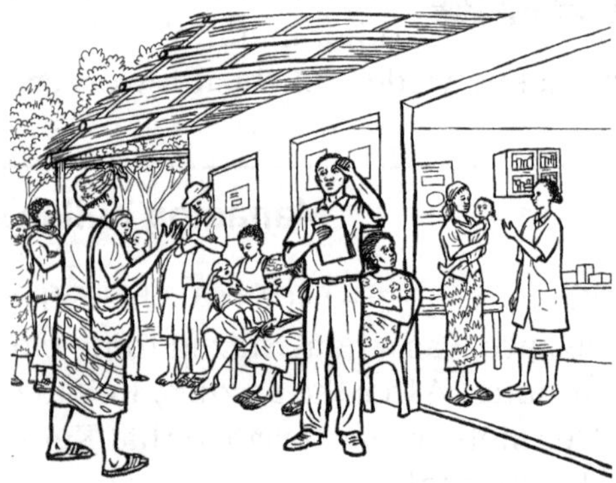

The nurse produced a keto cookbook with recipes made from ingredients commonly found in Ugandan homes.

For some ketogenic diet recipes that include foods common in different cultures, see pages 197 to 200.

Food security: Healthy eating for all

Healthy diets are possible only when there is enough food—grown, bought, or traded—for everyone. When the right to food is denied, hunger, malnutrition, and many health problems follow. Some people may need a special diet, like keto, to help with epilepsy. This is often more expensive. A family with limited resources is forced to decide between a healthy diet for one person or a healthy diet for other family members. This is not fair for the family or the community.

Food security means every person in a community has enough safe and nutritious food all year round to lead an active and healthy life. Although ensuring food security is the responsibility of every government, governmental corruption and actions by large corporations often prevent people from having access to the land and food needed to make sure that no one goes hungry.

Strengthening food security is possible in communities with little or no government support. Some ways to do this are:

Grow vegetables and fruits in family, school, and community gardens. Even if they do not own land, people can grow food to support families, restaurants, and farmers' markets.

Food cooperatives owned by the workers and the people who buy food there do not have to charge high prices to generate profits. Many food coops buy and sell locally grown food.

Farmers' markets let farmers sell directly to people. This can mean lower prices for food buyers and better income for farmers. It also can help farmers and food buyers learn about each other and the challenges they face.

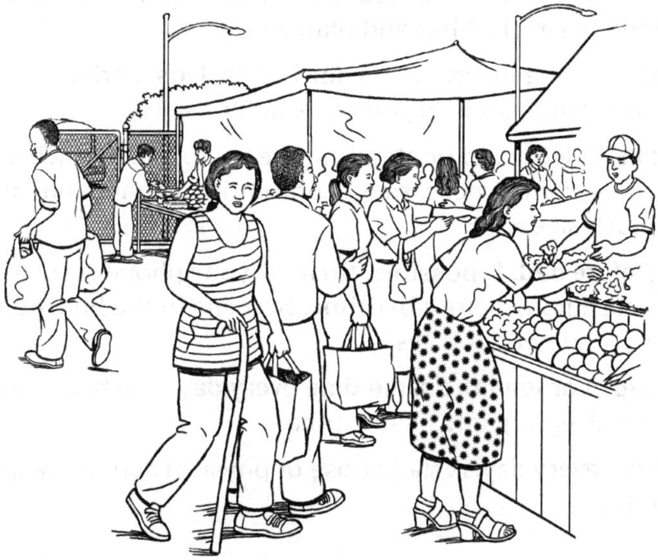

Sleeping well with epilepsy

Sleep is when our brains and bodies rest and recharge. Sleeping enough and sleeping well is a way to make seizures less likely to happen.

Sleep or lack of sleep does not cause epilepsy. But sleep problems and being tired can trigger seizures for a person with epilepsy. There are many ways sleep can be disturbed.

SIGNS **Disturbed sleep**

- Not sleeping long enough
- Waking up frequently
- Not having a regular sleep pattern (by working nights, changing shifts, traveling, or the demands of a newborn)
- Not being able to fall or stay asleep (insomnia)

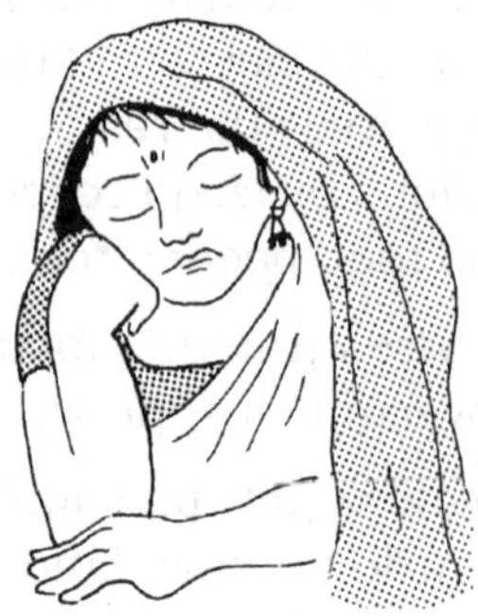

Managing disturbed sleep

Make your bedroom comfortable, neither too hot nor too cold. Cool temperatures help many people sleep better. In hot, dry weather, sprinkle a few droplets of water on your bed or wear a damp shirt to help keep yourself cool. Use light cotton bedding and sleep with a fan or air cooler turned on. In cold weather, cover ears, head, hands, and feet with warm clothing and blankets.

If you like massage, a gentle massage to your hands, legs, and feet with sesame or coconut oil (or no oil at all) can help you relax before sleep.

Avoid drinking alcohol. Reducing or stopping the use of alcohol when taking antiseizure medicines is often necessary. Combining alcohol and most antiseizure medicines can disturb sleep.

Limit screen time before bed. If possible, turn off your phone screen, television, or other screens at least 1 hour before bedtime. Screens in the bedroom can make it harder to fall asleep and get good rest.

Go to bed and get up at around the same time every day. The brain can train itself to go to sleep and stop sleeping at the same time.

Stay physically active every day. A daily dose of physical activity helps us grow tired and rest well at night.

Take your daily antiseizure medicine. Take your antiseizure medicine at the same time every day. Ask your health worker how you can avoid waking up in the middle of the night to take it.

Use gentle alarms. If you use an alarm on your phone or other electronic device, choose a pleasant sound to wake you more naturally.

Make sleeping comfortable while traveling. If you have trouble sleeping while traveling, bring something that reminds you of home, perhaps a small pillow. Stick to your regular sleep routine as best you can.

Take naps. If you do not sleep well at night, a short nap during the day can help you feel more rested. Napping for 20 to 30 minutes not too late in the day is best—it will not interfere with your sleep at night.

Yoga pose to relax and get ready for sleep

Yoga can improve our minds, our bodies, and our epilepsy. It can also help the body prepare for sleep. The traditional resting pose in yoga is called corpse pose, or *Savasana*. To get into this relaxation pose:

- Lie on your back on the floor or a bed, arms at your sides and palms facing up. Close your eyes and relax your shoulders and jaw. Take a few deep breaths.
- Hug your knees to your chest and take a deep breath in. Breathe out as you stretch out your legs without lifting any part of your body. Do this 3 to 5 times.
- Lie flat without stretching, your body fully relaxed.
- If any part of your body feels tight or painful, take a deep breath and, in your mind, breathe out into that part of the body.
- Silently count from 1 to 4 as you breathe in, and then again as you breathe out.
- Counting helps you focus on your breath.
- Keep breathing and let yourself drift into sleep.

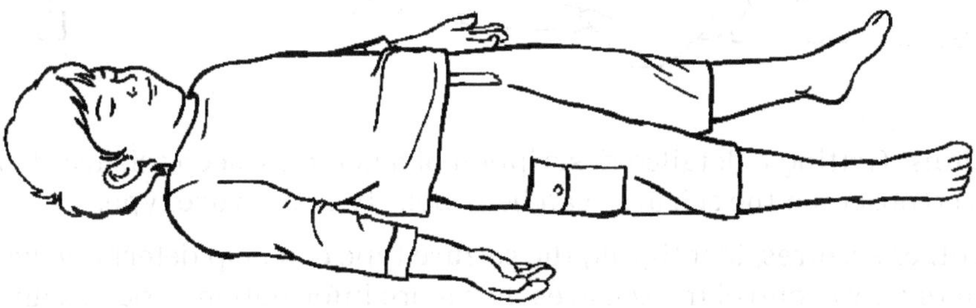

Seizures during sleep

Some people have seizures during sleep which they may or may not be aware of. They may learn about them from others who observe unusual movements, sounds, or behaviors as they sleep.

SIGNS Seizures during sleep

- Yelling or crying sounds
- Strong movements of arms and legs
- Random movements from side to side
- Waking for no obvious reason more than once a night

Identifying sleep seizures

Seizures during sleep can be difficult to discover or describe because the people around the person having seizures may also be sleeping or may not be fully awake.

To collect information:

Make a video. Filming while a person sleeps can capture their movements during a seizure. This will help identify the seizure type. Aim a mobile phone or other camera so the person's whole body can be seen.

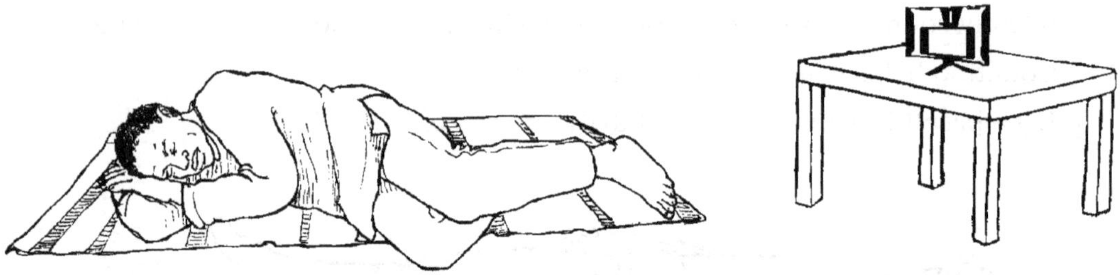

Ask questions. Getting a detailed description of a person's sleep seizures from someone who observed the seizures can help identify the seizure type.

As with other seizures, identifying the seizure type can help determine what medicine might best control the seizures. For more information about seizures during sleep, see Chapter 3, page 58.

Manta's sleep seizures

I was in my second year of university, writing papers and studying hard for final exams. I only had a few hours of sleep for 3 days and I was beyond tired. I took a nap, and that's when I had my first seizure.

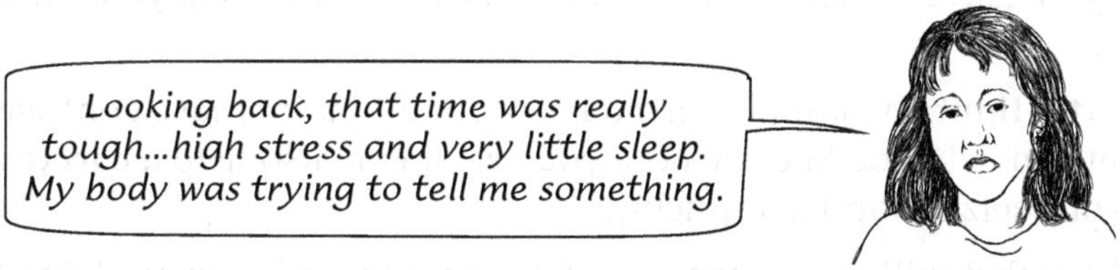
Looking back, that time was really tough...high stress and very little sleep. My body was trying to tell me something.

My roommate was studying in our room and saw me moving in bed. She did not say much about what she saw, except that it seemed to last only a few seconds.

We called my parents, and they told me to go to a hospital. After a brief exam, the health worker sent me home. I was still so tired. I went to bed but woke up again with jerking movements.

I was so frightened I went back to the hospital. This time I saw a brain specialist who asked me questions about what happened and took a brain scan.

The doctor said I had all the signs of epilepsy and that there seemed to be a connection between my seizures and sleep. She asked me to keep a diary and write about my seizures as soon as they happened.

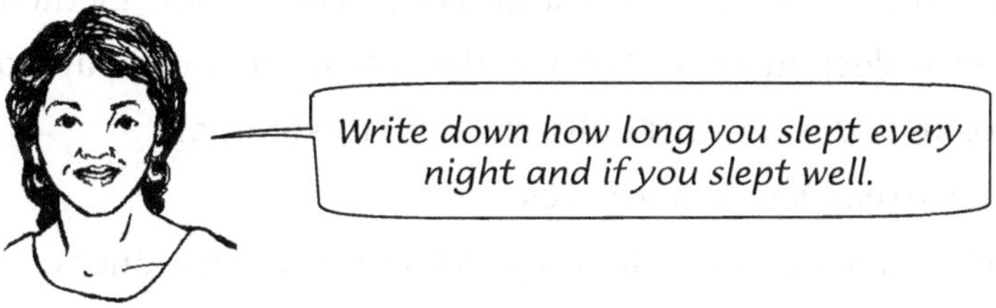
Write down how long you slept every night and if you slept well.

Keeping the diary helped me learn that my seizures are more frequent when I am tired and almost always happen while I am sleeping or right upon waking. The doctor gave me an antiseizure medicine for epilepsy. It helps. But the most important thing for me is to get enough sleep.

Preventing injuries from sleep seizures

Remove sharp objects or other dangerous things from near the bed.

Sleep close to the floor on a low bed or mattress. Place pillows or pads next to the bed to cushion a fall.

Share a bedroom. Have someone nearby who knows how to help you if a seizure happens.

Sleep with a little light. Waking up in a dark room might increase confusion after a seizure—light can help you know where you are. It can also help a caregiver be more alert to your seizure and act quickly.

Use a firm pillow that will not prevent you from breathing if you are lying face down during or after a seizure.

Avoid sleeping on your stomach. This increases the risk of inhaling vomit or other fluids during a seizure, causing breathing problems. Sleep on your side or back to allow for easier breathing.

If possible, sleep in a room on the ground floor. Not all seizures during sleep happen while a person is still in bed. Some people get up and move around during a seizure, which can lead to falls or injuries. If you cannot sleep on the ground floor, at least keep your sleeping area away from stairs.

Effects of antiseizure medicines on sleep

Side effects from antiseizure medicine often affect sleep. Some medicines:

- cause people to sleep more and may make people feel tired during the day.
- do the opposite and cause difficulty sleeping (insomnia).
- cause strange dreams or nightmares.
- cause anxiety, which can lead to sleepless nights and tiredness.

Sleep usually improves over time as the body gets used to the medicine. If the side effects of an antiseizure medicine are too strong, talk with a health worker to see if a different dose or medicine might work. People with frightening dreams may also find it helpful to talk about them with a friend, family member, or health worker.

The ways medicines affect sleep differ from person to person. Antiseizure medicines that are known to have more effects on sleep include phenobarbital, levetiracetam, and valproic acid.

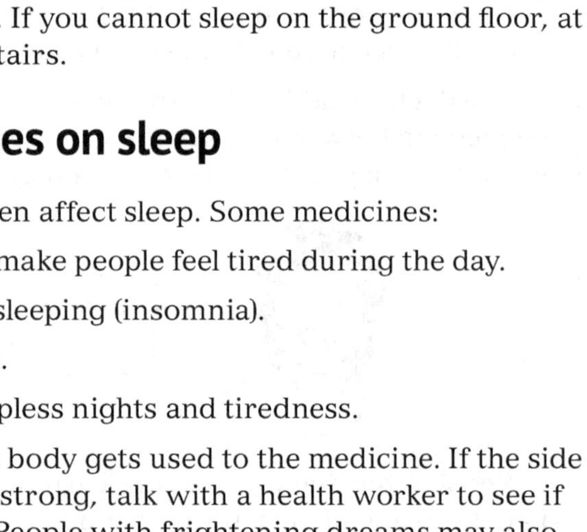

Recipes for a ketogenic diet

These recipes include approximate quantities of ingredients for 3 or 4 servings, to give a general idea of how easy and delicious a ketogenic diet can be. Talk to a health worker who knows about epilepsy and keto diets to help calculate more exact amounts that match a specific person's nutritional needs and seizure triggers.

Many people are used to measuring ingredients by sight rather than using tools like measuring spoons or scales. For best results in controlling seizures and meeting nutritional needs with a keto diet, measuring ingredients is important.

Simple Mackerel

This simple recipe for fish does not require an oven. Mackerel is a fatty fish and valuable source of energy in a keto diet. You can substitute mackerel with another local fatty fish, for example: sardines, hilsa (also called ilish or pulasa), trout, tuna, or Nile perch.

Ingredients:

- Fresh mackerel fillets (1 to 2 fillets per person)
- Sauce (soy, tamari, teriyaki, fish, or tomato, or miso paste), 15 to 30 ml (milliliters) or 1 to 2 Tbs (tablespoons)
- Oil (15 to 30 ml or 1 to 2 Tbs)
- Garlic cloves, finely chopped (1 to 2)
- Ginger, grated, 5 to 10 g (grams) or 1 to 2 tsp (teaspoons)
- Lime or lemon, sliced

How to make:

1. Mix sauce, oil, garlic, and ginger in a bowl.
2. Rub both sides of the mackerel fillets with mixture. Marinate the fish in the mixture for 15 to 30 minutes. The longer the time, the more flavorful.
3. Put a pan on medium to high heat.
4. Cook the mackerel fillets for 3 to 4 minutes on each side until the outside is browned and slightly crispy. Cooking time varies based on fillet thickness.
5. Squeeze lime or lemon slices over the mackerel. Then it is ready!

Lettuce wraps with chicken

This is a keto version of shawarma, a popular Middle-Eastern dish. The keto recipe replaces traditional bread with fresh lettuce leaves.

Ingredients:

- Chicken thighs, cut into easy-to-bite pieces, 1/2 kg or 1 lb (pound)
- Oil (30 ml or 2 Tbs)
- Onion, finely chopped (½)
- Garlic clove, finely chopped (½)
- Ginger, finely chopped (30 g or 2 Tbs),
- Cumin seeds or cumin powder (1 g or ½ tsp)
- Turmeric powder (1 g or ½ tsp)
- Salt and pepper (to taste)
- Lettuce leaves (2 large)
- Cucumber and tomatoes, chopped (½ of each)
- Coriander or cilantro, finely chopped (2 to 3 stems)

How to make:

1. In a bowl, mix oil, cumin seeds or cumin powder, chopped coriander, onion and garlic, salt and pepper.
2. Add chicken pieces to bowl and rub each piece of chicken with the mix.
3. Let the spiced chicken sit 15 to 20 minutes. Refrigerate it for a few hours for an even better flavor.
4. Heat oil in a pan over medium to high heat.
5. Cook the chicken pieces until fully cooked and slightly browned on the edges.
6. Put a few pieces of cooked chicken in the center of a large lettuce leaf.
7. Add chopped cucumber, tomato, and coriander.
8. Wrap the lettuce leaf around the chicken-cucumber-tomato-coriander.
9. Eat it fresh!

Cauliflower upma

Upma is a savory Indian dish. This recipe replaces the traditionally used semolina wheat with cauliflower.

Ingredients:

- Cauliflower, grated or finely chopped (1 medium-size head)
- Ghee (clarified butter) or oil (30 ml or 2 Tbs)
- Carrot, chopped (½)
- Green beans, chopped (5 to 7)
- Peas (a handful)
- Onion, finely chopped (½)
- Coriander or cilantro, finely chopped (2 to 3 stems)
- Mustard or cumin seeds (2 g or 2 tsp)
- Turmeric powder (1 g or ½ tsp)
- Red chili powder (1 g or ½ tsp)
- Salt and pepper (to taste)

How to make:

1. Grate or finely chop the cauliflower until it is the size of grains of rice.
2. Heat half of the ghee or oil in a pan.
3. Add cauliflower and cook for 5 to 7 minutes, stirring often. Once cooked, remove from the pan and set aside to cool.
4. In the same pan, add the remaining ghee or oil.
5. Add the mustard or cumin seeds so they pop.
6. Add chopped onion and cook until it turns golden brown.
7. Add carrots, green beans, and peas. Cook for a few minutes until soft.
8. Add salt, pepper, turmeric, and red chili powder.
9. Add cooked cauliflower to the pan.
10. Mix everything together to combine spices and cauliflower.
11. Top with chopped coriander or cilantro.
12. Enjoy! This dish can be refrigerated for 1 to 2 days.

Chicken suya

Suya is a popular West African street food known for its spicy and flavorful grilled meat, often served on skewers (sticks). This version can be cooked in a pan.

Ingredients:

- Chicken breast, cut into thin strips (½ kg or 1 lb)
- Onion, finely chopped (½)
- Garlic clove, finely chopped (½)
- Salt and pepper, to taste
- Oil (30 ml or 2 Tbs)
- Thin wooden skewers (2)

How to make:

1. Rub oil on chicken strips.
2. In a bowl, mix onion, garlic, salt, and pepper to create the spice mix.
3. Add the chicken pieces to the bowl and toss until they are well coated with the mix.
4. Let the chicken marinate for 20 to 30 minutes (or longer for more flavor).
5. Thread the chicken onto skewers.
6. Heat oil in a pan to medium to high heat.
7. Put the chicken-on-skewers on the heated pan. Cook 3 to 4 minutes on each side, or until the outside is browned and slightly crispy. Cooking time will vary based on the thickness of the chicken pieces.
8. Remove the sticks from the pan. Let them rest for 2 to 3 minutes before eating.

Chapter 7

In this chapter

Pregnancy and epilepsy **204**
Getting ready for pregnancy 204
If a pregnancy is unexpected. 205
Regular pregnancy checkups **205**
Take folic acid. 207
Pregnancy and antiseizure medicines **207**
Safe use of antiseizure medicines during pregnancy 208
Changing or adjusting antiseizure medicine: How to decide 210
Tiredness and nausea during pregnancy **213**
Why am I so tired? 213
Why am I so nauseous? 213
Pregnancy complications **215**
Seizures during pregnancy. 215
Physical injury from falls during seizures 216
Pre-eclampsia. 216
Eclampsia is an emergency!. 218
Placenta complications. 219
Labor and birth **219**
Birth emergency: Seizures that happen during labor 220
Breastfeeding for people with epilepsy **221**
Breastfeeding and antiseizure medicines 222
Helping mothers feel confident about breastfeeding. 224
Caring for your baby **225**
Birth control and antiseizure medicine **226**
Improving local epilepsy care for mothers **228**
Story: Neurology on Wheels takes epilepsy care to the village 228
Story: Epilepsy care far from cities. 229

Pregnancy and birth with epilepsy

A person with epilepsy can get pregnant, have a healthy pregnancy, and deliver a healthy baby. Eating well, getting enough rest and sleep, having regular checkups, and receiving the support and love of people around you make pregnancies healthier. A person with epilepsy has a few additional things to consider, and advice from your health worker can guide you in evaluating your antiseizure medicine to see if it is safe to use during pregnancy, if the dose needs to change during pregnancy, and if you need to take other precautions during pregnancy, delivery, or after birth to prevent injury to yourself or your baby.

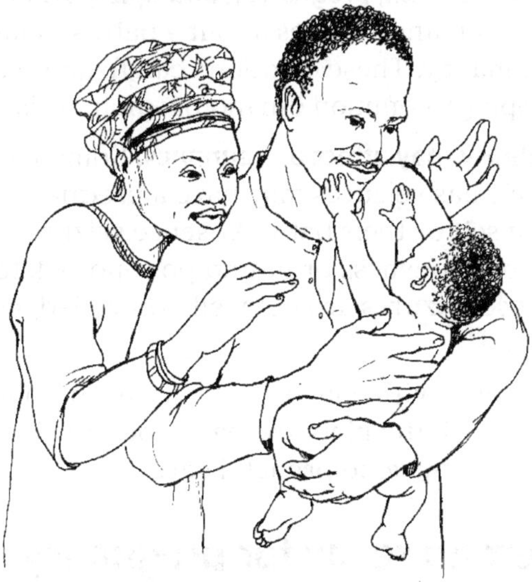

While most pregnancies are unplanned, planning for pregnancy can be especially helpful for a person with epilepsy. Planning can give you the time to make any needed changes to your antiseizure medicines as comfortably as possible. But whether your pregnancy is planned or not, you can still be healthy and deliver a healthy baby.

Although some types of epilepsy, including generalized and focal epilepsy, sometimes run in families, the chances a child will inherit epilepsy from a parent is very low. Most children of people with epilepsy do not develop epilepsy.

This chapter includes information about pregnancy and birth that is specific to people with epilepsy. For general information on how to make your pregnancy healthier, scan the QR code to access Hesperian's Safe Pregnancy and Birth mobile application or see Chapter 6: Pregnancy and Birth, in Hesperian's *Where Women Have No Doctor.*

Pregnancy and epilepsy

Every pregnancy is different. For people with epilepsy, pregnancy can affect how epilepsy presents or is managed, and epilepsy can influence the experience and management of pregnancy.

Pregnancy affects people with epilepsy in different ways. Some people have fewer seizures during pregnancy. Others have seizures triggered by the physical and mental changes that pregnancy causes. Antiseizure medicine that is safe for you and your baby can help make your pregnancy seizure free (see page 207).

Mental health, pregnancy, and epilepsy. Feelings of anxiety, stress about becoming a parent, and worries about a baby's health are all common experiences during pregnancy. These emotions can trigger seizures for some people. Insomnia (trouble sleeping), common during pregnancy, is also a common seizure trigger.

Epilepsy may affect a pregnancy. Someone who has well-controlled epilepsy and rarely has seizures may have a pregnancy that progresses with no extra risks for themself or their baby. Absence seizures or other seizures that do not include loss of consciousness or falling pose no risk to pregnancy. Risks are higher for people whose seizures are not well-controlled, especially when their seizures involve falling.

People with epilepsy may have a higher chance of getting pre-eclampsia (see page 216) or giving birth too early (before 37 weeks of pregnancy). These risks can be lowered by good prenatal care.

Getting ready for pregnancy

Most pregnancies are unplanned. In a perfect world, your pregnancy would happen when you feel physically, emotionally, and financially ready for it and have the family and social support everyone needs during pregnancy and after birth. If you are controlling your seizures with medicines, planning also gives you time to change or adjust your medicine to make your pregnancy healthier and safer. For more information, see "Pregnancy and antiseizure medicines," page 207.

Talk with a health worker about any medicines you use, including antiseizure medicines, and how often you have seizures, what kind they are, and if you have ever been hurt during a seizure. Together, you can make a plan to keep you and your baby safe.

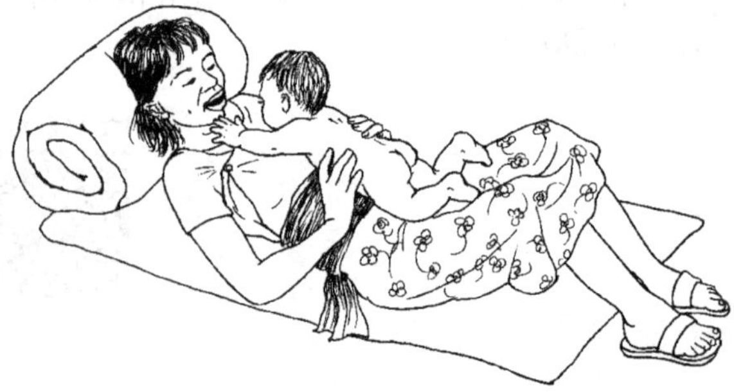

If a pregnancy is unexpected

If you find out you are pregnant and want to continue the pregnancy, talk with a health worker or midwife as soon as possible about how to have a healthy pregnancy. If you need to change your antiseizure medicine, beginning that process right away will promote better seizure control and a healthier pregnancy. A health worker can also help you to adjust your medicine dose, if needed, and work with you to make a plan for what to do if you have a seizure during your pregnancy.

If you do not want to continue the pregnancy, talk to a health worker or midwife about how to end the pregnancy with safe abortion. Abortion is safe when done with the proper medicines, and with support from an experienced accompanier, or by a trained health worker, depending on the type of abortion.

Abortion may be always legal or only sometimes legal, depending on where you live. Getting advice from a trusted health worker or community member who knows local laws and how to support you can help you make an informed decision and have a better experience.

For more information about abortion, scan the QR code to access Hesperian's Safe Abortion mobile application.

Regular pregnancy checkups

Whether or not you have epilepsy, and whether your pregnancy was planned or unexpected, checkups during pregnancy are important to help keep both you and your baby healthy.

Checkups allow you and a midwife or other health worker to:

- discuss how you are feeling.
- talk about how epilepsy and other health conditions may affect your pregnancy.
- check your health by measuring your body—your blood pressure, weight, belly growth, etc.
- find out how the baby in your womb is developing.
- ensure healthy eating and physical activity.
- address any questions or concerns you may have about your pregnancy.
- understand and prepare for the birth.

During checkups, a health worker can watch for signs of problems, such as severe pain, swelling of the hands or face, fever, bleeding, or headaches. Acting quickly if any of these signs appear can help keep both the pregnant person and baby safe.

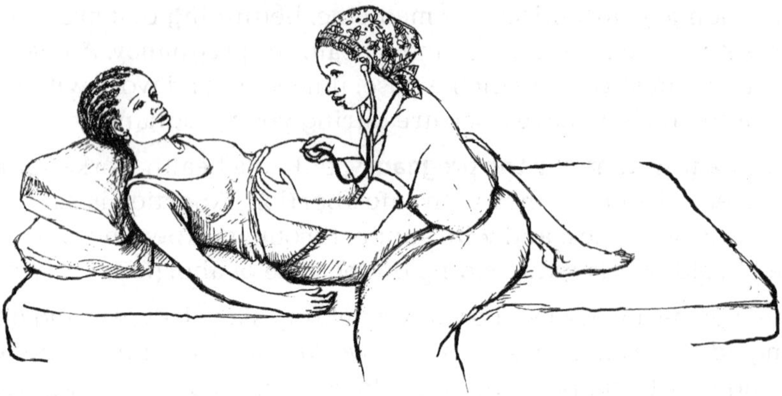

For a complete list of health issues to cover during a pregnancy checkup and information about what to do if there are problems, scan the QR code on page 203 to access the Safe Pregnancy and Birth mobile application or see Hesperian's *A Book for Midwives*.

If possible, a person should have 10 to 15 checkups during their pregnancy—one every month up to 6 months, two during months 6, 7, and 8, and then one each week during the last month. A midwife or other health worker may recommend more frequent checkups for a person with epilepsy than for someone without epilepsy. Frequent checkups can allow adjustment to your antiseizure medicine dose when needed.

At a minimum, 3 checkups during pregnancy are essential:

1. as soon as a person finds out they are pregnant
2. again around the 6th month
3. about a month before the baby is due

Checkups can happen at home or in a clinic or medical center if access to testing equipment and technology is needed.

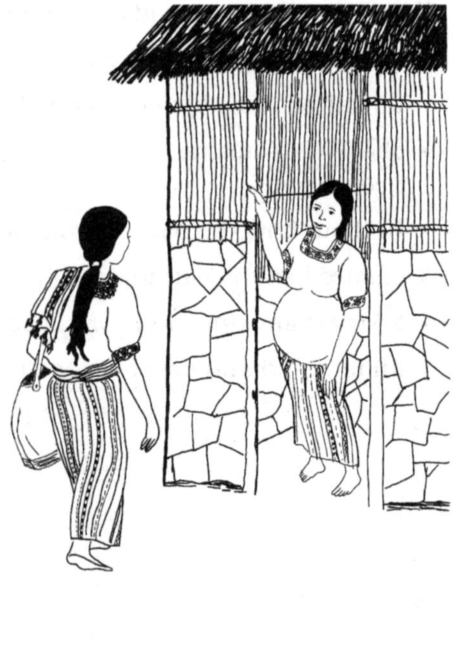

Take folic acid

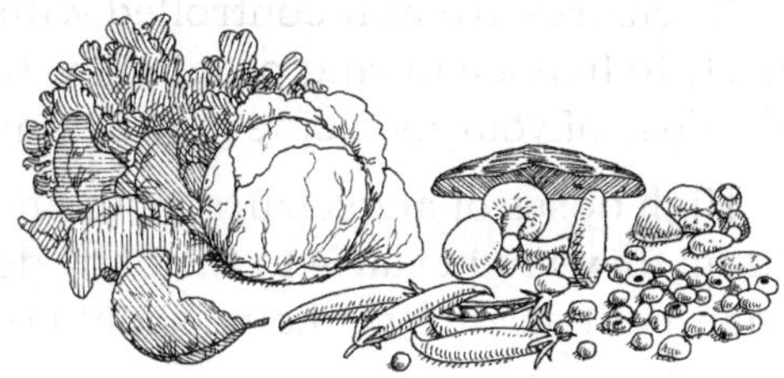

Some foods contain folic acid, but taking a daily supplement ensures sure you get enough.

Taking folic acid every day supports a healthy pregnancy. Folic acid is a form of vitamin B9 that supports a baby's healthy development in the first weeks of pregnancy. Maintaining good levels of folic acid in the body helps prevent early birth, pre-eclampsia, and low birth weight, and prevents harm to the baby's developing nervous system.

It is best to begin taking folic acid 3 months before trying to get pregnant, or start taking it as soon as you learn you are pregnant. Keep taking it throughout pregnancy and stop when you give birth.

In the past, higher doses of folic acid were recommended for people taking antiseizure medicines because of concerns that they lowered the amount of folic acid in the body. New research shows that too much folic acid may not be safe for the baby in the womb. So, the advice now for people taking antiseizure medicines is to take the same amount of folic acid taken by anyone trying to get pregnant or already pregnant—0.4 mg every day.

Pregnancy and antiseizure medicines

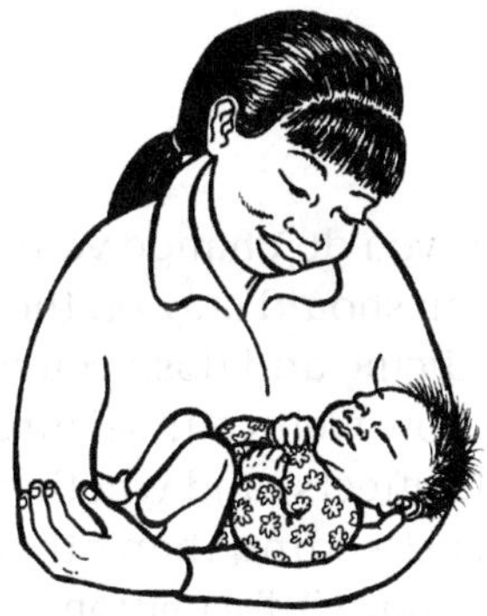

Some antiseizure medicines are safe to use during pregnancy and breastfeeding, and others are less safe. Some should not be used at all. But stopping antiseizure medicine increases the risk of seizures during pregnancy, making pregnancy more dangerous for both mother and baby. Talk to a health worker to make sure your antiseizure medicine is one that will have the least possible effect on your pregnancy and baby.

If a change in medicine needs to be made, try to do this before you get pregnant. Finding a medicine and dose that are safe and effective for you often takes 6 to 12 months, and sometimes longer. For more information about medicine safety and dose changes during pregnancy, see pages 208 to 212.

No matter what medicine you use, the dose may need to be adjusted to keep up with how your body changes during pregnancy. For instance, changes in your hormones during pregnancy can affect the way your body responds to medicines. (Hormones are the chemicals your body makes to help control and support your body's needs and your baby's growth and development.)

If seizures are well-controlled with medicine before pregnancy, they are less likely to happen during pregnancy. If they do happen during pregnancy, adjusting the dose of your medicine may bring them back under control.

High doses of antiseizure medicines sometimes need to be reduced to prevent harm they might cause to the baby developing in the womb. People using more than 1 antiseizure medicine should review their medicines and doses with a health worker.

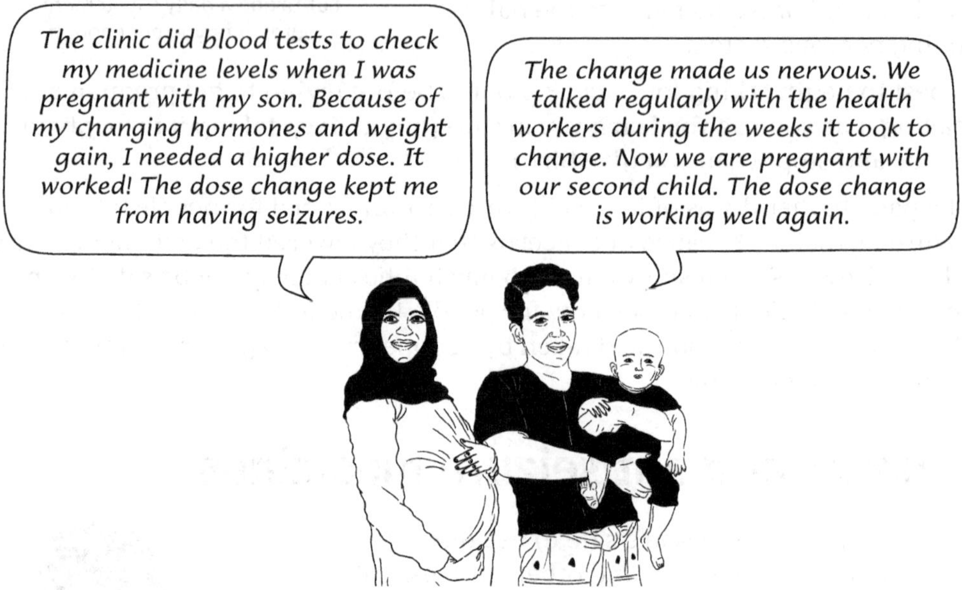
The clinic did blood tests to check my medicine levels when I was pregnant with my son. Because of my changing hormones and weight gain, I needed a higher dose. It worked! The dose change kept me from having seizures.
The change made us nervous. We talked regularly with the health workers during the weeks it took to change. Now we are pregnant with our second child. The dose change is working well again.

If you do change your medicine or dose, you and your health worker can decide if you should stay on the new medicine or dose after pregnancy or return to the medicine and dose you were taking before pregnancy. This decision will depend on how well your seizures were controlled both before and during pregnancy, side effects, and whether you plan to breastfeed (some medicines are safer for breastfeeding than others). Ask your health worker to help you with these decisions. For more information, see pages 221 to 223.

Safe use of antiseizure medicines during pregnancy

Some widely used antiseizure medicines increase the risk of physical disability in newborns and may cause developmental delays in growing children. The medicines valproic acid, carbamazepine, phenobarbital, phenytoin, and topiramate can affect the baby in the womb. The medicines lamotrigine and levetiracetam are safer during pregnancy, but they are not as widely available and may be more expensive. Other medicines considered safe are still being studied for their long-term effects.

It can be difficult to know what to do if the medicine you are using is not safe during pregnancy, but other, safer medicines are not affordable or not available where you live. Stopping medicine suddenly will probably cause you to have seizures, which may be dangerous for you and your baby. It may be safer to continue taking a less safe medicine than to have uncontrolled seizures while you are pregnant.

Talk to a midwife or other health worker about antiseizure medicines that are safe for pregnancy and what your options are.

Recommended	**Some problems, use a low dose**	**Avoid**	**Do not use**
Lamotrigine Levetiracetam	Oxcarbazepine	Phenytoin Phenobarbital Carbamazepine	Valproic acid

Lamotrigine and Levetiracetam are the safest options during pregnancy. Their standard doses do not harm a baby's development. These medicines may not be as readily available as other medicines.

Oxcarbazepine* can be used safely during pregnancy, but it is less well studied and may carry some risk for the baby, compared with lamotrigine and levetiracetam. Use at the lowest dose that controls seizures.

Carbamazepine has a higher risk to the developing baby than lamotrigine or levetiracetam, but it is widely available and may be necessary to use. Use the lowest dose that controls seizures. Avoid carbamazepine if safer options are available.

Phenobarbital and Phenytoin have a higher risk of developmental problems for babies. Avoid phenobarbital and phenytoin during pregnancy if safer options are available. Use only if they are the only options available that control seizures.

Valproic acid presents a high risk for developmental disorders to babies in the womb. Do not use during pregnancy. If it is the only option available that controls seizures, work very closely with a health worker who can talk with you about the risks to your baby and your health and watch your health closely during pregnancy. Do not stop taking medicine suddenly as this may cause seizures.

Find more information about antiseizure medicines in Chapter 4, pages 98 to 108.

*This medicine is not included in Chapter 4: Medicines for epilepsy and seizures, because it is not available in many communities. Where it is available, this information is useful to know.

HOW TO **Choose an antiseizure medicine for pregnancy**

- Find an available medicine that is safe for the developing baby.
- Make sure it controls the person's seizures.
- Find the lowest dose that controls seizures.

If the medicine has already been controlling seizures (no seizures for 1 year), see if it can be slowly reduced to a lower effective dose to have the least possible effect on the baby's development. Begin this process as early as 1 year before pregnancy or as soon as possible during pregnancy.

Changing or adjusting antiseizure medicine: How to decide

You may have concerns about changing a medicine or dose that works well to control your seizures. After all, the confidence and ease your medicine provides can help you avoid the stress and anxiety of an unexpected seizure. On the other hand, disabilities that antiseizure medicines might cause in a developing baby can be very serious.

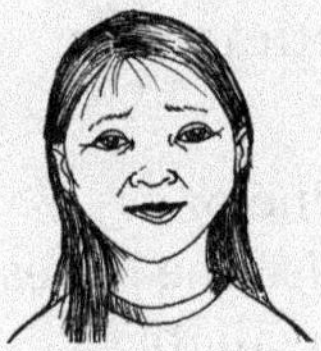

I am not sure I should change my antiseizure medicine. The last time I tried, I had a seizure in the kitchen and got burned. That was awful! But I should do it for the baby. This is so confusing! I need help deciding...

If you are planning a pregnancy, give yourself enough time to find a midwife or other health worker who understands pregnancy and birth for people with epilepsy. If you are already pregnant, talk to your midwife or health worker about your concerns and ask questions that can help you make a decision you feel comfortable with.

Although changing or adjusting antiseizure medicine is your choice to make, getting support and advice during and after your decision-making process can be helpful. Epilepsy support groups are a good place to share your experience and concerns, and to learn from other people's experience about the effects (good and bad) and risks of different medicines.

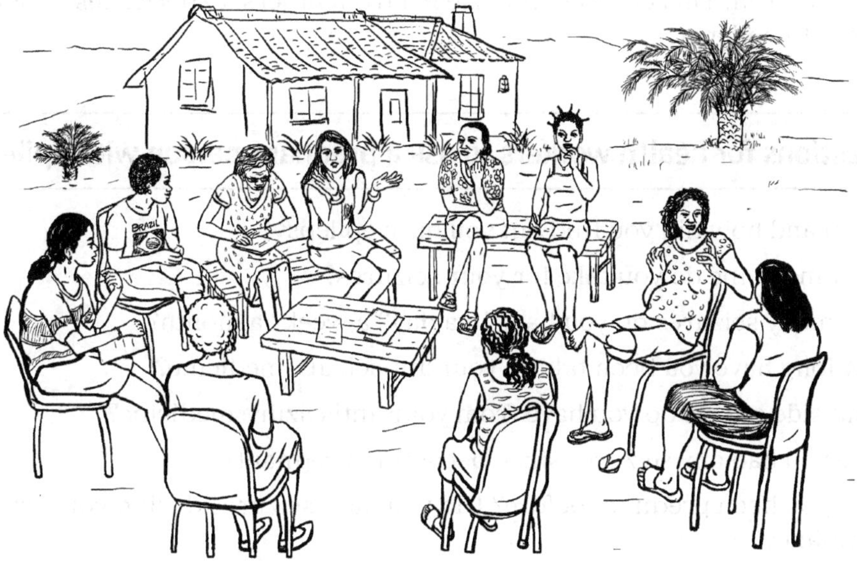

Since different medicines affect people differently, the advice you get from an epilepsy support group should not take the place of medical guidance from a health worker.

Questions about pregnancy for people with epilepsy to ask a health worker

- Is the antiseizure medicine I am taking safe for pregnancy?
- If my medicine is safe, will my dose need to be adjusted?
- If my medicine is not safe, what other medicines are available? How much time will I need to try a new medicine and get to the right dose?
- If I have seizures, will they harm the baby? What can I do to lessen any harm?
- How often do I need to see a health worker during pregnancy? When should I call or come to see you?
- What else should I be aware of to have a healthy pregnancy?

For the health worker. A person with epilepsy may be embarrassed or shy to talk about epilepsy. When you talk about pregnancy and birth to a person with epilepsy, show you are there to listen and help them, not to judge or criticize. This can help them feel safe sharing their worries and difficult choices. As they talk more, people often find they have the answers to their own problems. Encourage pregnant people with epilepsy or those trying to get pregnant to talk to other people with epilepsy who have children. This can help them learn from others' experiences about being pregnant with epilepsy.

Questions for health workers to ask a pregnant person with epilepsy

- When and how did you find out you have epilepsy?
- What medicine do you take for your seizures?
- How many seizures do you have in a day? a week? a month?
- How long have you been taking your antiseizure medicine?
- What side effects do you have from your antiseizure medicine?
- Have you had any seizures since becoming pregnant?
- Have you been pregnant before? Did you have seizures during your previous pregnancy?
- What questions or concerns do you have about your pregnancy and epilepsy?

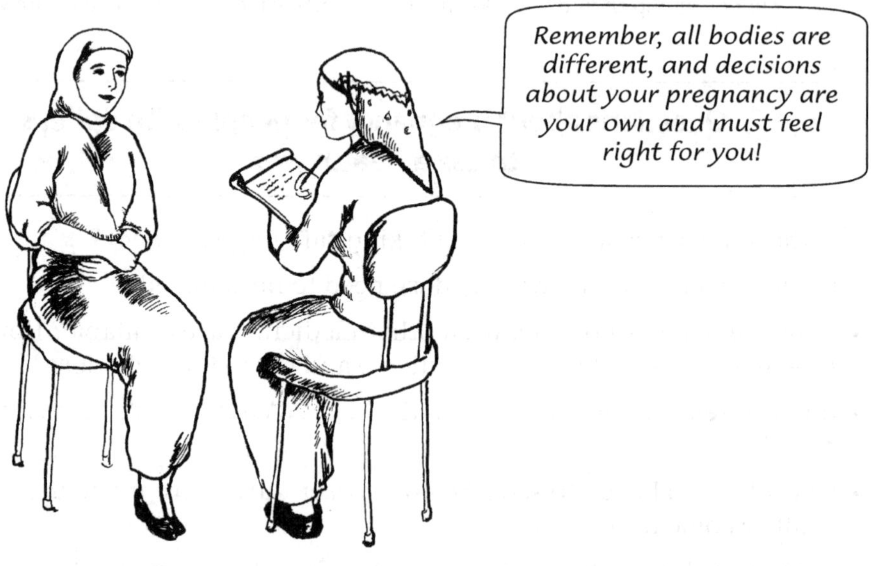
Remember, all bodies are different, and decisions about your pregnancy are your own and must feel right for you!

Tiredness and nausea during pregnancy

Tiredness and nausea are common complaints during pregnancy. For pregnant people with epilepsy, it can be difficult to know whether these signs are caused by pregnancy, by an antiseizure medicine side effect, or by a combination of both.

Why am I so tired?

Tiredness is a common side effect of many antiseizure medicines. It can also result from the process of changing a medicine or adjusting a dose. Tiredness is also a typical sign of pregnancy—growing a baby is extra work for the body, so people need more rest than usual. It can also be a sign of anemia (not enough iron in the blood), a common problem in pregnancy.

If your tiredness suddenly increases right after you have changed your antiseizure medicine or its dose, then the medicine is likely to be a cause. If your tiredness increases as you begin to feel other signs of pregnancy, such as nausea, frequent urination, or trouble sleeping, the pregnancy is likely a cause. But in either case, it is difficult to know for sure. Luckily, tiredness often lessens as your body adjusts to both pregnancy and changes in medicine.

To feel better, get extra rest during the day and try to sleep longer at night. Do not forget to drink enough water throughout the day. If tiredness becomes so intense that it gets in the way of daily activities, or makes you dizzy, faint, or unable to eat, drink, or take your medicine, talk to a midwife or other health worker.

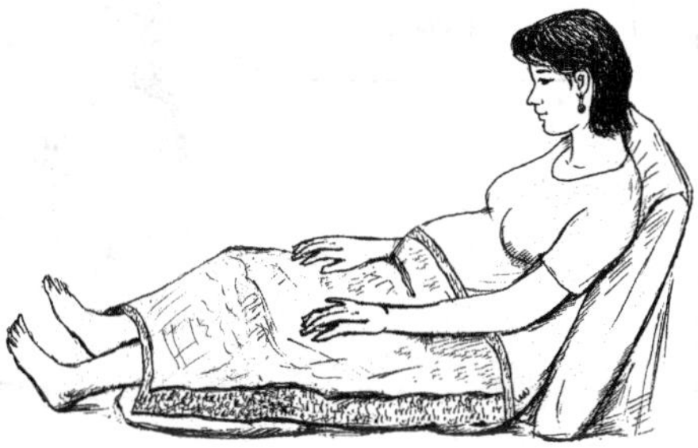

Why am I so nauseous?

Nausea is a common side effect of several antiseizure medicines. It can also result from increasing a medicine's dose. Sometimes called morning sickness, nausea is especially common during the first 3 months of pregnancy.

If your nausea suddenly increases right after you have changed your antiseizure medicine or raised its dose, then it is likely to be caused by the medicine. If your nausea increases as you begin to feel other signs of pregnancy, such as tiredness, frequent urination, or trouble sleeping, the pregnancy is likely a cause. In either case, it is difficult to know for sure. Nausea often lessens as your body adjusts to the medicine and after about 3 months of pregnancy.

HOW TO Feel less nausea

For many people, changes in eating can reduce feelings of nausea. Try any of these remedies:

- Eat small amounts of dry grain foods (crackers, bread, tortillas, chapatis, etc.) upon waking up.
- Eat small amounts of foods with protein (beans, nuts, cheese, etc.) before going to bed or if you wake up with nausea at night.
- Eat several small meals daily instead of 2 or 3 large ones. Sip liquids throughout the day.
- Drink a cup of ginger, mint, or cinnamon tea 2 or 3 times a day or before meals.

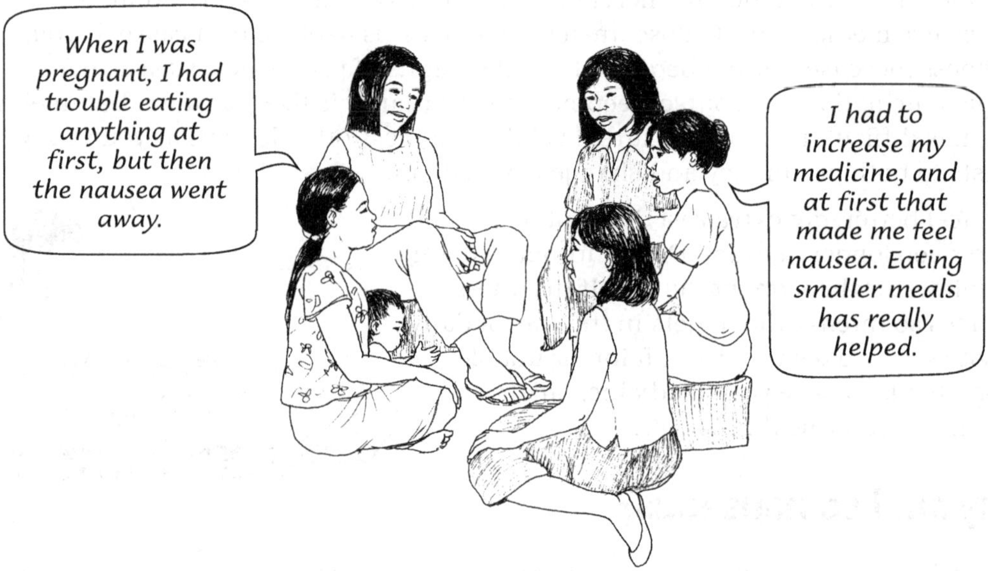
When I was pregnant, I had trouble eating anything at first, but then the nausea went away.
I had to increase my medicine, and at first that made me feel nausea. Eating smaller meals has really helped.

What to do when vomiting happens after taking antiseizure medicine

If you vomit less than 1 hour after taking your antiseizure medicine, repeat the dose. If vomiting happens again, wait until the next scheduled dose and try again.

If you vomit more than 1 hour after taking your antiseizure medicine, wait until the next scheduled dose to take it again.

If vomiting continues, see a midwife or other health worker.

Pregnancy complications

Pregnancy can be healthy and safe for people with epilepsy, but they do face some epilepsy-related risks and complications. Understanding these helps you prepare, get support, and better care for yourself and your baby. Complications like high blood pressure (pre-eclampsia), early labor (preterm birth), or changes in the placenta may be slightly more common in people with epilepsy. Seizures during pregnancy, especially if they cause falls or injuries, also add risk. Support and planning can reduce or prevent many of these risks.

To protect your health and the baby's health, take your antiseizure medicine every day, get regular checkups, rest often, eat nutritious food, and avoid alcohol and tobacco. If something does not feel right, talk with a midwife or other health worker. Reaching out sooner rather than later can make a big difference.

Seizures during pregnancy

Seizures during pregnancy may cause physical injuries, which may also prevent oxygen from reaching the baby in the womb. Try to avoid situations that trigger your seizures. This can be difficult because common physical and mental changes caused by pregnancy are seizure triggers for many people.

Changes in sleeping patterns

Growing a baby is hard work, and it can be difficult to get enough rest. Feeling anxious about a pregnancy and becoming a parent can also be tiring. As your body size increases, it may be difficult to find a comfortable sleeping position. Try to get as much rest as you can, especially if lack of sleep is a seizure trigger for you.

Body changes during pregnancy

The amount of blood in the body increases during pregnancy, and the heart, liver, and kidneys all work harder and faster. These changes can cause your body to clear seizure medicine more quickly, lessening the amount of medicine in your blood to a level where it may no longer control seizures. Pregnancy can also change how your stomach and intestines absorb medicine, especially if vomiting increases. Increases in body weight can affect how well your dose of antiseizure medicine works to control your seizures.

Regular checkups can allow your dose of antiseizure medicine to be adjusted so it continues to prevent seizures.

Physical injury from falls during seizures

The risk of injury from falls during pregnancy is high, especially for people whose seizures are not well-controlled. Some injuries caused by a fall may be easy to see, such as a cut or a bruise. But when an injury happens inside the body, it may not be visible. These injuries can cause internal bleeding or harm the baby growing in the womb.

WARNING SIGNS If you suspect internal injuries or if any of these signs are present, get the person to a medical center immediately:

- heavy and continuous vaginal bleeding
- abdominal pain after seizure ends
- dizziness, tiredness, or difficulty breathing

Pre-eclampsia

Pre-eclampsia is a serious high blood pressure problem that happens later in pregnancy, during labor, or a few days after birth. If not identified and treated, pre-eclampsia can lead to eclampsia, which causes seizures (a different type than epileptic seizures) and can cause death (see page 218).

While most people with epilepsy do not get pre-eclampsia, they do have a higher risk of getting pre-eclampsia than people without epilepsy.

Blood pressure should be measured at all pregnancy checkups, whether a person has epilepsy or not. High blood pressure can be a sign of pre-eclampsia.

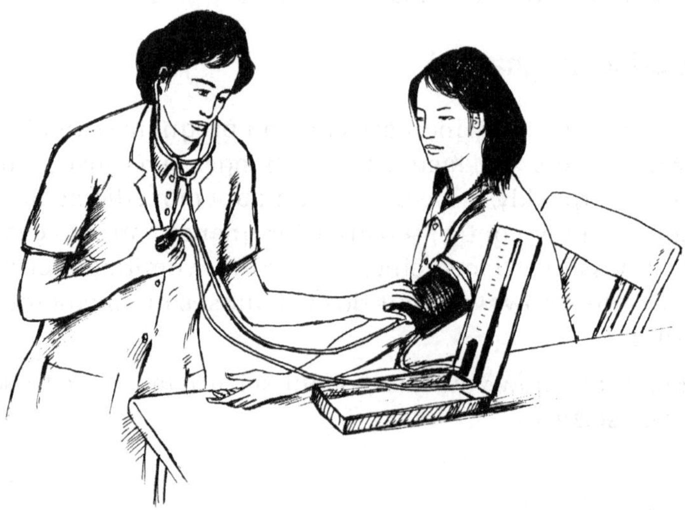

SIGNS Pre-eclampsia

High blood pressure. Healthy blood pressure is between 90/60 and 140/90 and does not go up much during pregnancy. High blood pressure is when the top number is above 140 and the bottom is over 90.

Protein in the urine. Test strips (brand names: *Uristix, Albustix, Labstix,* and others) change color when they measure too much protein in urine. Check the date on the box to make sure the test strips are not expired.

A pregnant person with high blood pressure and any of these signs probably has pre-eclampsia and needs help at a medical center:

- strong headaches that do not go away with medicine
- vision changes such as spots, blurriness, or double vision
- steady, severe pain in the top of the belly or the right side under the ribs
- overactive reflexes

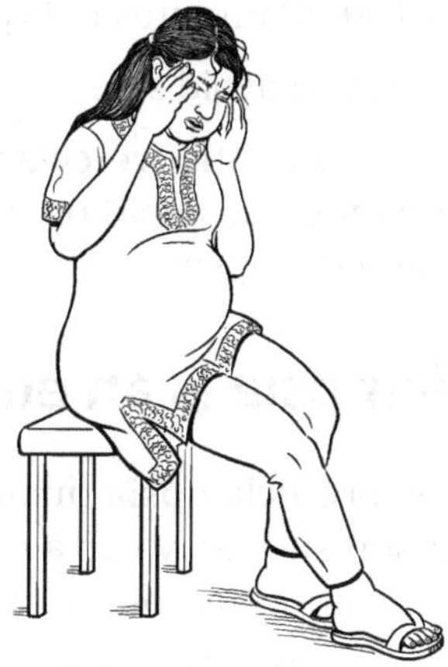

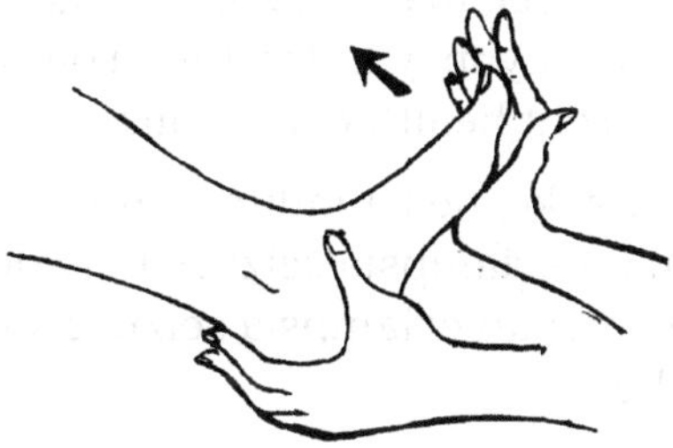

To check for overactive reflexes, have the person lie down and hold their foot like this. Give a quick push, then let go.

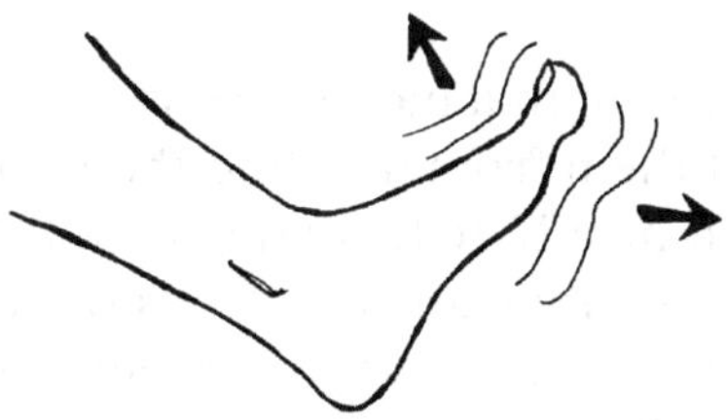

If the foot jerks 2 times or more, it is an overactive reflex. This is a danger sign.

On the way to a medical center, have the pregnant person lie on their left side. Someone should accompany them in case they have a seizure.

Preventing pre-eclampsia

A low-dose aspirin (75 mg or 81 mg) taken daily can help prevent pre-eclampsia. Activities and habits that help keep blood pressure in a healthy range also support prevention. For example:

- Eat vegetables, fruits, legumes, and whole grains rather than highly processed, salty, or sugary "junk" foods.
- Limit the amount of salt you eat.
- Get 30 minutes of light to moderate physical activity every day.
- Try to avoid stress.

A person with pre-eclampsia is often told to rest in bed for the rest of their pregnancy and avoid physical activity that might cause early labor or trigger eclampsia.

Eclampsia is an emergency!

When pre-eclampsia turns into eclampsia, this is an emergency! Eclampsia is when a person suddenly has a seizure. It may happen during the final weeks of pregnancy, during labor and birth, or up to 6 weeks after delivery.

Eclampsia seizures look like tonic-clonic epileptic seizures—a person may have jerking movements, their body may shake, or they may fall to the ground unconscious. But epilepsy and eclampsia are different health conditions.

Eclampsia seizures can cause physical injury, stroke, heart failure, and death, both for the mother and the baby. A person with an eclampsia seizure may deliver a baby too early (preterm or premature birth). When an eclampsia seizure stops oxygen from getting to the baby, the baby can die.

Treating eclampsia

A person with eclampsia needs emergency treatment in a medical center immediately. Place them on their side to prevent them from inhaling their vomit. Immediately stop the seizure by giving magnesium sulfate through IV (in the vein) or IM (in the muscle) injections in the buttock. If magnesium sulfate is not available, give diazepam instead (see page 110). For information on how to give emergency medicine during a seizure, see Chapter 4, pages 109 to 113.

Placenta complications

The placenta is an organ that grows in the uterus during pregnancy. It provides the baby with all their oxygen and food and removes waste. Some placenta-related complications are a little more common in pregnant people with epilepsy.

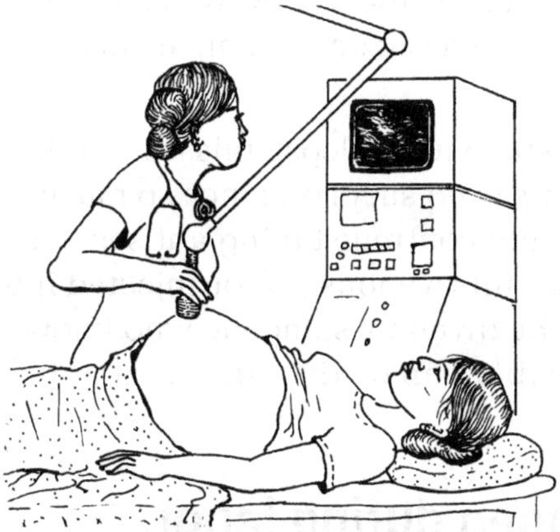

Placental abruption is where the placenta separates from the uterus too early. It may happen when a seizure causes an injury from a fall. Controlling seizures can prevent placental abruption.

Placenta previa is where the placenta attaches too low in the uterus and covers the cervix. It may be found during a checkup with an ultrasound (sonogram), a machine that uses sound waves to show the inside of your body and the baby in the womb. Or it may be diagnosed by bright red painless bleeding from the vagina after about 20 weeks of pregnancy, the main sign of placenta previa. If you have placenta previa, you will need to rest more, avoid heavy lifting and vaginal sex, and plan a hospital Cesarean (C-section) birth (the surgical delivery of the baby through a cut made in the abdomen and uterus).

Labor and birth

Having support can make labor and birth better for both parent and baby. Sharing observations with health workers about possible signs of illness or seizure activity, or information about seizure triggers, might help prevent problems during delivery. Family members can give emotional support by staying calm, kind, and encouraging. Remind the person in labor to breathe and to rest between contractions. Stay with the person in labor, hold their hand, and speak gently so they feel safe, cared for, and confident about the birth.

Many people with epilepsy plan to give birth at a medical center or hospital. That reassures them they can get help if a seizure or other unexpected situation develops during labor.

A person with epilepsy can have a vaginal birth just like someone who does not have epilepsy. Because giving birth is a physically tiring, stressful, and painful process, the person with epilepsy, her family members, and health workers should all try to reduce the impact of these or any other conditions that might trigger a seizure during labor. Seizures that do not cause a person to lose consciousness or fall, such as absence or some focal seizures, do not harm the pregnant person or baby in any way that affects birth.

Epilepsy and C-sections. Not all pregnant people with epilepsy need to deliver by Cesarean section. C-sections may be planned if the person had a tonic-clonic seizure or was injured during a seizure while pregnant. C-sections may be necessary for anyone, with or without epilepsy, whose baby is in a difficult position, who has a problem with the placenta or umbilical cord, whose baby has taken too long to be born, or who is in trouble in another way. If a person feels too sleepy, weak, or in any other way unable to participate in labor because of a seizure or antiseizure medicine, they will need a C-section.

A common problem during labor is that the person with epilepsy misses or takes an incorrect dose of their antiseizure medicine. This is no surprise since so much is happening! But even during labor, it is important to continue taking antiseizure medicine. If medicine cannot be taken by mouth, an intravenous (IV, or injected into the vein) option may be called for, but should only be given by someone who knows how to do so. The effect of missing a dose during labor can be the same as at any other time—it may cause a "breakthrough seizure."

Birth emergency: Seizures that happen during labor

Seizures during labor are rare, but they can happen if a person is tired, dehydrated, stressed, or misses a dose of antiseizure medicine. Seizures may be dangerous if they slow the baby's heartbeat or cause a decrease in oxygen to the baby.

In the unlikely event that a seizure happens during labor or delivery, protect the person from injury, turn them on their side, and make sure their airway is clear. If they are still in early labor, after the seizure ends, consider taking them to a medical center where they can be supported by a health worker with emergency training. If they are about to deliver or in the middle of delivery, wait for the seizure to end, deliver the baby, and then consider taking them both to a medical center.

If a seizure during labor lasts more than a few minutes or repeats, an emergency medicine like lorazepam may be needed.

Give 4 mg lorazepam through an intravenous (IV) drip for a generalized tonic-clonic seizure. If lorazepam is not available, diazepam or midazolam can be used. For information about rescue medicines, see Chapter 4, pages 109 to 113.

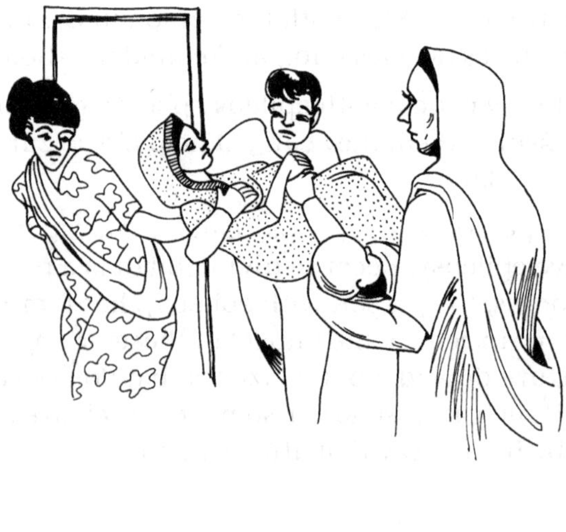

HOW TO **Adjust antiseizure medicine after delivery**

If a person's antiseizure medicine dose was increased during pregnancy to better control seizures, the medicine can be reduced in the first 3 days after giving birth. The goal is to reach the dose the person was taking before pregnancy, within 1 week after birth. Reduce it by half or to the pre-pregnancy level, whichever is less. Wait a few days if it needs to be reduced again.

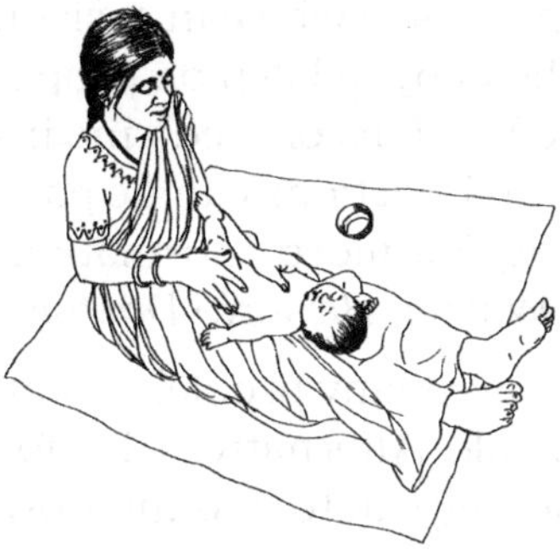

Breastfeeding for people with epilepsy

Breast milk gives babies all the nutrients and fluids they need for healthy growth and development. It is the best food for a baby, especially during the first 6 months of life. It is fresh, ready-to-use, at the right temperature, and it protects children against many infections and diseases. Breastfeeding is considered safe and is encouraged for mothers with epilepsy, just as it is for all mothers.

It is impossible to pass epilepsy to a baby through breast milk. Concerns about passing antiseizure medicine through breast milk should not stop the mother of a newborn from breastfeeding. The benefits of breastfeeding far outweigh any possible harms from your antiseizure medicine. So breastfeed as often as you are able.

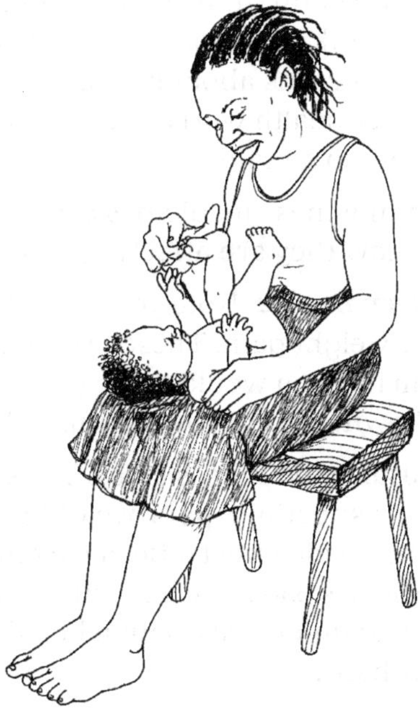

For the health worker. Talk to families and encourage them to give nothing but breast milk, not even water, for the first 6 months and to continue breastfeeding for at least 1 year.

It is not enough to just talk about breastfeeding. Some people may need support to learn how to breastfeed successfully. Help them find a neighbor, relative, or health promoter who can assist in learning how to hold the baby correctly, how to get the baby to latch on properly, and to provide emotional support. They may also need creams or medicine if skin problems develop on their nipples or breasts. Some skin infections can be passed from mother to baby and make breastfeeding a challenge. For more information about breastfeeding, see Chapter 7 of Hesperian's *Where Women Have No Doctor.*

There are many problems that can make breastfeeding difficult, and occasionally not possible. Alternatives like formula are sometimes necessary. Help all families do the best they can to find their own ways to care for and be close with a new baby.

Breastfeeding and antiseizure medicines

A small amount of antiseizure medicine passes to a baby during breastfeeding. While there is not yet 100% certainty that the breastmilk of people who take antiseizure medicine is totally safe, no studies show negative health effects on children breastfed as infants by mothers taking antiseizure medicine. All studies highlight the benefits of breastfeeding for mother and baby.

Medicines that pass at higher levels in breastmilk are phenobarbital, levetiracetam, zonisamide, and ethosuximide. That there is more of it in your breastmilk does not necessarily mean it will cause problems for your baby. If you have concerns about how breastfeeding is affecting your baby, talk with a midwife or other health worker. If you want to change your medicine, talk with them about how to do so safely.

While these medicines are considered safe for breastfeeding, pay attention to if and how they are affecting your baby.

Carbamazepine. Note your baby's signs of sleepiness, vomiting or upset stomach, or poor weight gain. These are side effects of carbamazepine on the baby. Keep track of them like you would track your own side effects. If the baby shows signs of jaundice (yellowing of eyes and skin), talk to a health worker immediately.

Ethosuximide causes side effects in some babies, such as sleepiness, lack of interest in breastfeeding, poor weight gain, irritability, and vomiting. Keep careful track of these side effects. Because ethosuximide is often used with other antiseizure medicines, side effects could be caused by the combination of medicines, not just ethosuximide. Talk with a health worker about any side effects you see in your baby.

Lamotrigine rarely causes side effects except for skin rash. Talk to a health worker if the baby develops a rash.

Levetiracetam only occasionally causes sleepiness in babies.

Phenobarbital can cause sleepiness and poor weight gain in infants, especially if used with other antiseizure medicines that have similar side effects. Breastfeeding may need to be stopped if the baby's drowsiness or poor growth does not improve, especially if the baby was born early and small, making them more sensitive to phenobarbital.

Zonisamide.* A health worker may suggest supplementing breastfeeding with bottle feeding and breastmilk with formula if side effects like lack of interest in breastfeeding, dehydration, irritability, and poor weight gain continue. If there are other options, they may suggest changing your antiseizure medicine. If other options are not available, a lower dose of zonisamide may be considered.

*This medicine is not included in Chapter 4: Medicines for epilepsy and seizures, because it is not available in many communities. Where it is available, this information is useful to know.

Tips for breastfeeding when taking antiseizure medicine

If you take antiseizure medicine once a day, take it just before the baby sleeps the longest, usually after the bedtime feeding.

If you take antiseizure medicine more than once a day, breastfeed your baby just before you take a dose. This is when the amount of antiseizure medicine in your body will be lowest.

Disrupted sleep and tiredness can trigger seizures. Removing breastmilk with your hand or a pump and then keeping it cool allows another caregiver to feed your baby so you can rest or get a good night's sleep. For information about removing milk by hand, see Chapter 7 of Hesperian's *Where Women Have No Doctor.*

Take precautions while feeding your baby to prevent injury from seizures that occur without warning. For example, sit on a low bed or mattress with your back to the wall and surround yourself with cushions.

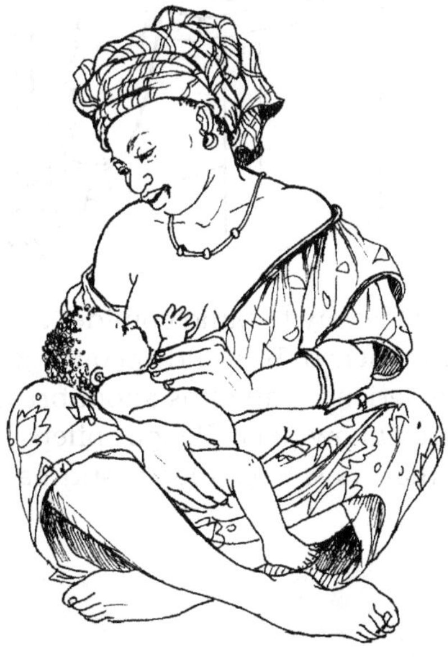

Helping mothers feel confident about breastfeeding

There will be less stigma against people with epilepsy breastfeeding when families and communities have correct information about epilepsy. Help people learn that breastfeeding cannot cause epilesy and seizures. Let others know that epilepsy cannot be passed through breastmilk to the baby. Encourage mothers with epilepsy to have confidence in their ability to breastfeed.

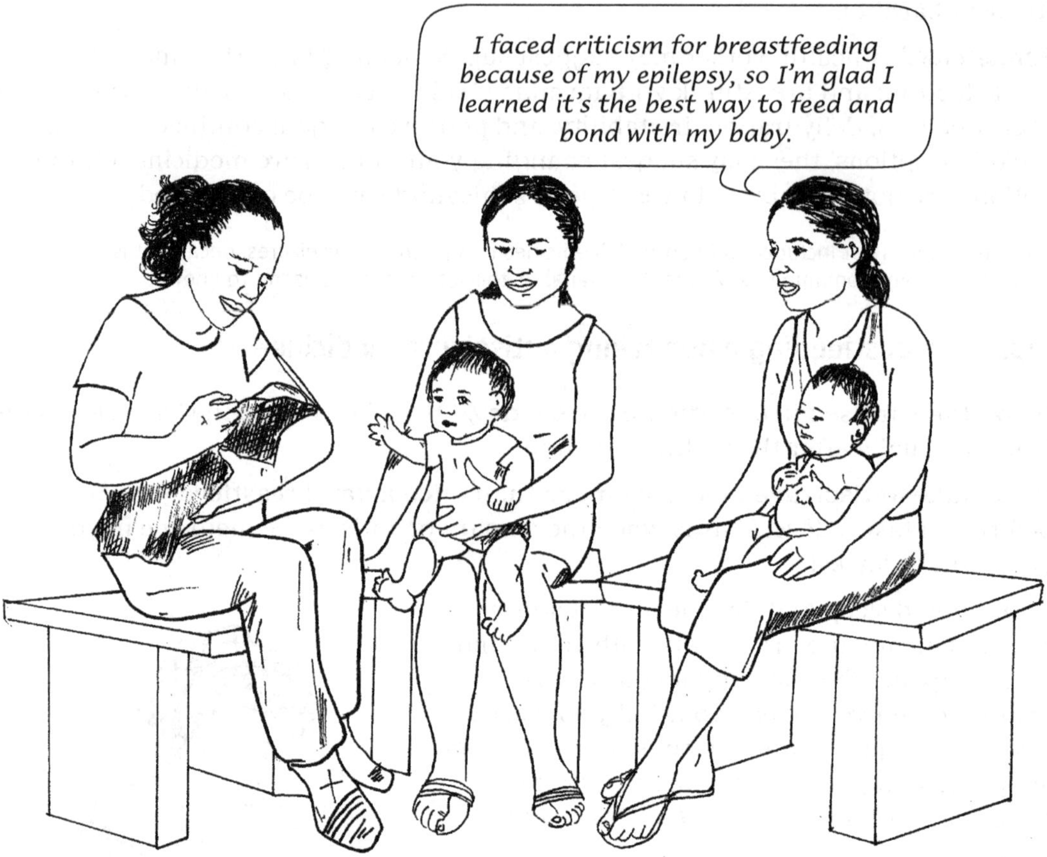
I faced criticism for breastfeeding because of my epilepsy, so I'm glad I learned it's the best way to feed and bond with my baby.

One way to build confidence is to bring together a group of mothers with epilepsy and their babies and encourage them to enjoy each other's company. As they share experiences and tips about breastfeeding and parenting, they can also share ideas about how to challenge epilepsy myths and stigma. For more information about other ways to challenge stigma, see Chapter 5.

Caring for your baby

Bathing and changing your baby. If you have seizures that make you lose consciousness or control over your movements, or your seizures are not controlled by medicine, try to have another person around when you bathe or change your newborn baby. Having assistance ensures both you and your baby are safe if a seizure happens. A support person can move you and your baby away from danger, provide any needed first aid, or get help in an emergency.

Change your baby's diapers (nappies) on a mat or blanket on the floor, to avoid any problems if you have a seizure.

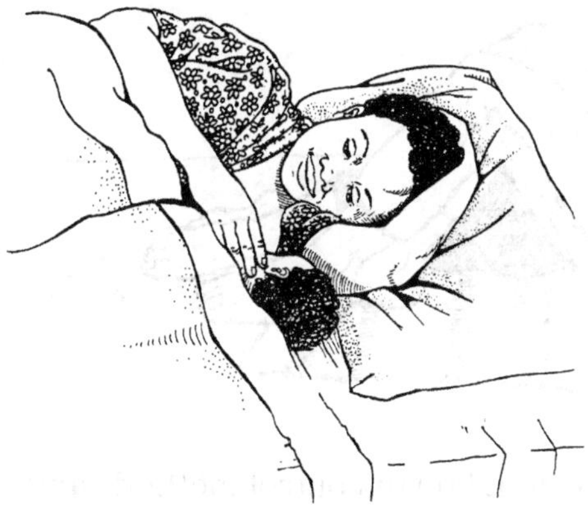

Sleeping with your baby. After having a baby, getting enough sleep can be hard, especially when you are feeding your baby every few hours at night. Try to prevent lack of sleep from triggering your seizures. Rest when your baby sleeps and ask family and friends for help so you can get as much rest as possible.

If you have sleep seizures, movements caused by a seizure might injure your small baby sleeping next to you. Instead, have your baby sleep nearby in a bassinet or crib.

Carrying your baby in a sling. If your seizures are well-controlled, a sling for your small baby can be used safely. The sling should keep the baby secure and close to your body, but make sure the baby's face is visible so they have no difficulty breathing. Because babies do not have neck control until they are about 3 months old, avoid carrying very young babies on your back. Babies carried in front get bounced around less and have less trouble breathing.

If your seizures are not well-controlled, consider using a stroller or pram instead.

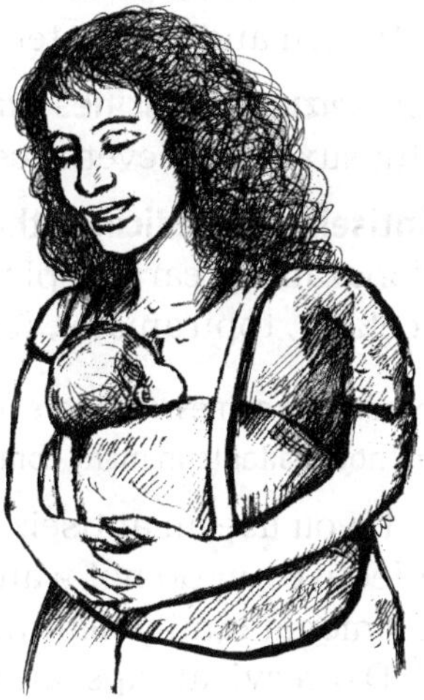

Birth control and antiseizure medicine

The ability to decide when to get pregnant and when to prevent pregnancy is central to staying healthy for everyone, including people with epilepsy. Family planning lets you get pregnant when you want and have the number of children you want. It puts you in control instead of leaving pregnancy and its responsibilities up to chance.

Family planning methods prevent pregnancy in different ways. Some contain hormones similar to those produced by your body. Hormonal methods include pills, injections, implants, patches, vaginal rings, and some IUDs (intrauterine devices).

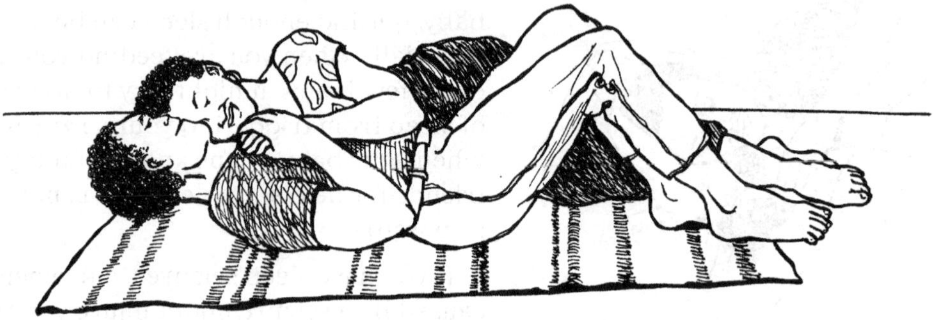

Many antiseizure medicines interact with hormonal birth control methods and make them less effective or not effective. This is true for methods that contain both estrogen and progesterone as well as for methods containing progesterone only.

Antiseizure medicines that do not affect hormonal birth control: clonazepam*, ethosuximide, levetiracetam, valproic acid

Antiseizure medicines that make hormonal birth control less effective: carbamazepine, clobazam, oxcarbazepine*, phenobarbital, phenytoin, primidone*, eslicarbazepine acetate*, topiramate*, felbamate*

*Medicines names with * are not included in Chapter 4: Medicines for epilepsy and seizures, because they are not available in many communities. Where they are available, this information is useful to know.

If you use an antiseizure medicine that makes hormonal birth control less effective but do not want to get pregnant now, talk to a health worker about non-hormonal family planning methods, such as condoms, diaphragms, non-hormonal IUDs, cervical caps, and other methods that can always be used effectively by people with epilepsy who are taking any antiseizure medicine.

The opposite can happen too—hormonal methods of birth control can make some antiseizure medicines less effective.

Lamotrigine and valproic acid can be less effective at controlling seizures when used with hormonal birth control methods. If this happens to you, talk to a health worker about finding a different birth control method or about adjusting the dose or changing your antiseizure medicine.

Valproic acid, phenobarbital, and carbamazepine can reduce a person's desire to have sex. This may make getting pregnant more difficult.

Starting birth control after giving birth. Because you can get pregnant again soon after giving birth, talk to a midwife or other health worker about starting or restarting birth control. For more information, scan the QR code below to access Hesperian's Family Planning mobile application.

Emergency contraception (EC) when taking antiseizure medicine. Emergency contraception (EC) is a way to avoid pregnancy after unprotected penis-in-vagina sex, but it is only effective if used soon after having sex.

A person taking antiseizure medicines can use EC pills safely. However, some medicines for HIV or tuberculosis (TB) lessen the effectiveness of EC pills. If this is a concern, talk to a health worker about using a higher EC dose or a copper IUD to prevent pregnancy.

For the health worker. People are often shy or embarrassed to talk about birth control because a conversation about birth control is also a conversation about sex. The stigma faced by people with epilepsy—especially women—regarding sex, relationships, and pregnancy can make it even harder for them to learn about and get the birth control they need.

By discussing family planning and its benefits with the people you treat, including those with epilepsy, you can be sure they will get correct information they can use to increase their control over their life and health.

Remember that people with epilepsy may have other health conditions (high blood pressure, HIV, TB, etc.) that can affect their options for safe, effective family planning options. Also, try to be sensitive to the social and family pressures that may affect their choices around family planning. This will help you offer care, information, and options that better fit each person's needs.

For more information about family planning, scan the QR code to access Hesperian's Family Planning mobile application.

Improving local epilepsy care for mothers

When health services, education, and antiseizure medicines are made available nearby, pregnant people with epilepsy can get the care they and their babies need. Local programs get information out more quickly and help the community help itself.

Neurology on Wheels takes epilepsy care to the village

In India, the community health program Neurology on Wheels delivers care for people with epilepsy to support safer and healthier pregnancies.

Neurology on Wheels is a traveling clinic that visits villages in the state of Andhra Pradesh to provide services to people who cannot easily get to hospitals or clinics. A medical team led by a neurologist offers epilepsy checkups and gives free medicines. The program includes education for families to correct common misunderstandings, like the belief that women with epilepsy should not get married or have children, or that epilepsy is not treatable.

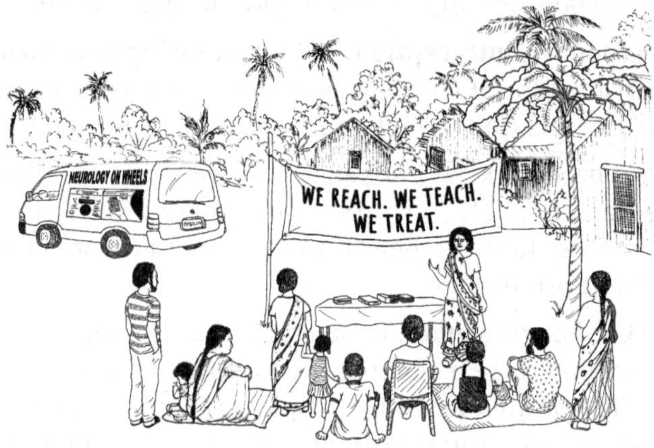

Neurology on Wheels works with the government's ASHA network of community health workers. ASHAs are trained female community health activists already involved with pregnancy care and women's health. By teaming up with ASHAs, the program adds epilepsy care and follow-up to the support available to rural women during pregnancy.

Neurology on Wheels shows how access to the right medicine and support enables women with epilepsy to have safe pregnancies and healthy babies:

- They get the medicines and health attention they need.
- They reduce fear and shame about epilepsy and pregnancy.
- Community health workers are trained to provide them with basic care and support before, during, and after pregnancy.

In rural areas where there is little or no organized government support for health, local health workers often step up to provide care. Then they need to involve the community in finding ways to make the care sustainable.

Epilepsy care far from cities

Nuru's labor pains had already started when she knocked on the door of the birth center in a small village in Uganda. Aisha was the midwife on call that night. She welcomed Nuru, gave her a little food and drink, helped her walk around and keep moving, and comforted her when her water broke. By sunrise, Nuru was the mother of a baby girl, Tomanika. She was exhausted by the delivery and quickly fell asleep.

Aisha noticed Nuru made jerking movements in her sleep. Even after she woke up, Nuru's face and arms moved uncontrollably. She had trouble holding and breastfeeding Tomanika because she felt so poorly. She was afraid she would drop her baby. Aisha saw Nuru was having different types of seizures—sometimes she lost consciousness, but other times she did not. She asked Nuru about her seizures.

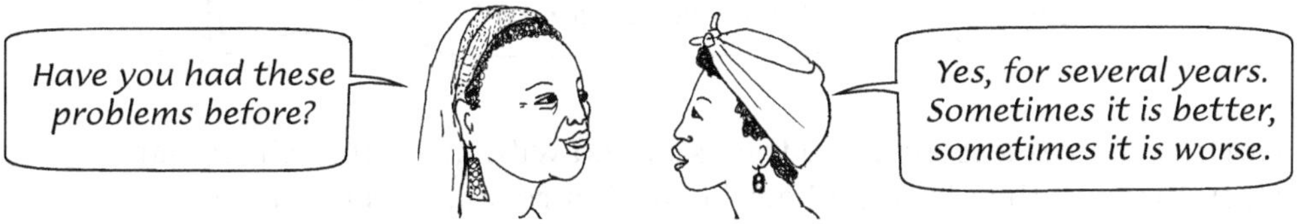
Have you had these problems before?
Yes, for several years. Sometimes it is better, sometimes it is worse.

Nuru explained her seizures began a few years ago after she fell and hit her head while working. When a health camp was held near her village, she talked to a visiting doctor. She even showed the doctor burn scars on her arm that she got during a seizure while cooking. The doctor gave her medicine to take every day—once in the morning and once at night.

The medicine made Nuru sleepy. Still, she took it every day as the doctor said. After some days, Nuru felt better. Her seizures happened less often. But her medicine ran out. Travel to the district health center was costly and Nuru had no money to buy medicine. All she could do was to wait for the next health camp.

continues

Epilepsy care far from cities *(continued)*

During the months she waited, Nuru's seizures returned. At the next health camp, she was given a different medicine. The new medicine slowed her seizures but gave her such terrible headaches that she stopped using it.

Shortly after this, Nuru got pregnant.

After hearing Nuru's story, Aisha phoned a doctor at the government hospital in the capital city who knew about epilepsy. She described Nuru's seizures—what they looked like, how many times they happened in a day, and how they left her feeling. She also told the doctor about Nuru's experiences with the 2 different medicines and how important it was that she be able to breastfeed her newborn.

The doctor agreed to send a 3-month supply of a different medicine by motorcycle to the birth center, at no charge. She explained the initial dose and then how to adjust it until it worked best.

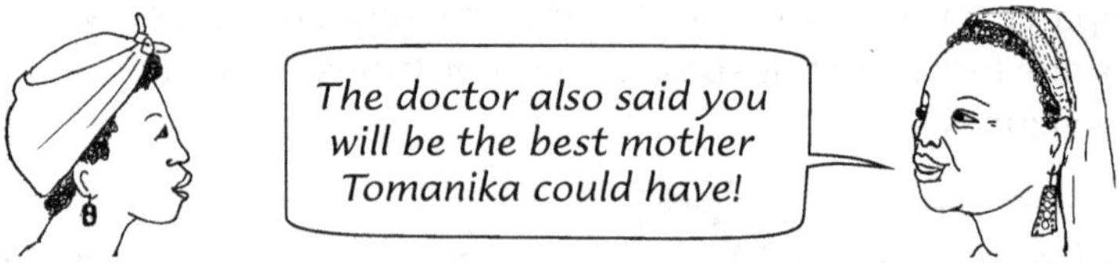

Nuru's seizures lessened and then stopped with medicine. She began to sleep through the night, and her health improved. Tomanika was breastfeeding and gaining weight. But Aisha was worried. She knew that Nuru's farm work would not allow her to pay for more medicine, even though the medicine did not cost very much.

Aisha decided to offer Nuru work at the birth center tending the garden, caring for the chickens, and sweeping the compound. The person doing these jobs was away for a few months and Nuru could take over until they returned. This would help cover the cost of Nuru's medicine for some months. Tomanika could stay in the nursery while her mother worked.

But how could they ensure Nuru continued to get the antiseizure medicine she needed every day? After all, the job at the birth center was temporary, and there were few opportunities for women in the village to work and earn enough to pay for the medicine.

continues

Epilepsy care far from cities *(continued)*

The midwives at the birth center started a community donation drive to people get necessary medicines they could not afford. They spoke at church and mosques. They got support from school children in the villages to go door-to-door and ask people to help their aunts, sisters, cousins, and daughters live a better life. They also started building relationships with community leaders who could help persuade political leaders to ensure a continuous supply of medicines safe for use by pregnant people.

Now their health center conducts a donation drive every 3 months and has created a small but growing fund for needed medicines.

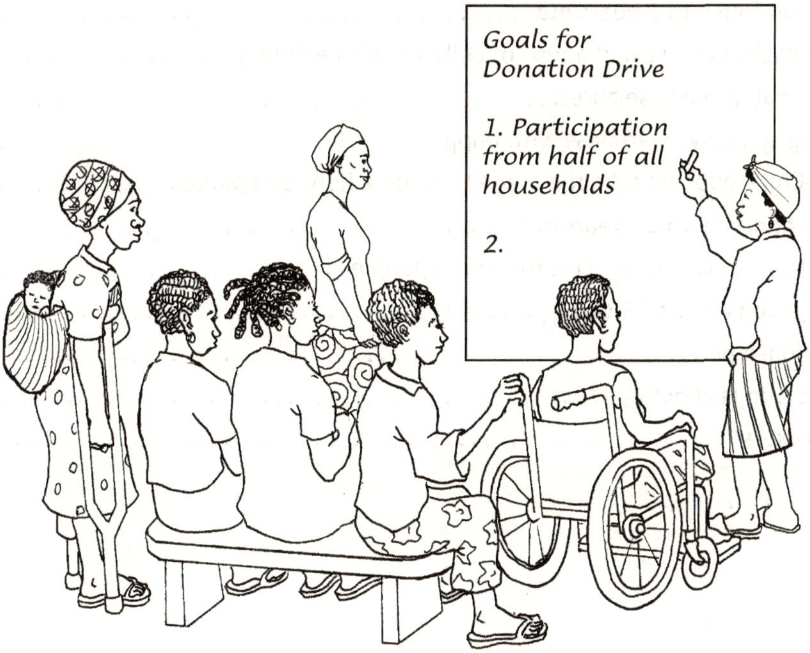

Chapter 8

In this chapter

Why talk with a child about their epilepsy and seizures? 233
Talk with children of all ages 235
Communicating with babies (birth to 2 years) 236
Talking with children 3 to 5 years old 238
How to talk about aura 240
Talking with children 6 to 8 years old 241
Prevent physical and sexual abuse of children with epilepsy 244
Talking about absence seizures 245
Promoting epilepsy awareness with puppets 247
Story: In Chile, puppets take the stage to shine a light on epilepsy 247
Talking with children 9 to 13 years old 249
How to stand up to bullies: Tips for young people 252
Talking with young people 14 to 18 years old 253
Sex and relationships 255
Talking with siblings about epilepsy 256
For health workers 259

Talking with children about epilepsy and seizures

Knowing about epilepsy and seizures helps children understand what is happening in their bodies. A child who knows they or someone else will be OK after a seizure is less likely to be scared or upset when they have one or see one.

When children learn that medicine can prevent their seizures, it may make them feel more comfortable playing with their friends. And it may also help them remember to take their medicine every day.

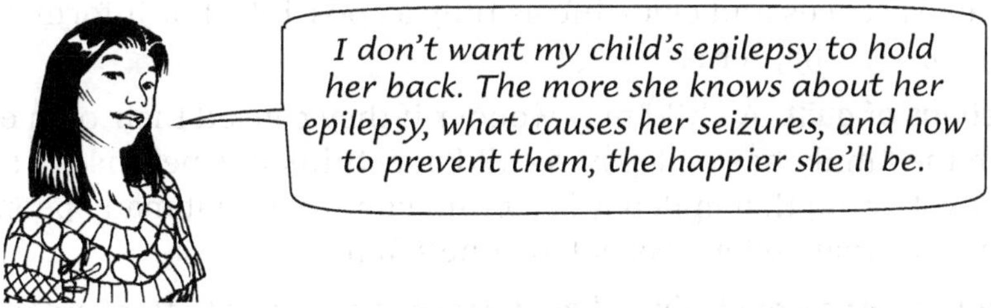

Family, friends, health workers, and others who encourage open and honest talking about epilepsy create an environment that better supports children who have seizures. At school, teachers can provide a child with support they may need and teach other students what to do if a seizure happens. Community education can highlight the benefits of accepting all children as they are, instead of focusing on what children with epilepsy cannot do and the problems they face.

Children with epilepsy can learn that even though they may face challenges, there is nothing "wrong" with them. Adults can help children accept themselves by explaining why stigma and bullying happen and taking a clear stand against it. This will help children with epilepsy develop confidence to stand up for themselves.

Why talk with a child about their epilepsy and seizures?

Safety. Understanding their epilepsy can help a child prevent injury to themself and others. If a child learns how to tell a seizure is about to happen, they can stay safe by sitting down, alerting someone nearby, or calling for help.

Less fear and worry. Children who know what to expect from their seizures and their recovery will feel less fear and worry and gain more confidence that they can handle their seizures. They will find reassurance and comfort when parents and others show concern and acceptance.

Taking daily medicine. Children who understand even a little about how medicine can control their seizures become more aware of its importance and more willing to take it every day. Helping children understand what medicine does, even if it tastes bad or makes them sleepy, can make it easier for them to feel good about taking it.

Reducing stigma. When people do not talk openly about epilepsy, fear of and discrimination against people with epilepsy can take root in the community and also inside the child. Adults talking with children about their epilepsy and children talking about their experiences with each other, caregivers, health workers, and community members, all contribute to fighting stigma. Parents and caregivers can support children to challenge stigma and misinformation by encouraging them to explore new experiences and enjoy life as fully as possible. For information about epilepsy stigma, see Chapter 5.

Reducing feelings of guilt. A child may wonder if they caused their own epilepsy. Or if someone in the family has epilepsy, a child may think it is because of something they did. By explaining that epilepsy is a brain condition that many people have, children can learn that epilepsy is not anyone's fault.

Building peer support through shared experience. As a child better understands their experience of living with epilepsy, they are better able to connect with other children who also live with the condition. By sharing stories and experiences, children support each other, building confidence and community.

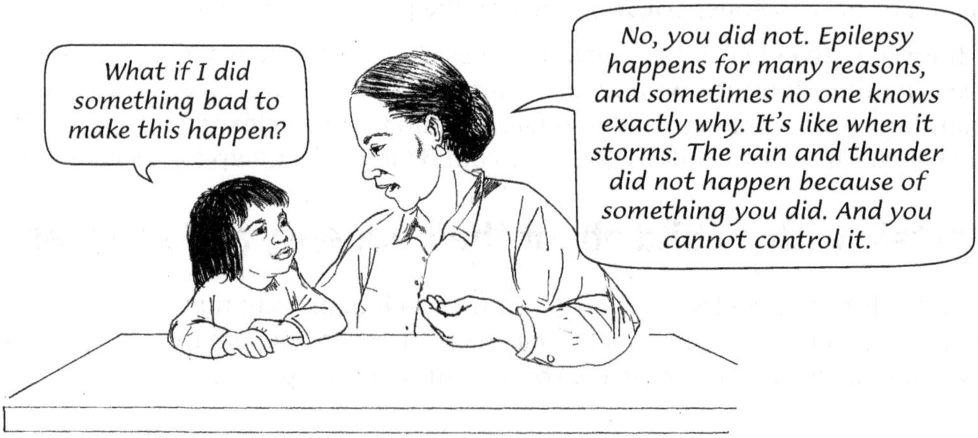
What if I did something bad to make this happen?
No, you did not. Epilepsy happens for many reasons, and sometimes no one knows exactly why. It's like when it storms. The rain and thunder did not happen because of something you did. And you cannot control it.

Benefits of talking to all children about epilepsy and seizures

Because children thrive through playing, learning, and just being together, all children will benefit from understanding more about epilepsy. When a child has a seizure, children around them can prevent them from getting injured. When children understand what a seizure is, they will not feel afraid when they see someone having a seizure. The more children understand about epilepsy as a health condition, the less likely they are to bully or exclude a child who has seizures.

Talk with children of all ages

What a child will understand about epilepsy and seizures depends on their age. Parents and caregivers know and understand their children better than anyone else, including what words they may or may not understand, how they take in new information, and what questions they may ask. Your knowledge of and love for your children will help you talk with them about epilepsy.

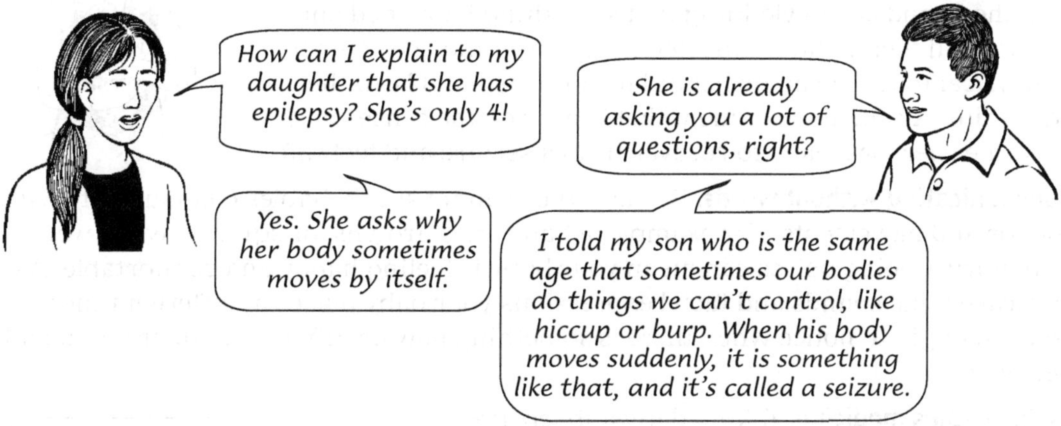

No matter their age, talking with a child about living with epilepsy does not mean you must have all the answers or share everything you know. Young children who are just learning to use words need small bits of information rather than everything all at once. As children grow and change, they will want to know more, including why they have seizures. It is OK to say you do not know. Together you will learn how to talk openly and honestly about epilepsy, and together you will learn how to best manage their condition.

Communicating with babies (birth to 2 years)

Seizures happen more often in babies and infants than at any other time in childhood. They can be caused by epilepsy or by fevers, difficult births, or other illness. Seizures in a baby can be sudden and short. Seizures with convulsions or other body movements can be hard to tell apart from other ways a baby moves their body, like flapping their arms, stretching their entire body, and eye movements.

By watching a baby's movements, parents and caregivers can get clues about possible seizures, so the baby gets the right treatment. For example, repetitive movements like chewing, smacking lips, and leg-bicycling that happen many times close together is a possible seizure. The same actions happening just once or occasionally are not likely to be seizures.

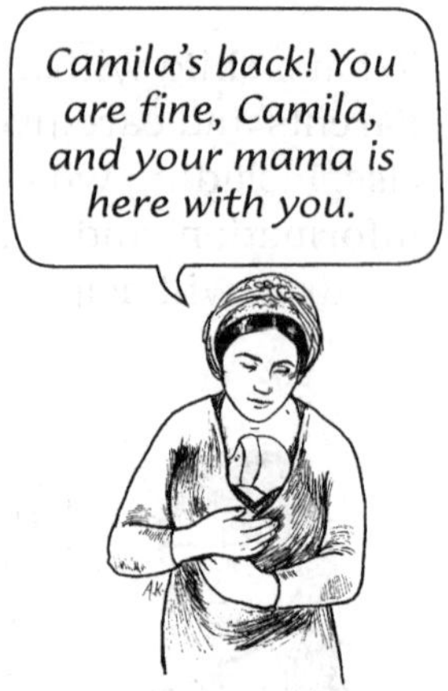
Camila's back! You are fine, Camila, and your mama is here with you.

Helping seizure recovery. We cannot know what a baby feels when they come out of a seizure, but they may feel anxious, confused, or uncomfortable. When a seizure ends and awareness returns, reassure them by holding them, speaking with them, and acknowledging that something happened and you are still there. Stay connected by maintaining eye contact or physical touch. It can be helpful to stay quiet and keep the lights dim. A calm environment that is easy on the senses may make it easier for a baby to recover from a seizure and feel safe.

Communicating without words. Because they cannot speak, babies communicate with sounds and movements. For example, a baby cries, frowns, or squirms when wet or hungry. Cooing noises can mean your baby is feeling happy and comfortable. As you learn what sounds and facial expressions your baby makes at different times, you will begin to notice when there is something new or different in their mood and behavior.

Giving babies medicine. Taking daily antiseizure medicine may make a baby irritable or uncomfortable. A baby may try to avoid taking medicine by turning their head away from it, coughing, or spitting it out. Distract or calm your baby with love, care, and attention by speaking softly, singing, or gently massaging them when you give medicine. Make up a simple, reassuring song that lets the child know it is medicine time.

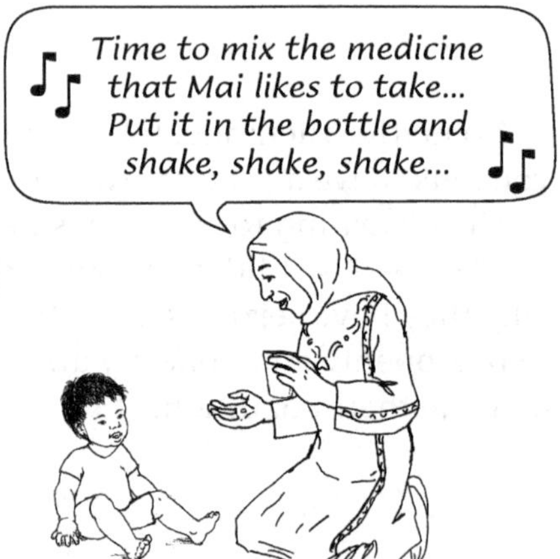
Time to mix the medicine that Mai likes to take... Put it in the bottle and shake, shake, shake...

Seizure first aid training. If you need to leave a baby who has seizures with an older child or another caregiver, make sure the person knows what to do when a seizure happens. For information about seizure first aid, see Chapter 2.

Caring for fever seizures. A high fever (above 38°C or 100.4°F) may cause a seizure in a newborn or infant. When the fever lowers, the seizures typically go away but may return if the baby has another high fever. For information about fever seizures, see Chapter 3, page 59. For information about medicines to reduce fever, see Chapter 4, page 114.

Finding support. Caring for an infant and toddler, whether they have epilepsy or not, can be tiring. Ask for help, take time to rest, and be patient with yourself and your child. Your child's epilepsy should not stop you from reaching out for support from family and friends, or from finding ways to enjoy the time you share with your baby.

For the health worker. When you care for a baby who has epilepsy or seizures, communicate as clearly as you can with parents and other caregivers. What causes seizures and how to care for a baby with epilepsy or seizures are complex topics. As you discuss these issues, share the most up-to-date medical information you have. When you cannot answer a question confidently, you can say, "I will find out and let you know"—and be sure to follow up. Make sure parents know how to reach you for advice or during an emergency.

It can also be helpful to arrange support from other parents of children with epilepsy. Identify or start support groups in your community to help connect people. For information about support groups, see Chapter 5, page 136.

HOW TO Communicate with children who have rare epilepsy syndromes

Parents and caregivers of children with rare childhood epilepsy syndromes, such as Dravet syndrome, Lennox-Gastaut syndrome (LGS), and West syndrome, among others, need additional support. These usually require lifetime care and management. Children with these syndromes may have delays learning to speak, difficulty speaking, or may remain nonverbal, but not all children will have the same level of disability. You can support their attempts to communicate with gestures, facial expressions, and signs. Guidance from a speech pathologist may help. Teaching them (and you!) the sign language used in your country will help their mental and social development. For information about rare childhood epilepsy syndromes, see Chapter 3, page 60.

Talking with children 3 to 5 years old

Children usually begin to notice and question things happening in their bodies after their third or fourth birthdays. They often know when they are sick and can understand explanations about what is happening and why. Listen closely to a child's questions and respond simply and clearly. Although a child may not understand words like "epilepsy" and "seizures," parents and caregivers can begin using these terms so they become familiar.

Why seizures happen. Explain to the child that seizures happen to many people because of different health problems, and sometimes nobody knows why they happen. Let them know seizures are not something to be afraid of and that having seizures does not have to stop them from doing what they love. Children with seizures can still do things they enjoy, like playing, drawing, and learning. Encourage the child to ask you any questions they may have or tell you if they are worried about something. Remind them that you love them and that their seizures are just one way they are special.

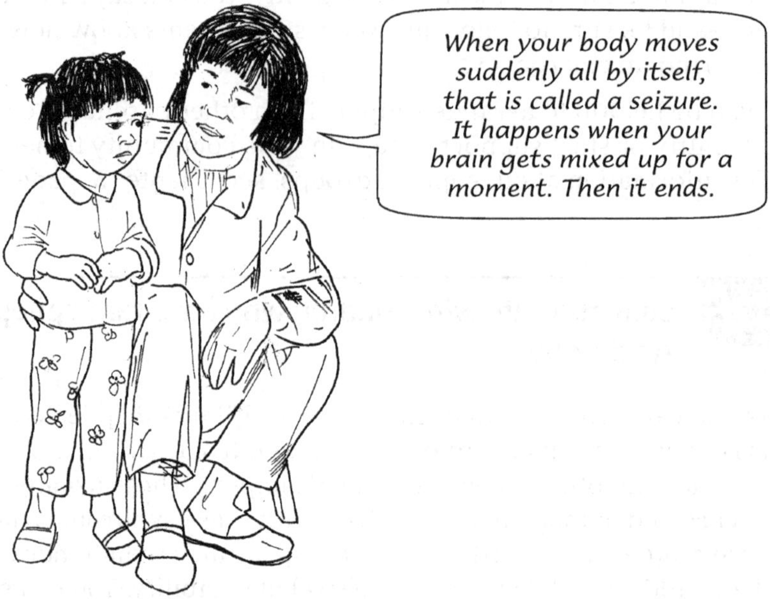
When your body moves suddenly all by itself, that is called a seizure. It happens when your brain gets mixed up for a moment. Then it ends.

Asking for help. By age 4, children can understand that they might get hurt if they have convulsions that make them fall. It is a good time to share simple information about seizure first aid. Explain basic ideas, like listening to their body for warning signs, and sitting down or telling someone if they feel they are about to have a seizure (see "How to talk about aura," page 240). Be sure they understand that there is nothing shameful about having a seizure, and if they need any kind of help afterwards, they should ask an older child or adult.

What happens during their seizures. Drawings and pictures can get a child's attention and help them understand the brain and seizures. Share a picture or make a drawing that gives an idea of what is happening in the child's brain during a seizure.

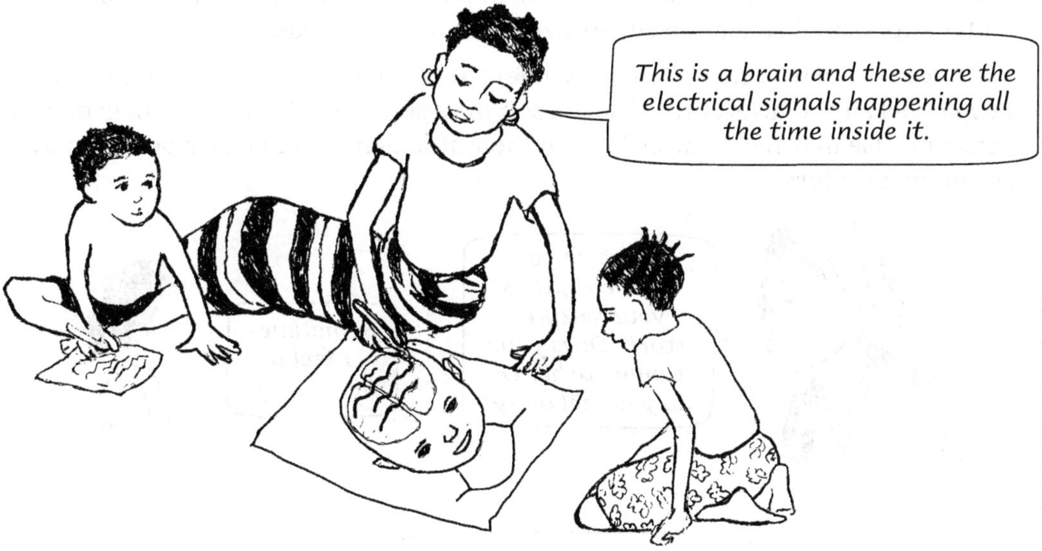
This is a brain and these are the electrical signals happening all the time inside it.

Helping your child's community understand seizures. Just as you teach your child about epilepsy and seizures, you can also talk with their siblings, cousins, and other playmates. Children understand at a young age that people's bodies don't all look or act the same way and differences do not stop them from playing together. With support from adults or older children, young children are good at learning how to care for each other. Introducing basic steps of seizure first aid can be both helpful and fun (see Chapter 2).

Families of a child's friends and neighbors may not have experience with epilepsy and may have wrong or strange ideas about it. Help them learn the basics about epilepsy so they do not pass misinformation to others. All parents and caregivers can teach children to speak up and give correct information when they hear a person say something about epilepsy that is not true.

HOW TO **Talk about aura**

An aura is a sign or physical sensation that is considered the beginning of a seizure, but may be felt minutes before a seizure happens. A child who can feel, understand, and tell others about an aura can often avoid getting hurt during a seizure. Parents, teachers, caregivers, and community members can provide better support when a child recognizes an aura and speaks up.

Not everyone who has seizures will feel an aura, but it is helpful if they do. People feel auras differently. One person may get a certain taste in their mouth, someone else may feel "butterflies" in their stomach, and another person may see unusual colors.

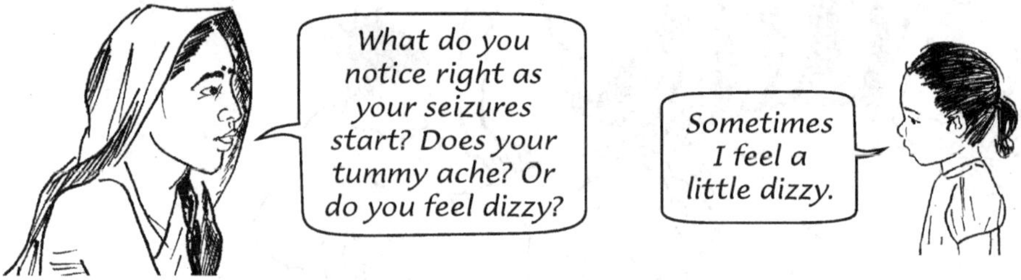

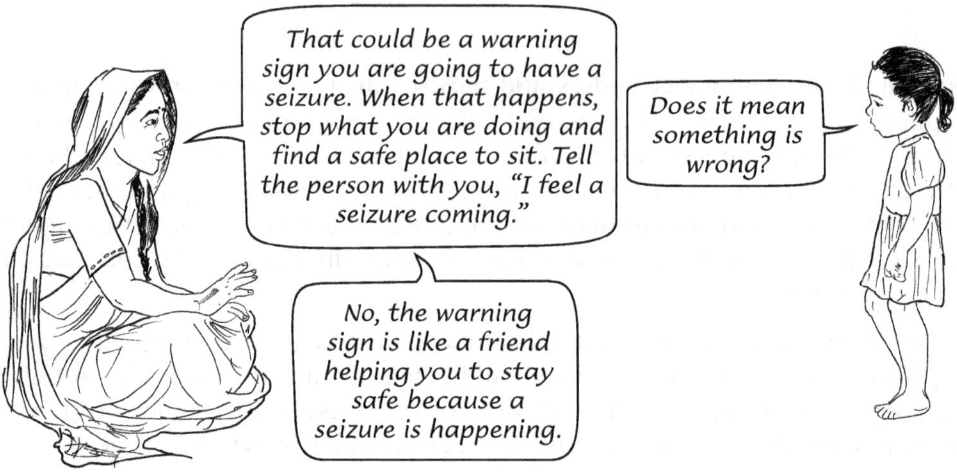

Many children enjoy drawing. Invite a child to draw the unusual feelings their aura causes.

Talking with children 6 to 8 years old

As children get older, they are able to understand more about their bodies in general as well as more about their brain, epilepsy, and seizures. Parents and caregivers can expand on the simple information they shared earlier. Children at these ages are better able to take their medicine properly, avoid things that trigger their seizures, protect themselves from injury, and help when they see someone having a seizure.

What happens during their seizures. Children at this age need to know what happens so they can protect themselves, know what they can ask of others, and what to do after they have a seizure. Make sure they know if they may fall or drop things they are holding so they and others around them can try to make the seizure as safe as possible.

A child is likely to feel embarrassed if their seizures cause them to wet or soil themself. Help the child understand this is part of their seizure, not because they are "babies." Speak openly with your child's teachers, school nurse, or administrator about how some people lose bladder or bowel control during a seizure. Ask them to avoid drawing attention to your child if it happens to them. Pack an extra set of clothes in your child's backpack or leave clothes with a teacher so they can help your child change after a seizure.

If the child will need to sleep or rest quietly after a seizure, make sure they and their teacher know it is OK to need this. Encourage the child to explain to their friends that resting helps them recover.

Avoiding seizure triggers. If you know what triggers a child's seizures, talk together about how to avoid those triggers. For example, depending on the trigger, you might suggest that the child not eat too much sugary food, not exercise so much they get out of breath, avoid too much time in the sun, stop playing when they feel tired, or rest more when they have a cold or infection.

Why seizures happen. Find a way to explain that your child will understand. Here are some examples that might work for you and your child:

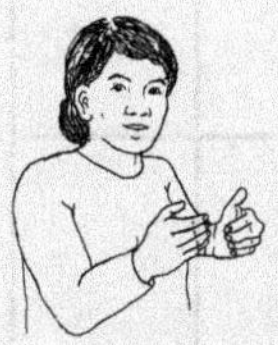

Our brains send electrical signals that tell our bodies what to do. It's like watching television, when sometimes the picture and sound suddenly stop. When the signals start flowing properly again, everything goes back to normal.

Something like that happens during a seizure. Electrical signals in the brain get mixed up and make the body shake and fall. Then, after a minute, it wakes up again.

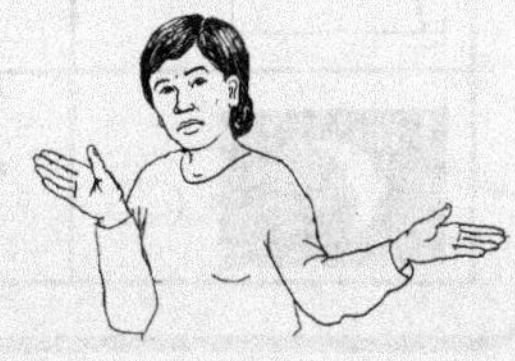

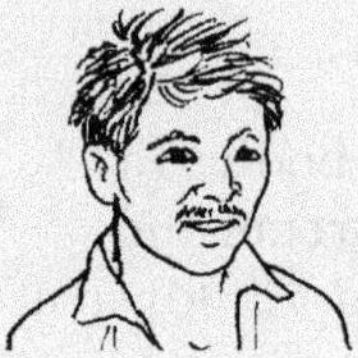

It is like a mobile phone. Sometimes, you are talking to someone and the call drops. Then they call again and you continue talking. That's sort of what happens with your body and brain during a seizure—it drops off, and it comes back.

It's like heavy traffic, but instead of too many cars, it's too many messages in your brain all at once. Everything stops, and then it starts going again.

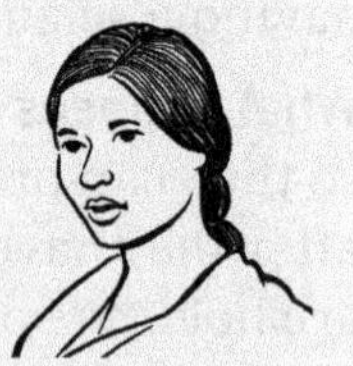

Taking medicine. Children at this age tend to like and depend on routines. Parents and caregivers still have to remind and support them, but can encourage children to take responsibility for remembering to take their antiseizure medicine.

ACTIVITY **Make a chart: Medicine superstars**

Draw a simple chart with rows and columns for each day of the week (see example below).

Explain to your child that every time they take their medicine on time, they get to mark the chart with a star or other shape.

When your child earns 7 marks in a row, offer a small reward such as an extra story or a weekend activity, anything that works for your family.

Ira's medicine chart

	Sun	Mon	Tue	Wed	Thu	Fri	Sat
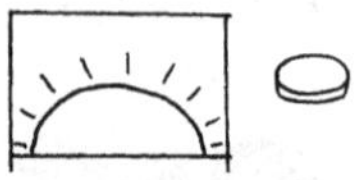	★	★	★	★			
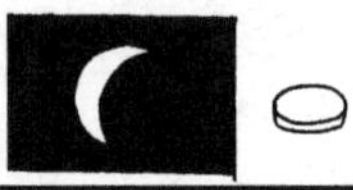	★	★	★	★			

Asking for help. Having a seizure is nothing to be ashamed of. If the child knows they are going to have a seizure, they can ask for help to stay as safe as possible. If they are feeling poorly while recovering from a seizure, they can also ask for help to get what they need to feel better—a drink of water, dry clothing, a quiet place to rest. The more people who know about a child's epilepsy and what they need to recover, the easier it will be for them to avoid harm and regain comfort.

Fighting stigma and wrong ideas. If a child tells you that someone has treated them poorly because of their epilepsy, offer words of comfort and remind them that not everyone understands epilepsy. Explain that people are often afraid of things they do not understand and will make things up or repeat things they have heard others say, even if they are not true. Talk with the child about how they can speak up against teasing and bullying, and let them know you will support them. Help them think about and practice what they could say to a person who insults them (see "How to stand up to bullies: Tips for young people," page 252).

Ask your child if they would like you to talk about epilepsy with other parents or reach out to teachers or a neighborhood group to organize a seizure first aid training. Be sure to follow through on what you offer to do. Invite them to help if they want to.

Speaking out against stigma is not the responsibility of a child with epilepsy or their family alone. Children learn by watching adults around them, and parents and caregivers need to prevent bullying and instead act to create communities where kindness and respect are the norm. Accept differences among people, pay attention when others speak, oppose bullying, and praise your child when they share toys or help another person to model behaviors you would like them to develop.

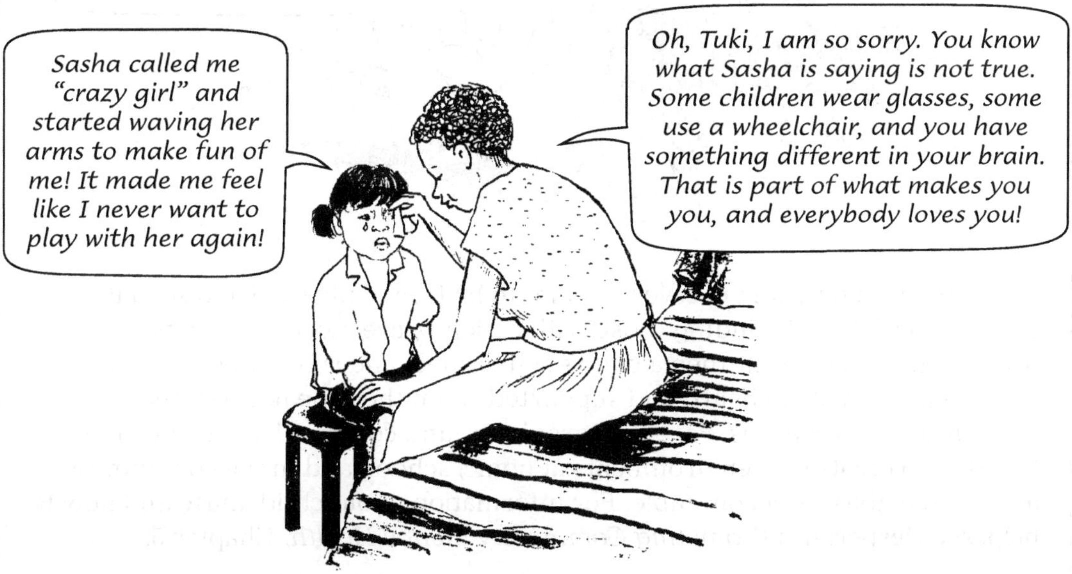
Sasha called me "crazy girl" and started waving her arms to make fun of me! It made me feel like I never want to play with her again!
Oh, Tuki, I am so sorry. You know what Sasha is saying is not true. Some children wear glasses, some use a wheelchair, and you have something different in your brain. That is part of what makes you you, and everybody loves you!

Prevent physical and sexual abuse of children with epilepsy

Children with epilepsy are at a higher risk of being physically and sexually abused than other children. Because they are often seen as weak or different, others may try to control, frighten, or exploit them. When they lose consciousness during a seizure, or need time to recover from a seizure, they become more vulnerable to abuse. Usually, abuse happens in secret and is carried out by someone the person knows.

Talk to children about their right to keep their bodies private and say no. Be aware of signs of physical and sexual abuse:

- unexplained bruises or strange marks on skin
- fear of certain people
- sudden changes in behavior
- a child becoming quieter or withdrawn

Pay attention when a child shows fear or asks for help. If you suspect a child is being harmed, talk with a health worker or another trusted adult about what to do.

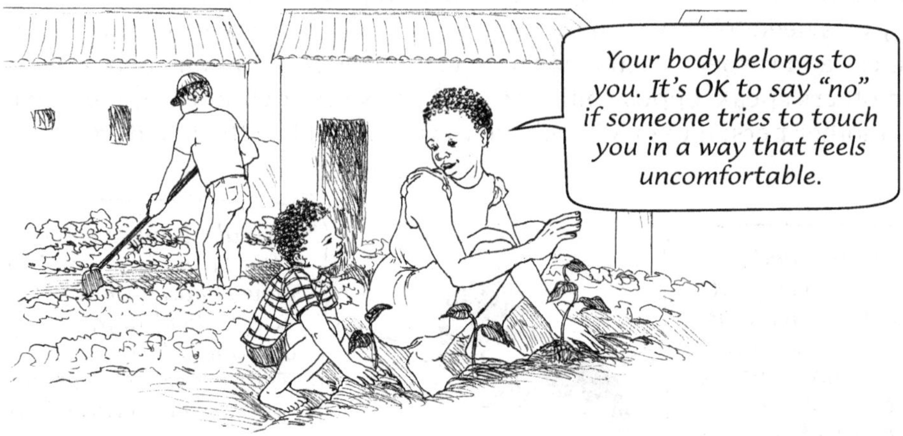
Your body belongs to you. It's OK to say "no" if someone tries to touch you in a way that feels uncomfortable.

By openly addressing everyone's right to be free of physical and sexual abuse, all children, including those with epilepsy, are more likely to be protected. As you strengthen a child's self-respect and self-confidence, they learn that they will be heard and supported when they speak about their feelings and experiences. Parents, caregivers, and community leaders can work together to create safe environments at home, school, and in the community, and to hold abusers accountable. For information about child abuse and how to help, see Hesperian's *Promoting Community Mental Health,* Chapter 5.

Talking about absence seizures

While absence seizures can happen at any age, they are most commonly recognized when children are between 6 and 8 years old.

What happens during their seizures. Children who have absence seizures may suddenly stop moving, stare blankly, or smack their lips. These episodes usually last only 3 to 15 seconds, but they may happen many times during a day—sometimes even hundreds of times! Usually, a child having an absence seizure will not know it is happening.

Helping a child with absence seizures. First, explain to the child that their absence seizures are a health condition and not something they can control. When you notice an absence seizure happening, guide the child away from any danger and stay with them until they are alert again.

Then begin to organize a safety net and support system by telling people close to the child—siblings, neighbors, the child's friends and their families—what an absence seizure is and what to do when one happens.

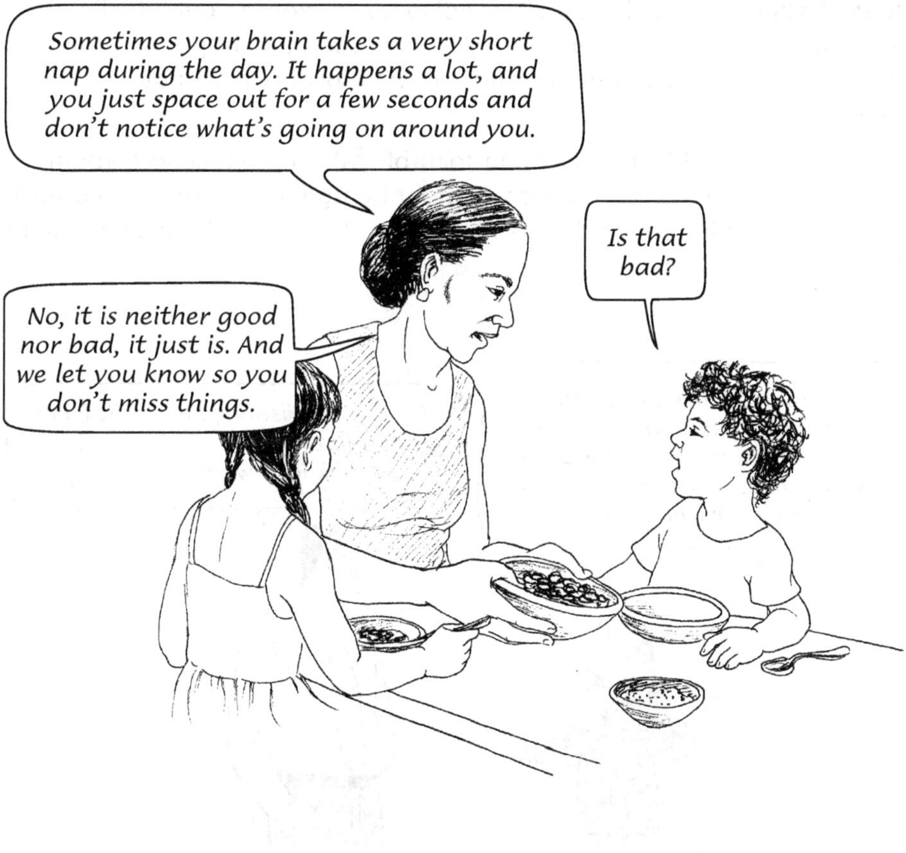
Sometimes your brain takes a very short nap during the day. It happens a lot, and you just space out for a few seconds and don't notice what's going on around you.
Is that bad?
No, it is neither good nor bad, it just is. And we let you know so you don't miss things.

What you see during an absence seizure. If you are looking at a child having an absence seizure, you might mistakenly think they are not paying attention. It may take a while before you recognize that a child's blank stare could be a type of seizure.

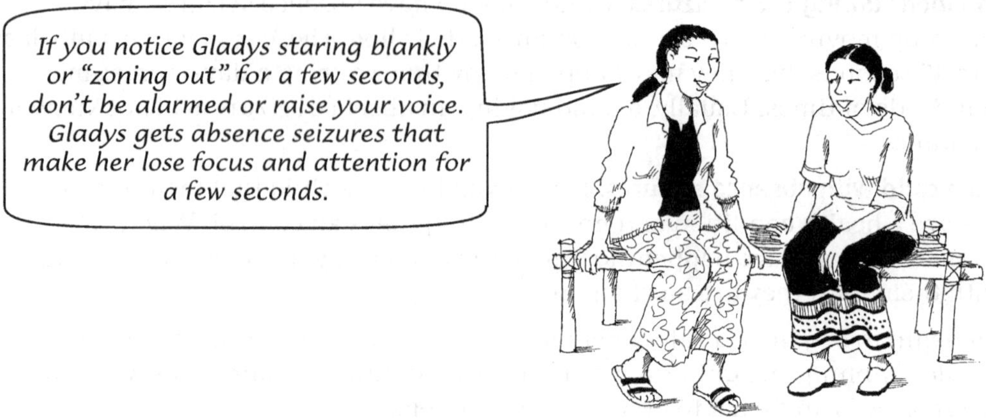
If you notice Gladys staring blankly or "zoning out" for a few seconds, don't be alarmed or raise your voice. Gladys gets absence seizures that make her lose focus and attention for a few seconds.

Absence seizures at school. The brief, painless episodes of "zoning out" during absence seizures are typically followed by a rapid recovery. It is important for parents to talk to teachers so they understand it is not a problem of "not paying attention."

Parents can encourage children to feel comfortable talking to teachers about what they experience. When teachers listen without being judgemental and offer to help rather than dismiss what the child has to say, they help to build trust and safety in the school.

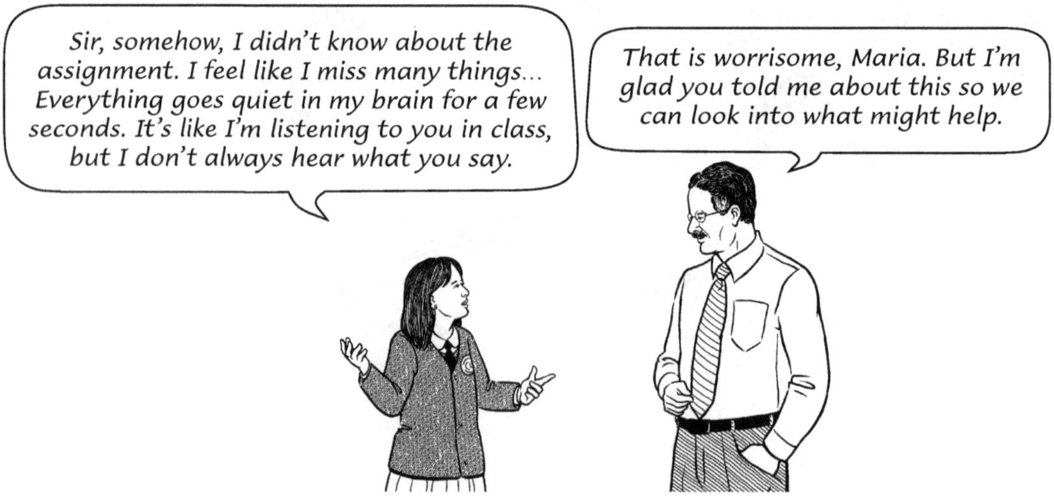
Sir, somehow, I didn't know about the assignment. I feel like I miss many things... Everything goes quiet in my brain for a few seconds. It's like I'm listening to you in class, but I don't always hear what you say.
That is worrisome, Maria. But I'm glad you told me about this so we can look into what might help.

Promoting epilepsy awareness with puppets

Puppets are a great way to teach children about epilepsy. Children (and adults!) are attracted by the entertainment of a puppet show. A good story and a few memorable characters make it much easier to communicate about and understand difficult or sensitive topics. Children with epilepsy who might not be able to talk about their feelings can learn from puppets that mirror their feelings, teaching them and others what it can feel like to have epilepsy.

In Chile, puppets take the stage to shine a light on epilepsy

Community health promoters in Chile created and filmed a puppet show to raise awareness about epilepsy in elementary and middle schools.

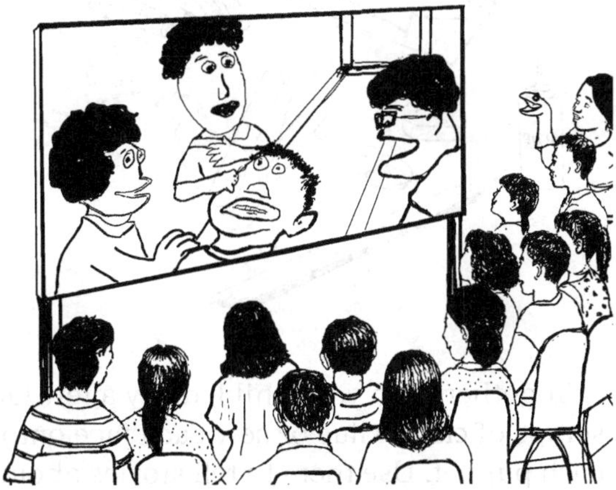

The video features puppet Juanito, who attends school with his friends and has a caring and supportive family. One day during recess, Juanito has a seizure on the school playground. His alarmed but quick-thinking classmates rush to tell their teacher that Juanito needs help. After making sure Juanito is safe, the teacher asks the students to describe what they saw. This not only helped the teacher understand the situation but also educated the children about seizure symptoms.

After Juanito recovers, the teacher speaks with him gently and calmly. She suspects Juanito may have epilepsy.

We follow Juanito as he visits the doctor with his parents, spends time at home with his grandmother, and plays with friends at the playground. In each setting, Juanito's experiences spark conversations about epilepsy, spreading awareness among different community members.

To see if the video helped children learn, the community health promoters asked students some questions about epilepsy before and after showing it. Even children who had not heard of epilepsy before knew what to do after watching it when asked, "What should you do if your friend has a seizure?"

HOW TO **Make puppets at home**

Simple puppets to entertain and teach children about epilepsy can be made at home. Puppet stories can describe familiar experiences, the adventures of epilepsy superheroes, and everything in between. Puppets can be made from paper glued onto sticks, using simple materials like something to draw with (markers, crayons, colored pencils), paper or cloth scraps, scissors, short sticks, and glue (or needle and thread). Or you can make sock puppets.

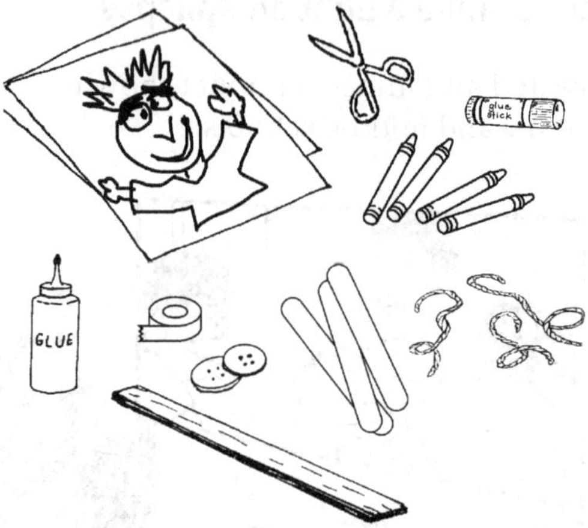

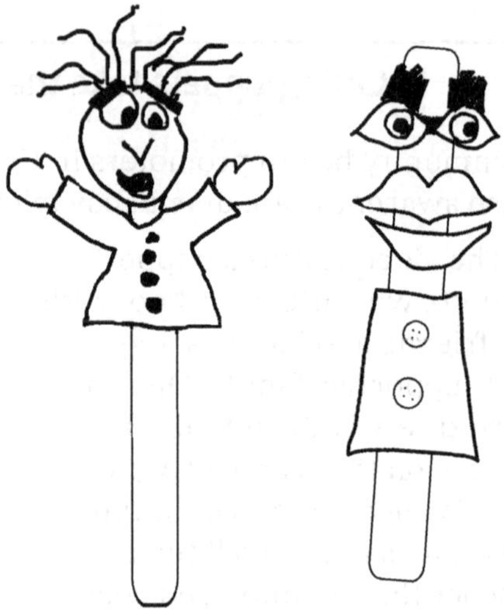

Together with your child, draw a few faces on paper or make them out of scraps of cloth. Glue or sew each face onto a stick or sock. Let the child name each puppet. Use them to tell stories about different topics, like what happens when a person has a seizure, what questions a doctor might ask about seizures, or how to help when someone is having a seizure.

A puppet made from a sock looks alive!

1. Fit the sock over your hand.
2. Make the mouth by pushing in the cloth between your thumb and fingers.
3. Add eyes, nose, and hair to the sock.

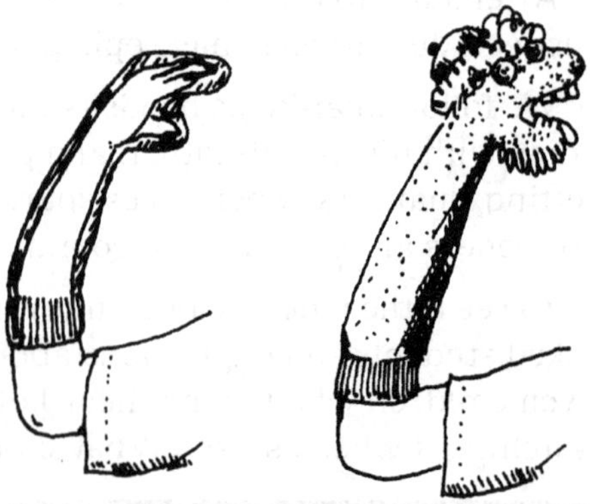

Talking with children 9 to 13 years old

Children these ages are developing more independence and are learning more from life outside the home—in school, with friends, from sports and other organized and informal groups, and from all forms of media. They may express themselves in new ways and look more to peers for support.

The physical changes of puberty also affect how children think and feel. Changes in height, weight, and hormones can affect their medication needs. If a child's seizures suddenly return after having been controlled, they may need a dose adjustment or a different medicine. Talk with children about how body changes might affect their epilepsy.

As a child with epilepsy grows more independent, talk with them about how their expanding social circle means they will meet people who do not know about their epilepsy and may have wrong ideas about it. Encourage them to wear an epilepsy bracelet (see Chapter 6, page 164) and help them practice explaining what it means to have epilepsy and seizures, so they feel ready when the topic comes up.

Being safe doing physical activities. Parents and caregivers may worry about and discourage or stop the participation of a child with epilepsy in sports and other physical activities. Instead of placing limits on your child, continue to treat epilepsy as just one part of their life that does not have to stop them from doing things they want to do.

Talk with your child about what they will do if a seizure happens during different activities. How can they prepare for a "breakthrough seizure" if one happens because their medicine stops working as well? What can they do if they feel aura? Will your child have a "buddy" with them or is there someone else who knows how to help them in case of a seizure? Do they need safety equipment, like a helmet? Talk with your child about how to avoid things they know might trigger their seizures, such as thirst (carry a water bottle), hunger (bring a snack), etc.

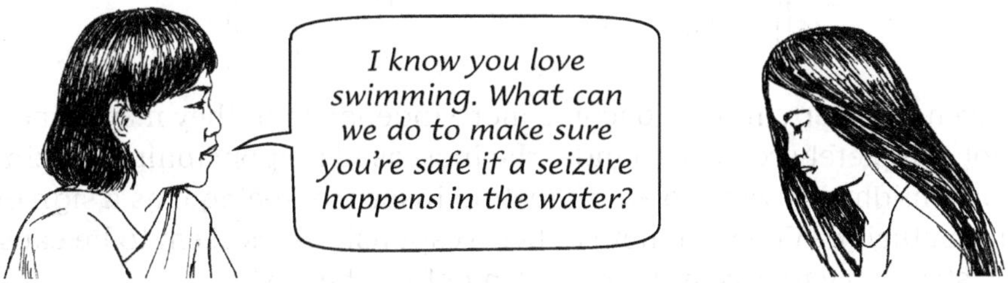

Help your child strengthen their self-confidence and creativity by problem-solving together.

Sometimes children may feel safety measures, such as wearing a helmet while bicycling or never swimming alone, draw too much attention to them or their epilepsy, or make the activities less fun. But often, these safety measures are good ways to protect everyone, not just people with epilepsy. Talk about safety during physical activities with everyone not just with your child.

Taking medicine. Children at this age can take on more responsibility for themselves, including taking their daily antiseizure medicine on their own. It is normal for people of any age to forget sometimes. Try to find a way to help your child remember without causing tension or nagging.

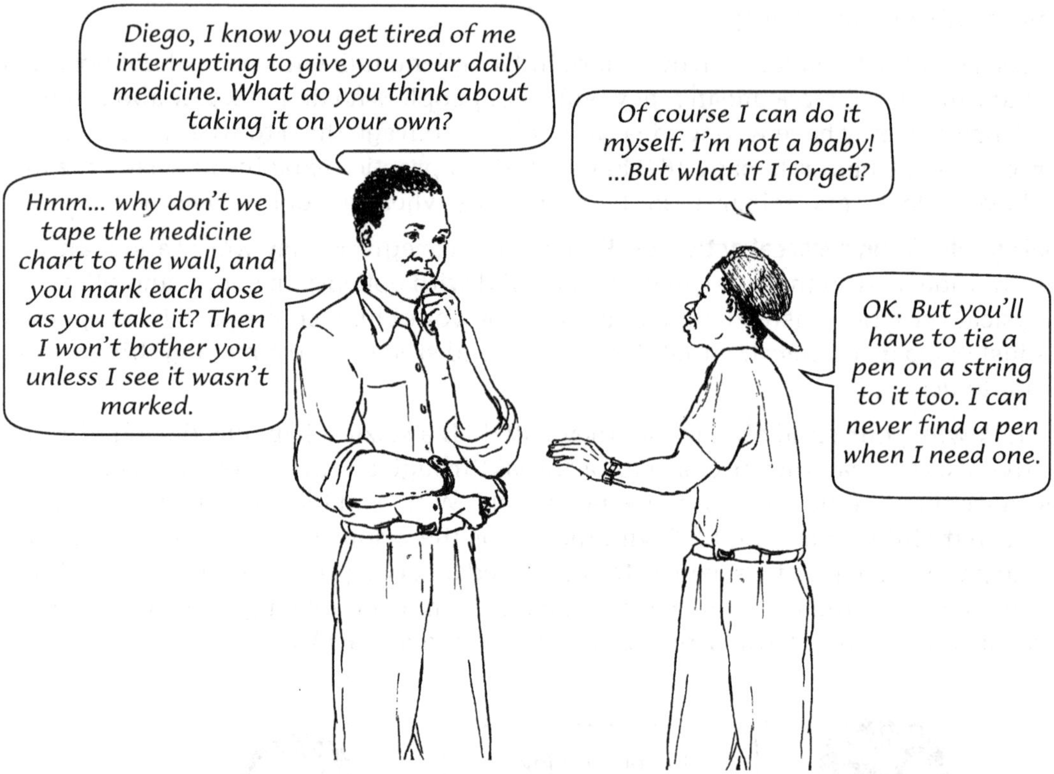

Offer to help. Even as older children become more independent, they may sometimes feel they are not completely ready to handle the increased responsibility of being "grown up." They might not want to admit feeling insecure, seeing it as a sign of weakness or immaturity. When you notice their responsibilities seem to be causing them too much stress, try to lessen their burden before they ask.

Navigating social relationships. As children approach their teenage years, fitting in with friends usually becomes more important to them. For children with epilepsy, these relationships can be especially challenging. A child may feel self-conscious about having seizures or needing to be extra careful. They may resent being treated like "the kid who needs special attention because of epilepsy."

Parents and caregivers often face the tricky challenge of supporting a child without getting in the way. At these ages, your child may want to handle their friendships and other social situations and relationships on their own. You can help by being a guide rather than taking over or making your child feel pressured into doing what you suggest.

For instance, be sure to talk with your child about any plans or ideas you have for community education about epilepsy, so they know what to expect. Listen to how they feel about this and ask if they might like to be involved, but do not pressure them if they prefer not to participate.

Bullying. Children and youth with epilepsy too often experience bullying and teasing from other children and adults. This can cause a child to withdraw from learning and social activities or drop out of school. Bullying creates stress, which is a common trigger for seizures. The more people know about epilepsy and its causes, the less likely they are to engage in or tolerate bullying and ridicule.

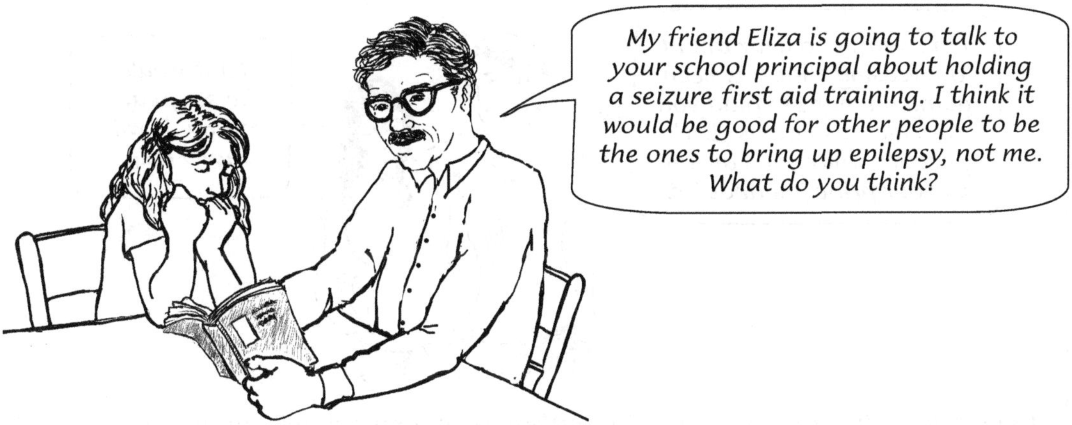
My friend Eliza is going to talk to your school principal about holding a seizure first aid training. I think it would be good for other people to be the ones to bring up epilepsy, not me. What do you think?

Everyone—parents, teachers, neighbors, and community members—has a role to play in handling bullies and creating an environment in which bullying is not OK. When adults take the lead, children can feel more confident standing up against bullying.

HOW TO Stand up to bullies: Tips for young people

No one has to accept bullying and teasing. Here are some ways to respond if you are bullied because you have epilepsy:

Be confident in yourself and remember that epilepsy does not define you. Focus on your strengths—your talents, the activities you enjoy and are good at, and the goals you are working toward.

Remember all the reasons why your friends and family love you. Let this awareness help you stay calm. Practice not showing you are upset. Bullies often seek a reaction. Not reacting can make them lose interest.

Confront a bully by being assertive. Tell the bully to stop what they are doing. For example, use your strong voice to say: "Stop teasing me about my condition. It is not OK. You are wrong and mean to treat me this way!"

Stay connected with supportive friends who appreciate you and will stand up for you.

Talk with an adult you trust who is good at listening. Share your experience and feelings with a parent, teacher, sports coach, or neighbor instead of keeping them to yourself. Practice what you might say if you are bullied again.

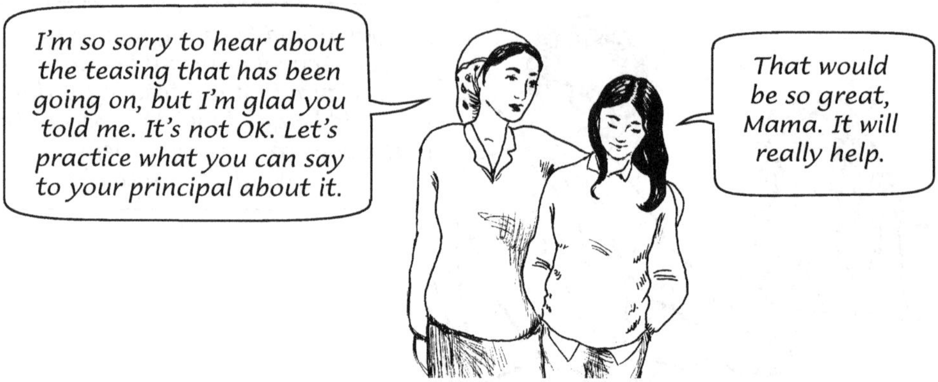
I'm so sorry to hear about the teasing that has been going on, but I'm glad you told me. It's not OK. Let's practice what you can say to your principal about it.
That would be so great, Mama. It will really help.

Report bullying to a person with authority at your school, community council, or church. Ask them to inform you of what action they plan to take to address what happened. Bring a friend with you so you feel supported and also have a witness to how they respond.

As long as you are not being physically attacked, standing up to bullies does not mean physically fighting back. It means speaking up confidently. If you think you are in danger, seek help from adults that you trust.

Talking with young people 14 to 18 years old

Happiness and safety for young people with epilepsy increasingly extends beyond the daily activities of home and school life. As they grow older, teens take on more responsibility—they set their own goals, solve problems themselves, and learn what they like and don't like. Still, they need adult support.

Help teens feel heard and supported. Give your teen space. This can mean letting them know you are there for them, but the decision to talk is up to them. While it is important to show interest in their life outside the home, asking too many questions can feel invasive and push them away. Teens often share less with parents than they did when they were younger. When they do open up, be prepared for lots of emotions, including anger, frustration, and sadness. Show the teen you are comfortable listening to them express their feelings and try to listen without judging, even when their views are different than yours. This helps build and maintain trust between you.

Peer pressure. Young people often feel they have to go along with what others their age are saying and doing. Peer pressure is social pressure to act as others do, in order to be liked, included, and respected. It can lead to behaviors that may be dangerous, such as using drugs or alcohol, because a person fears saying "no" will make their friends dislike them, reject them, or see them as unworthy of friendship. This is as true for teens with epilepsy as it is for other youth.

Talking with teens about alcohol and drugs is important. When a young person's brain is still developing, use of alcohol and drugs can be harmful. For someone with epilepsy, alcohol and drugs may trigger seizures or interact badly with antiseizure medicines, causing unwanted side effects and changing how well seizures are controlled. Using drugs or alcohol can also cause other problems, such as missing a medicine dose while "sleeping off" a hangover.

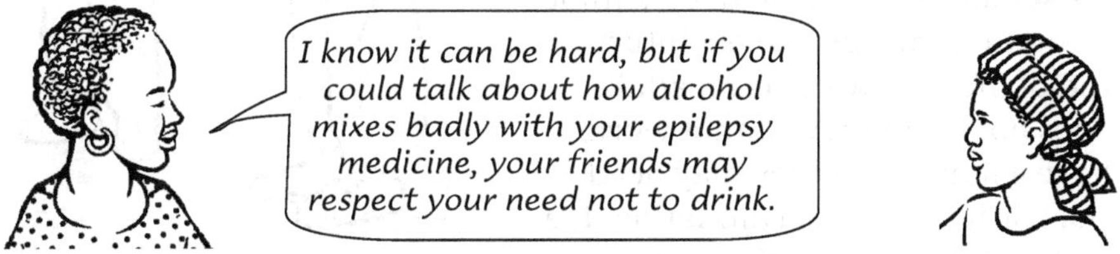

Peer pressure to physically look a certain way can also be challenging for teens with epilepsy. Some teens may feel pressured to lose weight, so they skip meals as a form of "dieting." This is particularly unhealthy if hunger is a seizure trigger. Others may feel pressure to build up their muscles, so they start a new or more intense exercise program. This may make the tiredness caused by some antiseizure medications even harder to manage.

Managing screen time. Young people with epilepsy are just as likely as anyone else to spend a lot of time on mobile or computer screens. The use of electronic devices can bring both positives (like learning and connecting with friends) and negatives (like lost sleep, stress, unsafe interactions, or even seizures, if their use is a trigger). Encourage your teen to talk with you about their experiences online and how they can navigate the digital world. If the teen is worried about telling friends they cannot spend time online, offer to practice having conversations about setting limits and finding alternatives. For information about ways to stay safe and protect your privacy online, see page 144.

Getting enough sleep. Because bodies and minds change so much during these years, young people also need more sleep. This can be difficult as the amount of schoolwork increases and teens want to enjoy time with friends later into the evening. Not getting enough sleep or enough good quality sleep can trigger seizures. Encourage 8 to 10 hours of nighttime sleep every day. For more information on sleeping well with epilepsy, see page Chapter 6, page 192.

Fighting stigma and wrong ideas. When your teen is feeling low about having epilepsy, supporting their connections with other young people can be especially helpful. Encourage teens to seek out peer groups or online communities where youth can share experiences, build friendships, and support one another with their challenges. Getting involved in community activities or volunteering to raise epilepsy awareness can help them feel included and valued as they develop new skills and confidence. For more on stopping epilepsy stigma, see Chapter 5.

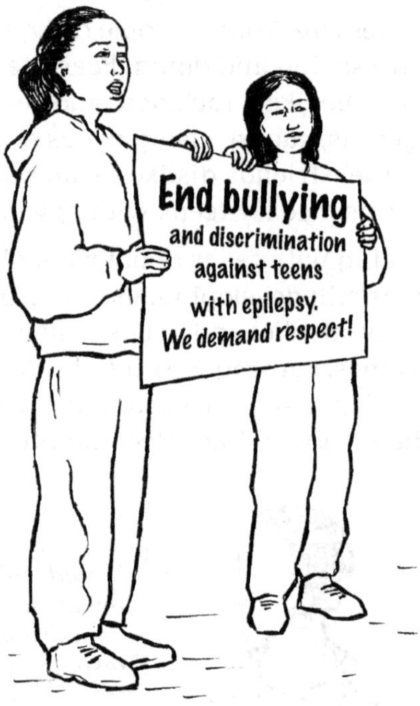
End bullying
and discrimination
against teens
with epilepsy.
We demand respect!

Planning for adulthood. Teens with or without epilepsy begin to think about their future and the kind of life they want as an adult. Epilepsy does not mean they cannot work, study, or have a family, but they may need extra support or face job discrimination due to their condition. Encourage the teen to talk about their interests and dreams, and to identify people they can rely on for guidance and friendship. Remind them that epilepsy is only one part of who they are and will not stop them from building a meaningful life.

Sex and relationships

Having epilepsy does not affect a person's ability to have feelings for other people or the desire to get closer to someone. Neither does epilepsy change the body's ability to experience and enjoy romantic or sexual feelings. Like everyone else, a person with epilepsy can decide if, when, and how they want to, or do not want to, explore sex or a romantic relationship.

For teens and young people

Telling someone you are interested in or already dating about your epilepsy does not mean you are sharing a weakness. It is just sharing part of who you are. It is natural to feel nervous about having these conversations, but talking openly can help build trust and understanding. As someone with epilepsy, you already have experience paying attention to and talking about your body and feelings. This may help you feel comfortable talking about relationships and sex with a potential sexual partner. You can decide what to share and when.

When you are ready, share basic information about:

- epilepsy as a brain condition... it is not contagious!
- what happens when you have a seizure.
- any seizure triggers you may have.
- seizure first aid.

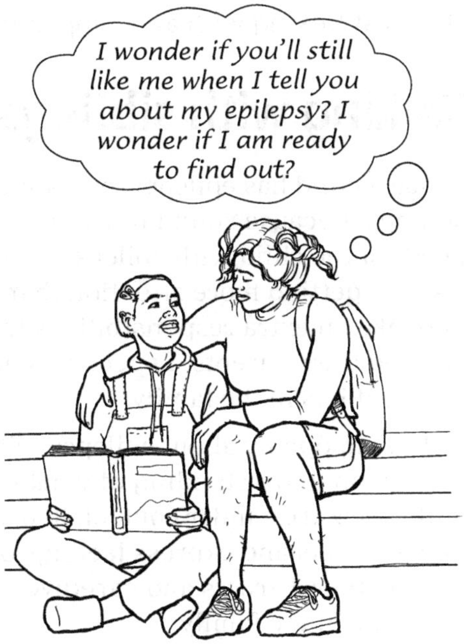

You have probably already experienced how epilepsy can affect relationships—sometimes it strengthens bonds between people, other times it frightens people away. When you open up about your epilepsy, you can expect questions and comments that will tell you something about what the person knows or thinks about epilepsy. How they respond to you may also help you decide to continue seeing this person or notice "red flags." If a person rejects you because of epilepsy or seizures, it means you would not have been able to trust a relationship with them anyway.

Safe sex. Sex can be as healthy and enjoyable for people with epilepsy as it can be for people who do not have epilepsy. However, some antiseizure medicines make some kinds of birth control less effective. Other medicines may lower desire, as can fear of having a seizure while being sexual. If you're feeling unsure about whether to have sex with someone, find an adult who understands these issues and is willing to discuss your decisions with you, perhaps a relative or someone in the community you trust who also has epilepsy. For information about how to protect yourself from unintended pregnancy or how to plan for a pregnancy with epilepsy, see Chapter 7.

For parents: Talking with your teen about sex and relationships

It is common to feel uncomfortable talking with your child about sex and relationships. But developing an interest in sex and romantic relationships is often a part of growing up, and knowing how to do that safely is important for everyone. If you find it difficult to discuss sex and relationships with your teen, you can encourage them to reach out to someone with whom they feel safe—a relative, family friend, teacher, counselor, health worker, or an adult who also has epilepsy. If your teen cannot find someone they are comfortable speaking with about sexuality and dating, ask a health worker to recommend a counselor or other adult who is skilled at talking with and supporting young people.

Talking with siblings about epilepsy

When a child has epilepsy, everyone in the family is affected, including the child's siblings. Because adult family members may need to take extra time to care for the needs of the child with epilepsy, the other children may resent that their brother or sister is getting more attention than they are. Or they may feel pressure to be "good" and take on extra responsibilities to make up for the challenges that epilepsy is causing their parents. Especially with young children, this can lead to "acting out" and conflicts in the family.

Talking openly about epilepsy with the entire family helps everyone develop a common understanding of what is happening and why it is important to get a child's seizures under control. It also gives other children a chance to talk about how they feel and express feelings of anger, fear, or sadness, as well as concern for one another. Parents and caregivers can share how much they love and appreciate everyone in the family.

Especially with the added stress that comes with an epilepsy diagnosis, it can be difficult for parents and caregivers to remain patient and caring with each child all the time. If possible, try to make regular times to do "special" activities with each child. They will appreciate the attention, and you can learn how epilepsy is affecting them and their needs.

Older siblings are sometimes expected to "watch out for" and care for younger children or a child with epilepsy. While this often happens naturally given the love among children in a family, it can also create tension. As siblings get older and want to spend more time with friends their own age, they may not always want to include a sibling, whether or not the child has epilepsy.

Acknowledge how much you value and appreciate the care siblings give the child with epilepsy. Help siblings understand how fear of epilepsy and social stigma make it harder for a child with epilepsy to spend time with playmates and friends their age. Also try to arrange for other caregivers so the older siblings have some days each week for social time free from babysitting.

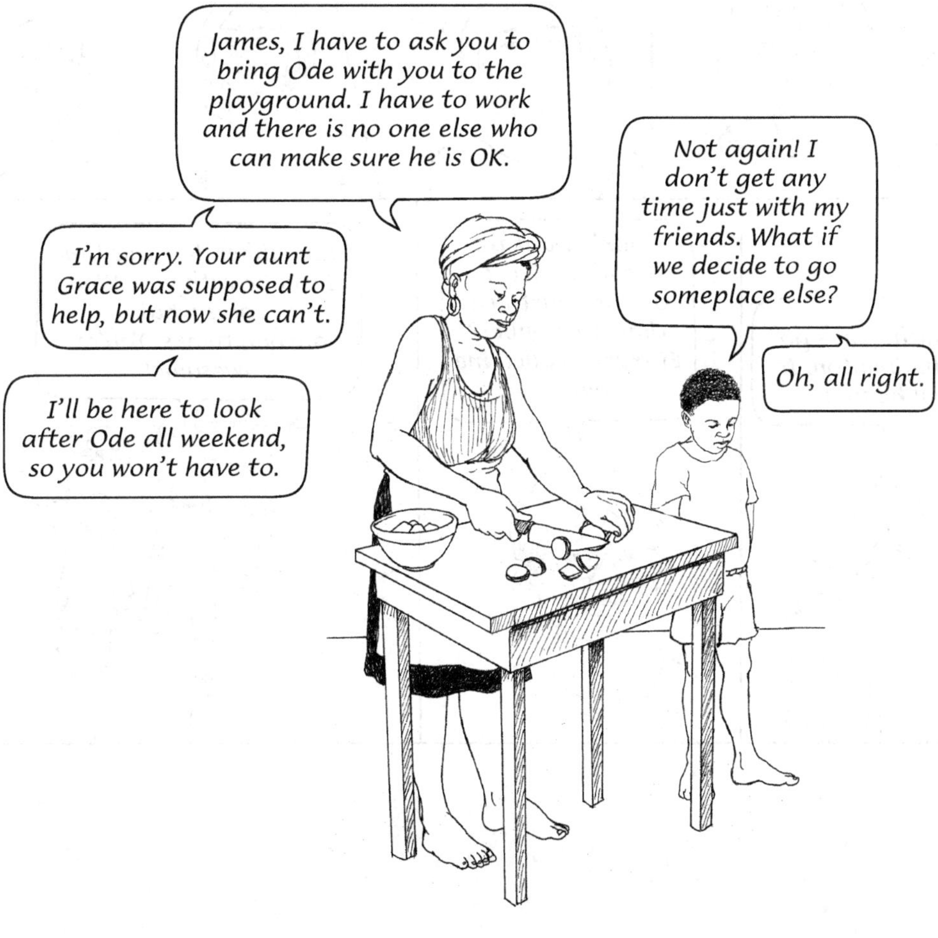
James, I have to ask you to bring Ode with you to the playground. I have to work and there is no one else who can make sure he is OK.
Not again! I don't get any time just with my friends. What if we decide to go someplace else?
I'm sorry. Your aunt Grace was supposed to help, but now she can't.
Oh, all right.
I'll be here to look after Ode all weekend, so you won't have to.

No one wants to see a child with epilepsy get hurt, either physically or emotionally. Like parents, the child's siblings may become so focused on protecting a child with epilepsy that they miss how the child's abilities increase with age. Protection is important for children, but being too protective can limit a child's growth and confidence. While keeping safety in mind, siblings can encourage a child with epilepsy to try new things like other children their age.

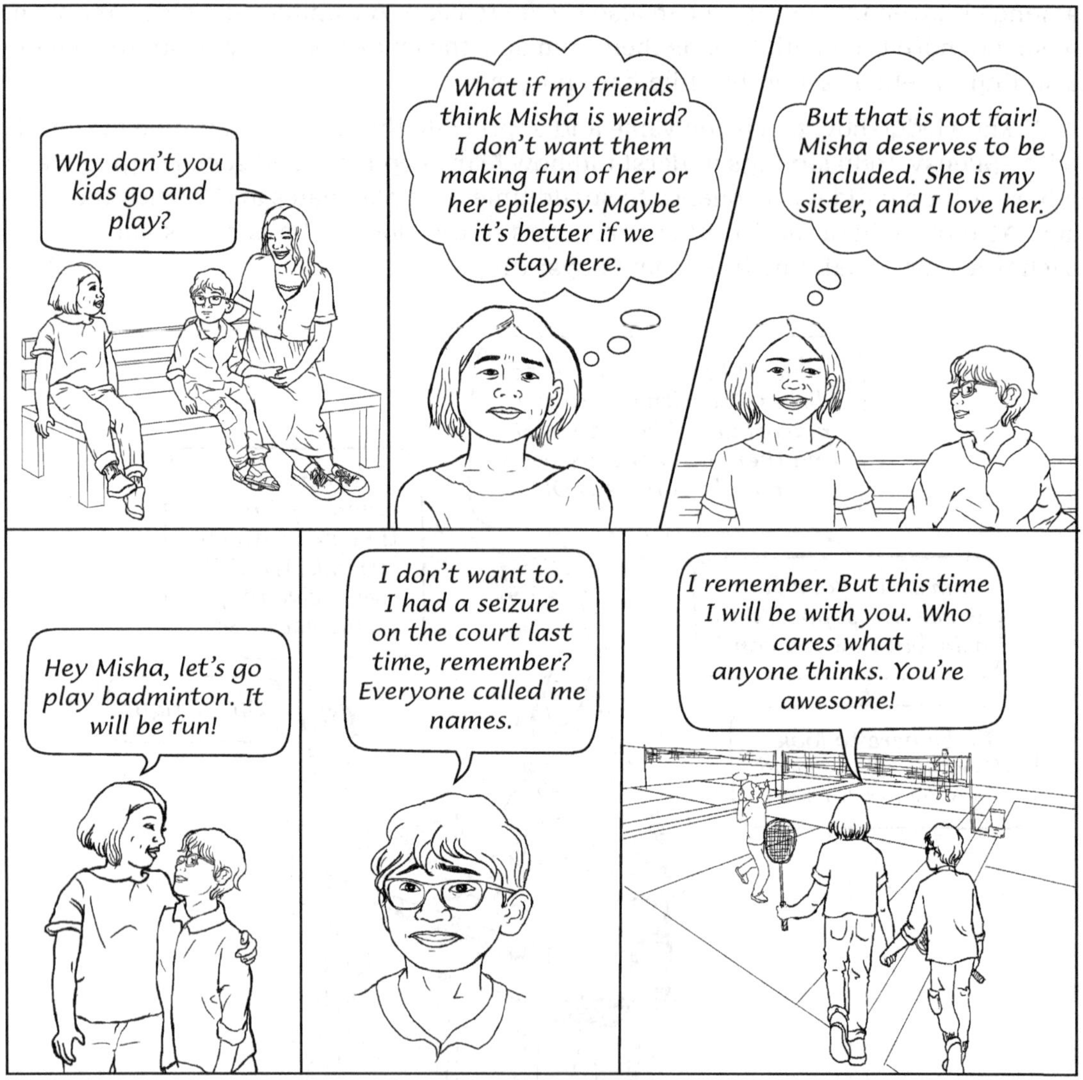
Why don't you kids go and play?
What if my friends think Misha is weird? I don't want them making fun of her or her epilepsy. Maybe it's better if we stay here.
But that is not fair! Misha deserves to be included. She is my sister, and I love her.
Hey Misha, let's go play badminton. It will be fun!
I don't want to. I had a seizure on the court last time, remember? Everyone called me names.
I remember. But this time I will be with you. Who cares what anyone thinks. You're awesome!

For health workers

Children with epilepsy can benefit greatly when health workers and adults outside the family develop relationships with them. Simple actions like making eye contact, waving hello, or stopping to talk even briefly can help them feel seen and know they are valued.

While wearing a white medical jacket might command respect from your coworkers, it may frighten children who only see people wearing them when something scary has happened with their health. You can help children with epilepsy feel more comfortable by wearing more colorful, casual clothes—which are also often easier to keep clean.

Showing a personal interest in the child in front of you helps builds trust. Starting health visits with questions like, "What grade are you in?" or "What games do you like to play with your friends?" can help a child feel comfortable talking with you for the first time, or as someone they have met before but not seen recently. Even though you may be pressed for time, it is worth building a relationship with your young patients.

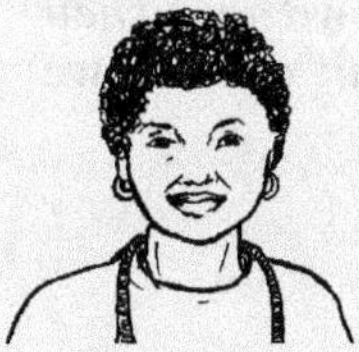

When I talk with a child, I want them to understand I care about them. I start by asking, "What do you like to do at school?" instead of asking about epilepsy or seizures.

Sometimes a child's answers will clue you in to how they are feeling about themself or what they are concerned about. By allowing a conversation to flow naturally, you may learn helpful information that a routine set of questions might not reveal.

For older children, you might also ask, "How do your teachers and classmates feel about your epilepsy?" or "Do you think epilepsy stops you from doing activities you enjoy or would like to try?"

When explaining things to children, think of ways to be as clear as possible. Because everyone communicates and understands things differently, you can increase understanding when you:

Use easy words, plain language, and speak slowly. Avoid medical words or complicated terms. Unfortunately, the language of epilepsy and seizures is filled with them! For example, instead of "seizure management," say "what to do when a seizure happens." Using common words helps a child pay attention to your message, rather than confusing them with information they must try too hard to understand.

Repeat key points and ask a child to repeat them back to you. After explaining something important, repeat it in the same simple way. Then ask the child to say it back to you in their own words. For example, when talking about aura, you can say, "If you feel dizzy, sit down right away. Can you tell me what you will do if you feel dizzy?"

Divide complex instructions into small steps. For example, instead of saying, "Take 1 pill with water, 10 minutes after a meal, every day," you can say, "One, eat breakfast. Two, wait 10 minutes. Three, pop one tablet out of this medicine strip and swallow the tablet with plenty of water. Now repeat that all back to me and count out each step using your fingers."

When it comes to learning about a child's health, you may need to rely on information from parents or other caregivers. But it is important to hear directly from children about how their seizures and medicines make them feel. With older children and teens, always include them in conversations about their health so they do not feel left out, undervalued, or invisible.

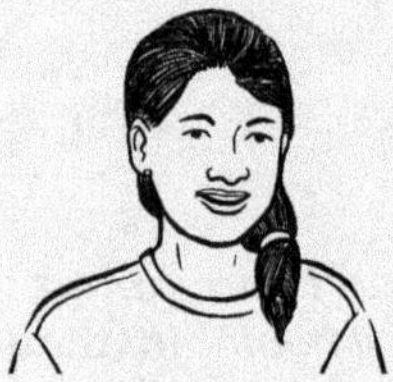

I want teens to understand I care about them and value their ideas. I start by asking to speak with them alone, without their parents. Then, if questions come up that they can't answer, we invite the adults in.

Chapter 9

In this chapter

Links between violence and epilepsy 263
Who is most at risk for violence? 264
Activity: Structural violence in your community 265
Story: Harriet Tubman 268
Seizures from stress and trauma 269
Prevent violence to prevent epilepsy **269**
Prevention strategies 271
Story: Convincing students to wear helmets 272
Story: Preventing epilepsy by promoting safer births at Nakivale Refugee Camp 273
Story: Making work safer 274
Story: Breaking the silence on gender-based violence 274

Preventing violence can prevent epilepsy and seizures

To prevent epilepsy, we must prevent what causes it. While sometimes it is genetic and cannot be prevented, for many people it is caused by violence—both physical violence and the structural violence built into our societies. This chapter is about understanding and preventing the violence, inequality, and discrimination that can cause and worsen epilepsy and seizures.

Links between violence and epilepsy

Injuries that harm the brain are some of the most common causes of epilepsy. Head injuries may be caused by falls, vehicle crashes, dangerous work, playing sports, or the effects of alcohol or other drugs.

Head injuries can also result from physical violence, including the use of weapons and the destruction in conflict zones, criminal assault, and police violence. At home, violence from a partner or family member may cause serious head injury. Severe head injuries can cause brain damage that may lead to seizures and epilepsy.

Other forms of violence that can cause epilepsy and seizures may be less easy to see. The way societies and communities are set up affects how and where we live, what educational opportunities and jobs are available to us, and how we are treated by government programs and institutions. When harm, threats, and unfair limits on our choices or opportunities are caused by an economy, social system, or government, this is structural violence. Structural violence results from systems of racism, sexism, class division, and homophobia. These unfair systems affect everyone's ability to enjoy life and have equal access to opportunity, and they harm some people more than others.

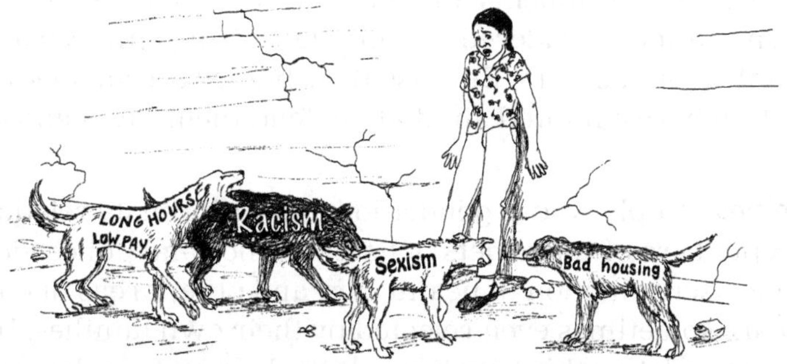

Social conditions that create division and discrimination are a constant source of structural violence in people's lives.

Structural violence can lead to epilepsy and seizures. For example, poverty may force a woman to marry at a young age and prevent her from being able to access help during a difficult birth. If her labor goes on for too long, the baby may not get enough oxygen or their head may repeatedly push against the mother's pelvic bones. These situations can injure the baby's head and brain and cause epilepsy. Another example is when poverty prevents a family from treating their child's malaria or meningitis. If a child does not receive treatment for these illnesses or if treatment is delayed, the child can have seizures that might develop into epilepsy.

But when girls are allowed more access to education, they often wait until they are older to marry or bear children. And when healthcare is made available to all who need it, people will not be prevented from getting treatment.

Who is most at risk for violence?

Physical and structural violence can affect anyone, but they cause more harm to people who have less power over their lives. To prevent people from being harmed in ways that can cause epilepsy and seizures, it is helpful to ask: Who is more likely to be injured by physical violence? Who is more likely to be involved in accidents? Who is more likely to be harmed by structural violence and discrimination?

People living in poverty. Poverty is structural violence. Substandard housing, unsafe transportation, dangerous jobs, poor nutrition, unaffordable health care, and lack of clean water may seem different than physical violence, but they cause physical harm just the same. For example, poor living conditions can lead to having tapeworms, which can cause brain infections and seizures (see Chapter 3, page 62). And when poverty causes health problems, it often also denies treatment.

Women. Women are more likely than men to be physically injured by intimate partners, including by sexual violence, and to be discriminated against in jobs and educational opportunities. When a woman is beaten during pregnancy, injuries to her or the baby can cause epilepsy.

Children. Poverty, debt, or the loss of parents may force children to leave school and work, often in unsafe environments and for lower wages. Physical and emotional abuse of children is often considered acceptable, putting children at risk of violence from family members and others. Because their bodies are smaller and less developed, children have a limited ability to defend themselves and get help when needed.

LGBTQ communities. People whose gender identity or intimate relationships are not socially accepted are often targets of hate violence and police violence. LGBTQ people often face discrimination in health care and other areas of community life. Sadly, they are sometimes even rejected by their own families. In some countries, same-sex relationships are against the law, and employment and housing discrimination against LGBTQ people is common.

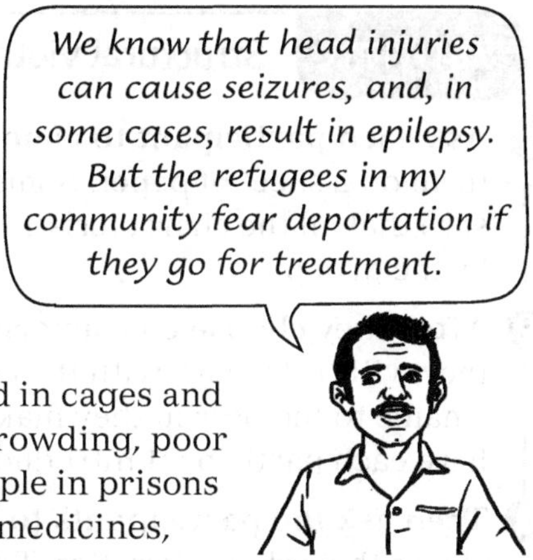

Migrants, immigrants, and refugees. Often forced by poverty and political violence to leave their homes or countries, migrants may be threatened with deportation or removal, forced to survive by working in dangerous and low-paying jobs, and crowded into unhealthy living spaces, often without access to health care, social supports, or personal safety.

People in prisons. In many prisons, people are locked in cages and controlled with violence. They are harmed by overcrowding, poor nutrition, lack of exercise, and poor health care. People in prisons who have epilepsy are regularly denied antiseizure medicines, which can lead to more frequent and worsening seizures.

ACTIVITY Structural violence in your community

This activity helps show that people with less power over their lives may be more vulnerable to violence. It works best with at least 5 or more people.

To prepare: Make 2 lists—one with words or characteristics that describe a person with more or less power (see below), and one that describes challenging things that may happen in a community. (see next page). Add or delete from the lists so they reflect your community.

Characteristics

MORE POWER		LESS POWER	
Man	Office worker	Woman	Factory or field worker
Adult	Citizen	Child	Immigrant
Rich	Dominant religion	Poor	Other religion
Light skin	High caste	Dark skin	Low caste
Boss	No disability	Worker	With disability
Majority ethnicity	Heterosexual	Minority ethnicity	LGBTQ

continues

ACTIVITY Structural violence in your community *(continued)*

1. **Ask each participant to choose 5 characteristics from the list** and write them on a sheet of paper. Some of their choices will overlap but try to make sure that all the characteristics show up at least once among the choices made by the group.

2. **After they choose characteristics,** ask each participant to make up a person they will "role play" with the characteristics they have chosen. Have them give a name to the person they make up and invent a few other details. One by one, have each participant introduce themself to the group.

3. **Then ask the participants to line up side by side,** holding the paper that shows their characteristics. Tell them that you will say out loud things that may happen in the community. If they think their character or their character's family would be affected by it, they should take a step forward. If not, they stay where they are. If they are not sure, they should say so and the group can discuss and decide.

4. **Read the "things that may happen"** (examples below) out loud one at a time. Remind people to take a step forward if they think their character would be harmed in the situation.

- School fees doubled for each child
- Principal decides schools will not accept or teach students with disabilities
- Local health clinic closes so nearest is now 10km/6 miles away
- Armed conflict breaks out; people must show identity papers to get a job, rent a house, get health care, etc.
- Politicians blame immigrants for crime
- Religious leaders say women should stay home and care for children
- Bus fares and fuel costs increase

- Agricultural chemicals pollute river where people get water
- Unemployment increases; men drink in the street
- Abortion is made illegal
- Groups protecting rights of women, minorities, LGBTQ people are shut down
- Police violence increases
- Sales tax/VAT increases
- Partner drinks, is abusive, but you feel you cannot leave
- Boss demands sexual favors
- Factory explosion injures many workers

continues

ACTIVITY Structural violence in your community *(continued)*

5 **Reflection:** Ask these and other questions for group discussion:

- Which of our characters have moved a lot or been harmed the most?
- What characteristics do they share?
- What does this say about how inequality affects our society?
- Which of the harmful situations might cause or worsen a person's epilepsy and seizures?

6 **Conclusion:** Lead a group discussion on the kinds of actions that might reduce or prevent physical and structural violence in your community, especially as they relate to conditions that can cause seizures. Emphasize the importance of people working together to help each other deal with the challenges they face.

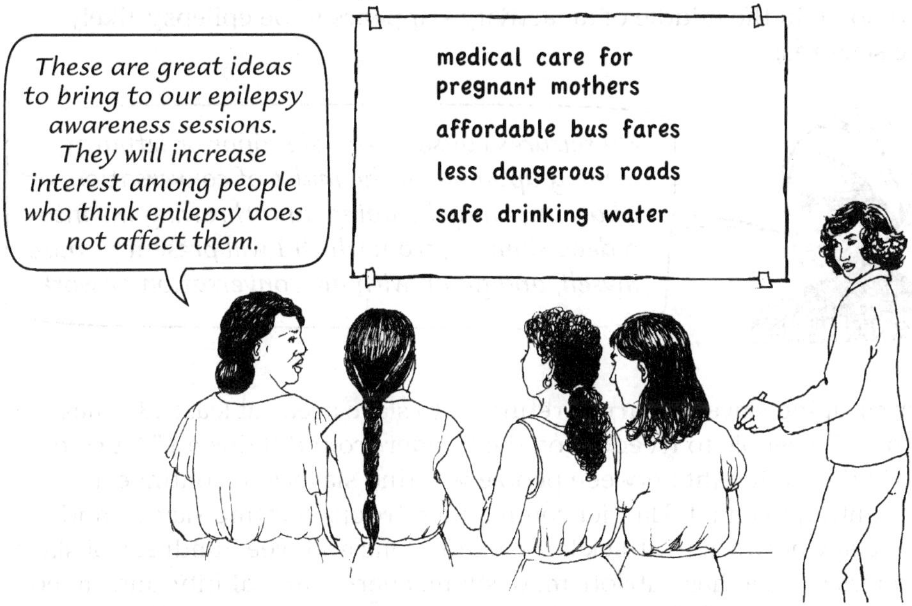
These are great ideas to bring to our epilepsy awareness sessions. They will increase interest among people who think epilepsy does not affect them.
medical care for pregnant mothers
affordable bus fares
less dangerous roads
safe drinking water

Harriet Tubman

Slavery is one of the most violent institutions imaginable. An enslaved person has had almost all control over the conditions of their life taken away from them.

Harriet Tubman, one of the great heroes of the United States, was born into slavery in 1820. When she was 12 years old, a white overseer attacked an escaping slave with a large iron weight. He missed his target but hit Harriet in the head, nearly killing her. As a slave, she got no medical treatment for her injury, but her mother nursed her back to life.

The violent blow to her head injured her brain and caused her lifelong pain, including headaches and seizures. Because people did not understand much about epilepsy 200 years ago, and any testing and treatment that did exist was denied to people in slavery, we cannot know for sure if Harriet Tubman developed epilepsy. But what Harriet describes in her biography—her brain shutting down in the middle of an activity—appears to be epilepsy, likely absence seizures.

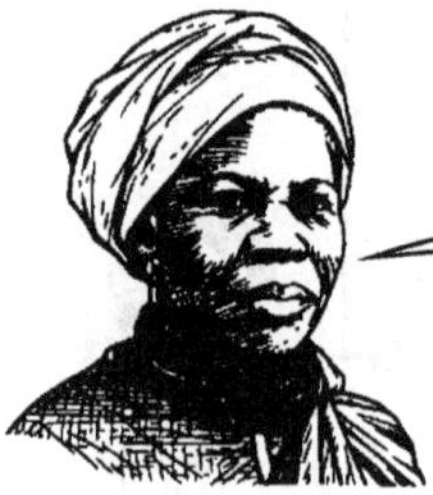

My seizures cause a sort of stupor or lethargy, coming upon me in the midst of conversation, or whatever I may be doing, and throwing me into a deep slumber, from which I will presently rouse myself, and go on with my conversation or work.

After escaping slavery, Harriet returned to slave areas at least 13 times to lead over 70 people to freedom on the "Underground Railroad." During the US Civil War, fought between people wanting slavery to continue and people wanting to end it, Harriet commanded troops fighting slavery and directed a spy network to attack large plantations and free hundreds of slaves. Newspapers praised her patriotism, wisdom, energy, and ability, and called her "General Tubman." This well-deserved praise was unheard of in that era for an enslaved person, for an African-American, for a woman, or for a person with epilepsy, much less for someone with all 4 characteristics.

Seizures from stress and trauma

Violence in any form can lead not only to physical injuries but also to stress, anxiety, and trauma. In some people, especially those who have been affected by war, rape, and childhood abuse, these psychological injuries can trigger seizures.

Seizures with psychological causes—often referred to as "psychogenic non-epileptic seizures" (PNES) or "conversion disorder"—are frequently mistaken for epilepsy. However, unlike seizures from epilepsy, which are caused by abnormal electrical activity in the brain, these seizures are a response to psychological distress. Because they are not due to a physical brain condition, psychologically-caused seizures do not respond to antiseizure medications. Instead, they are managed as a mental health issue. To learn how to recognize and treat these types of seizures, see Chapter 3, pages 70 to 79.

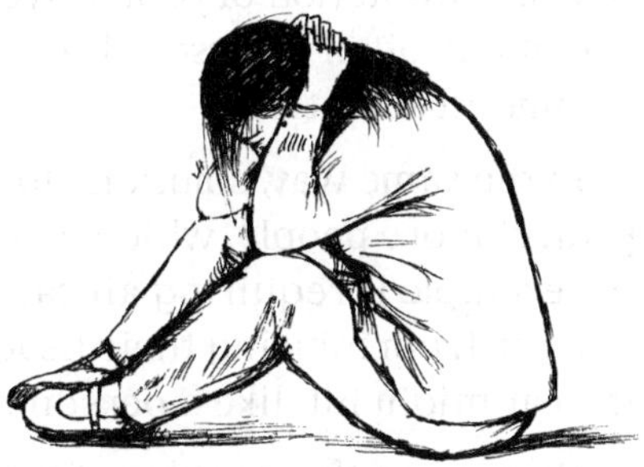

Seizures from psychological causes can be prevented in the same way that structural violence can be prevented—by improving living conditions, replacing stigma with acceptance, and making services and opportunities available to all.

Prevent violence to prevent epilepsy

Head injuries resulting in traumatic brain injuries (TBI)—whether caused by accident or by the physical violence of domestic abuse, police or criminal assault, or the destruction of war—can lead to seizures that may last a person's entire life. They are a leading cause of epilepsy.

Imagine you are at a peaceful demonstration with hundreds of people to oppose cuts in your country's health budget and to support more resources for people with health conditions like epilepsy. This angers the government, which calls out the police to break up your rally. As a policeman raises his baton, you realize it is too late to think about preventing the head injury that could cause epilepsy. However, there are various ways that violent injuries could have been prevented:

1. **Use of personal protective equipment:** Wearing a helmet could protect you.
2. **Change part of the situation**: Not arming the police or training police not to attack peaceful demonstrators could protect you.
3. **Remove the problem:** Full government funding of the health budget, which would eliminate the need to protest, could protect you.

Each of these actions suggests a way to prevent epilepsy-causing head injuries. And each kind of action has its benefits and limitations.

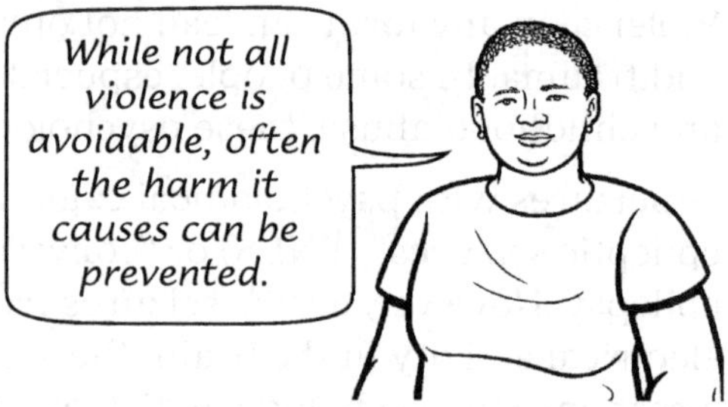
While not all violence is avoidable, often the harm it causes can be prevented.

A benefit of **personal protective equipment** is that it may be easy to get and use. For example, wearing a helmet when playing contact sports or putting a flashing light on a bicycle may be within a person's reach. A limitation of protective equipment is that it is often a personal solution, not a community solution.

In the same way, solutions to problems that **change part of the situation** can protect more people, which is good, but these solutions still do not protect everyone. An example is requiring all cars to have seatbelts. Using seatbelts can protect people in a car from injuring their heads during an accident, but they do not protect people the car might hit, like a person riding a bicycle or crossing the street.

Removing the problem for everyone is the most effective solution but also often the hardest to do. For example, if a child gets an infection in their brain and a high fever, they need immediate treatment. If their parents have good health insurance or enough money to see a doctor and buy the medicine they need, the child will recover. But if the family is denied health care because of poverty, there is a chance the child could get seizures and epilepsy. A government guarantee of the right to health would remove the problem for everyone.

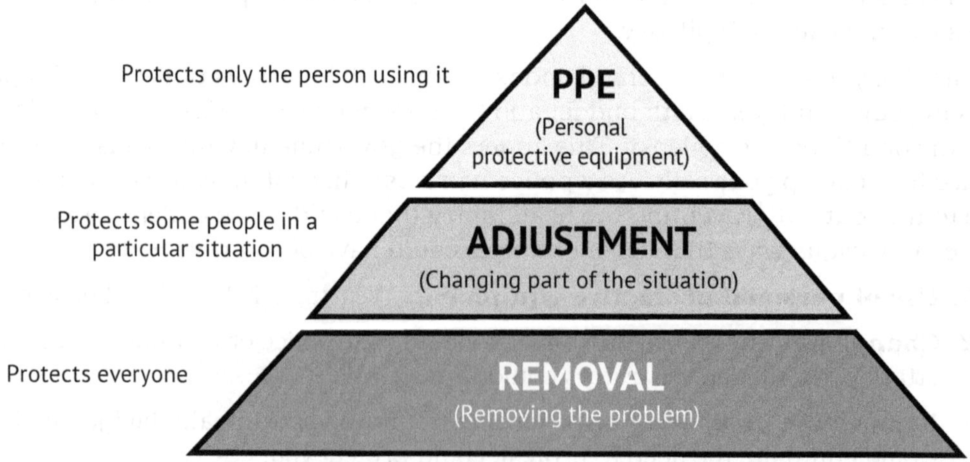

Prevention strategies

What can you do to stop the harm caused by physical and structural violence in your community before it leads to epilepsy and seizures? A good place to start is to examine the root causes. Bring together a group of people to create a list of what is contributing to violence, discuss which issues are most important, and identify the problems the group might be able to affect. Then you can begin to plan specific actions that can make change happen.

There are often many ways to solve a problem. For example, if your group decides to try to stop head injuries caused by violence in relationships, you might talk about how to help people learn that hitting their partner is never OK, how to limit the heavy use of alcohol that can make domestic violence worse, how to teach basic self-defense skills, or how to increase economic support for those who leave a violent relationship.

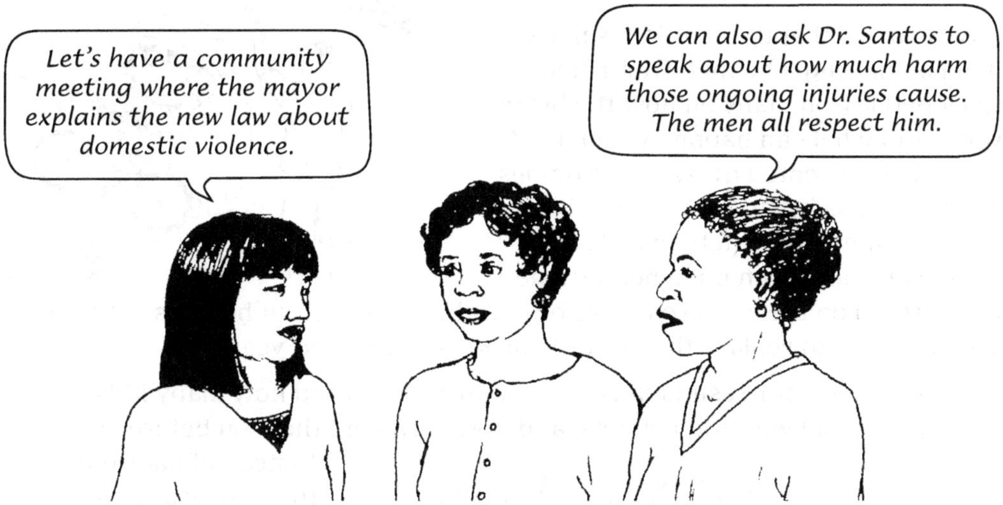
Let's have a community meeting where the mayor explains the new law about domestic violence.
We can also ask Dr. Santos to speak about how much harm those ongoing injuries cause. The men all respect him.

Creating a world that supports and improves our lives rather than harms us is the aim of prevention strategies and working for change. Ending the physical and structural violence that can cause epilepsy and seizures is a big goal that may seem overwhelming, but like all big problems, it can be broken down into smaller, more manageable pieces to work on over time.

These four stories show the ways that people in various communities—a school in Cambodia, a refugee camp in Uganda, a factory warehouse in Jamaica, and in different parts of India—identified a source of violence that can cause injuries that may lead to seizures and epilepsy. They each addressed physical and structural violence by developing prevention strategies, including community education and actions for change.

Convincing students to wear helmets

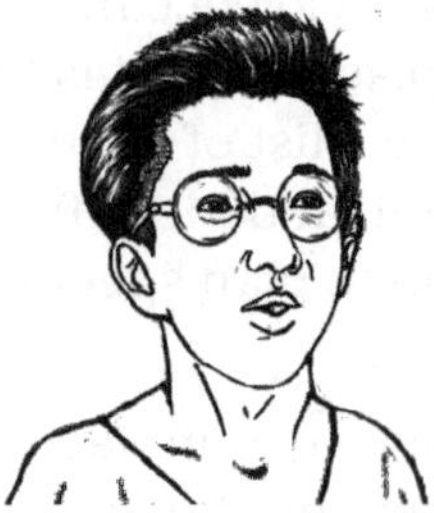

Where I teach in rural Cambodia, lots of students come to school on bicycles, scooters, or motorcycles on crowded, bumpy roads. Because the government does not maintain roads well in rural areas, too many students get hurt in traffic accidents. Hardly any students wear helmets. I spoke in class about the importance of wearing a helmet and even got helmets for kids who needed them. But it didn't work. After a few weeks, they stopped using them.

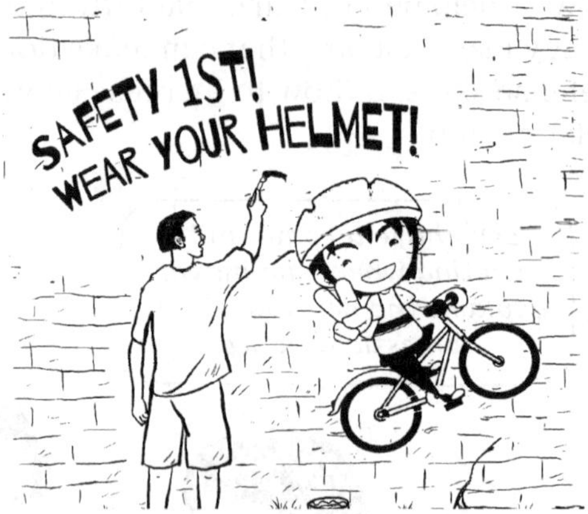

Then our school became part of the Cambodia Helmet Vaccine Initiative and the Helmets for Kids campaign. That succeeded where I had not. Why?

We learned that the solution is more than just getting a helmet. Our school developed lesson plans on how the brain works and what can happen when it gets injured. We invented quizzes and games about traffic safety to make it fun. Local artists painted bike safety murals on school walls and even put a helmet safety billboard up on the main road. We got funding to hand out helmets the first year, and then to replace the lost or broken ones the next year.

We measured our results during the year by counting how many kids arrived at school wearing helmets, and how many put them on before leaving.

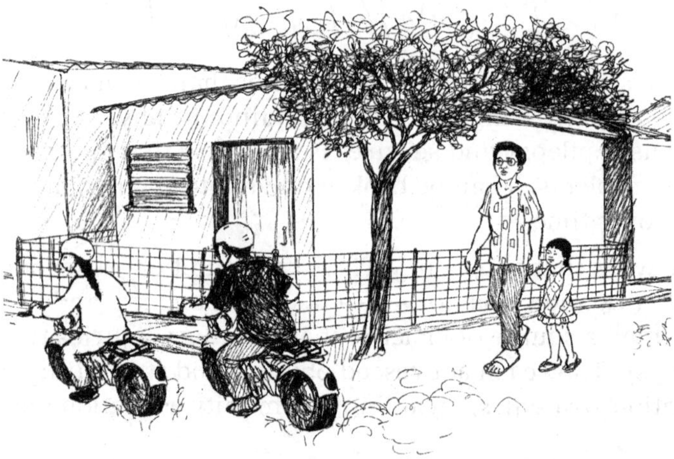

Instead of nagging them to wear helmets, we created a culture of safety to motivate helmet use when riding bikes or motorbikes! So now, even though the government still neglects the roads, our students are safer.

Preventing epilepsy by promoting safer births at Nakivale Refugee Camp

The huge Nakivale settlement area in Uganda houses more than 270,000 refugees who cannot safely return to their homes in Burundi, Democratic Republic of Congo, Eritrea, Ethiopia, Rwanda, Sudan, and Somalia. Refugees from war and conflict experience more epilepsy and seizures than others because they experience more head and brain injuries, untreated infections, and psychological trauma. To address this, aid organizations partnered with health workers and community leaders to start an epilepsy care project to help people who did not have access to the right antiseizure medicine, faced stigma, and could not consult epilepsy specialists. This project improved the lives of those with epilepsy in the camp.

But it did not explain why so many children born in the camp had epilepsy. A lack of trained health workers, long distances to the main camp hospital, and few ambulances together resulted in mothers not getting enough care during pregnancy, labor and birth, and after delivery. These were the preventable causes for 7 out of every 10 Nakivale children who were born with epilepsy.

The Nakivale epilepsy care project responded by promoting safer births and improving the identification and treatment of seizures in the camp. The team built a maternity ward with an operating room (operation theatre) for C-sections, trained more health workers in maternity care, seizure first aid, and epilepsy referrals, and improved training and conditions for birth attendants.

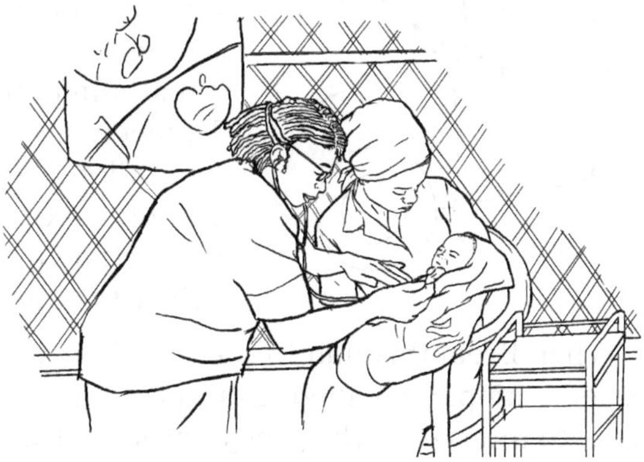

Village health team members from the refugee communities were also trained to recognize signs of epilepsy, like shaking, falling, loss of consciousness, and unusual sensations. Camp translators learned the right words to describe epilepsy and seizures in the languages people speak, which improved communication among health workers, people with epilepsy, and their caregivers. Health center nurses learned more skills to assess and treat epilepsy through an online course designed for them.

These improvements have reduced brain injuries during birth that can cause epilepsy and have also made safe and healthy births available to everyone in the Nakivale settlement area.

Making work safer

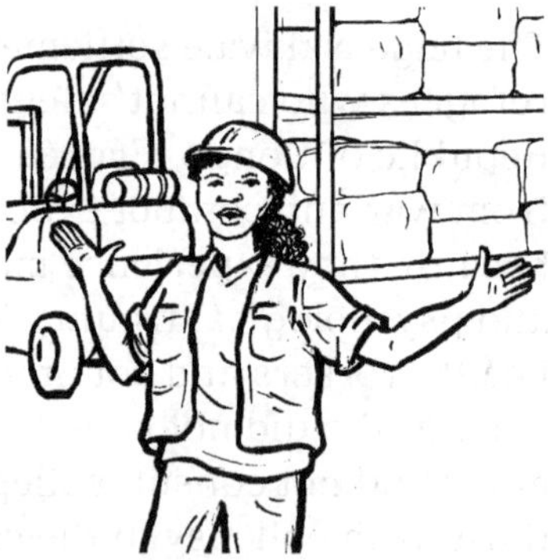

I work in a factory warehouse in Jamaica. We are not well paid, and the management did not care about making our workplace safe. When we had large shipments of supplies, we stacked everything on top of each other because there just wasn't enough room. Then the stacks would get too high and the boxes fell over. People got head injuries and materials were damaged. We explained to the boss how using industrial shelving would save money: fewer parts would break and fewer people would lose time recovering from accidents. He agreed and we got the shelves. There hasn't been a warehouse accident in months.

Breaking the silence on gender-based violence

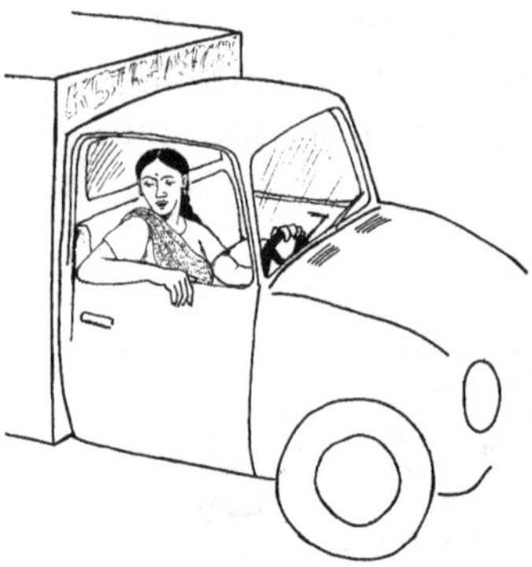

Breakthrough India, a non-governmental organization that works to fight gender-based discrimination and violence, created a large media campaign using radio, video, leaflets, bulletin boards, and town meetings to carry the message that women have the right to be free from violence. An album and music video called *Mann ke Manjeere (My Mind's Rhythm)* was heard and seen by millions of people and was especially popular among youth. They told the true story of a woman who left a violent husband and became a truck driver to support herself and her children.

Then Breakthrough India took their work to another level. They started a 2-year campaign called "Stand Up," during which they taught young people how to intervene when they witnessed sexual harassment and public crimes against women. And they taught those young people how to share what they learned with others. Campaign organizers reached hundreds of thousands of young people, as well as village leaders, law enforcement, and government workers with their community-based trainings.

Campaigns like Breakthrough India's not only improve conditions for women, they also unite communities to build a more just and less violent world.

It is impossible to know how much epilepsy these strategies were able to prevent, but by working together, people improved community life. As more people get involved, more meaningful change can be made, which will help everyone, with or without epilepsy.

Every piece of the problem we address leaves us better able to take on the next challenge, and being successful in one area strengthens our belief that greater changes are possible. Your commitment to change and your efforts to achieve it will inspire more people to participate. As your numbers grow, so does your power to make change happen.

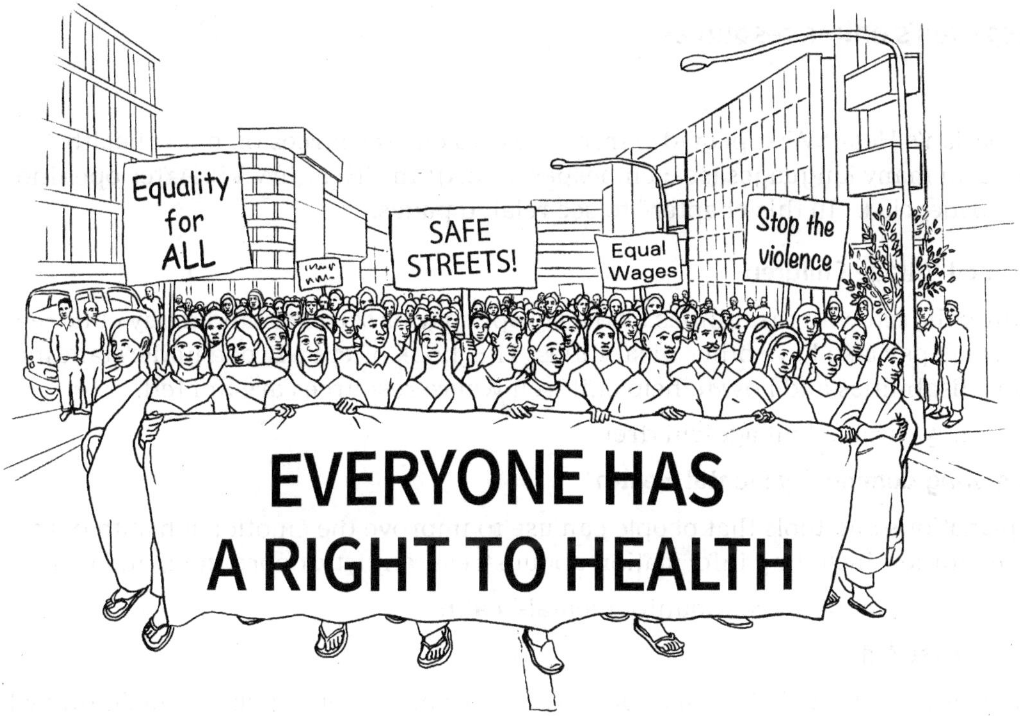
Equality for ALL
SAFE STREETS!
Equal Wages
Stop the violence
EVERYONE HAS A RIGHT TO HEALTH

Where to find more information

In writing this book, we reviewed many resources, published research, websites, and training guides. Here is a selection of epilepsy materials on education, care, and advocacy that we found helpful. Many are online and free to use.

To access this list of resources on Hesperian's website, scan the QR code on the right with your mobile phone camera or use this link:

- en.hesperian.org/hhg/Other_Resources:Epilepsy

Hesperian's online resources

Hesperian's HealthWiki provides free access to our resources on many health topics, in many languages (see: en.hesperian.org/hhg/HealthWiki). After opening each page, click "In this chapter" to see related pages.

Disabled Village Children

Many children with disabilities also have epilepsy or seizures; and many children with epilepsy also have other disabilities. This book offers a broad understanding of many disabilities and how to help children where resources are limited.

- bit.ly/disabled-village-children

Promoting Community Mental Health

Explanations and tools that people can use to improve the emotional health of their communities, including information about stress, anxiety, depression, and trauma.

- bit.ly/promoting-community-mental-health

Pocket First Aid

Provides basic first aid information covering a range of emergencies, including what to do if a person has a seizure.

- bit.ly/pocket-first-aid

A Book for Midwives

Covers the essentials of care before, during, and after pregnancy and birth.

- bit.ly/a-book-for-midwives

Helping Children Live with HIV

Includes information about child development and support for communicating with children of all ages.

- bit.ly/helping-children-live-with-HIV

Epilepsy organizations

The International League Against Epilepsy (ILAE) has chapters in 120 countries. Their website and newsletters provide up-to-date information on medical and social aspects of epilepsy. While the main language is English, information is available in many languages.

- ilae.org

The International Bureau for Epilepsy (IBE) has chapters throughout the world which focus on advocacy for social and legal rights for people with epilepsy.

- ibe-epilepsy.org

IBE also maintains a website focusing on women and epilepsy:

- womenandepilepsy.org

There are many national, local, and special focus epilepsy organizations. Here are two listings you may find useful:

- epilepsyfoundation.org.au/understanding-epilepsy/international-links
- ilae.org/patient-care/resources/links

General epilepsy information

Epilepsy: A public health imperative (2019)

This World Health Organization (WHO) report, done in collaboration with the ILEA and the IBE, explores the impact of epilepsy worldwide and outlines public health actions needed to improve care.

- who.int/publications/i/item/epilepsy-a-public-health-imperative

Intersectoral global action plan (IGAP) on epilepsy and other neurological disorders, 2022-2031

This WHO document sets policy goals to improve access to epilepsy treatment and reduce epilepsy stigma internationally. It is accompanied by an implementation toolkit for people working to turn the plans into reality.

- bit.ly/WHO-IGAP-document
- bit.ly/WHO-IGAP-toolkit

Free Access Epilepsy Journals

Many medical sources with research and information about epilepsy are very expensive to read. The 10 scientific journals listed on this website are free for everyone to read, although some may be difficult to understand.

- gfmer.ch/Medical_journals/epilepsy.htm

Seizure first aid

Seizure first aid videos

From the British Red Cross:

- bit.ly/BRC-seizure-first-aid-video

From the Apollo hospital group in India:

- bit.ly/Apollo-seizure-first-aid-video

Seizure first aid posters

Downloadable posters with simple, step-by-step guidance in multiple languages.

- epilepsy.com/tools-resources/forms-resources/first-aid

Online seizure first aid training

An on-demand seizure first aid training designed for school settings but appropriate for anyone seeking to learn the basics of epilepsy and how to recognize and respond to a seizure. From Epilepsy Alliance America.

- bit.ly/online-seizure-first-aid-training

Identifying seizure types

Epilepsy and Seizures

Developed by the US National Institutes of Health, this resource explains the different seizure types and includes information on childhood epilepsy, nonepileptic seizures, treatments, and more.

- ninds.nih.gov/health-information/disorders/epilepsy-and-seizures

Types of Seizures

An explanation of the new ILAE system for classifying types of seizures designed to support better recognition and management of epilepsy and seizures. For medical professionals.

- epilepsy.com/what-is-epilepsy/seizure-types

Psychogenic Nonepileptic Seizures (PNES)

A set of resources on seizures not caused by epilepsy, with links to articles, webinars, books, and films for patients, families, and health professionals. The FAQs (Frequently Asked Questions) are available in both English and Spanish.

- nonepilepticseizures.com/epilepsy-psychogenic-nes-reading-materials

Advocacy tools

IBE Advocacy Toolkits

Guidance, ideas, and inspiration for organizations working to:

Make Epilepsy a Priority in Africa:

- bit.ly/IBE-toolkit-Africa

Make Epilepsy a Priority in the Americas:

- bit.ly/IBE-toolkit-Americas

Reduce Epilepsy Stigma in Africa:

- ibe-epilepsy.org/stigmatoolkitafrica

The Community Health Worker's Training Curriculum for Epilepsy Self-Management

Developed by the Managing Epilepsy Well Network to train CHWs with some medical knowledge to support people with epilepsy in community settings.

- managingepilepsywell.org/community-health-worker

The Curse of Stigma (video)

A documentary film that shares stories of living with epilepsy and the pain, isolation, and harm suffered because of discrimination and deeply-embedded cultural beliefs.

- thecurseofstigma.org

What's Wrong with How We See Epilepsy

This short article reviews and counters 10 harmful myths about epilepsy.

- bit.ly/whats-wrong-with-how-we-see-epilepsy

Living well

Exercise and epilepsy: Research and myths (audio)

An ILAE podcast episode that discusses current research and myths about exercise for people with epilcpsy.

- bit.ly/ILAE-podcast-research-and myths-exercise

Self-Management Tools

These resources from the Managing Epilepsy Well Network explain epilepsy self-management as a team effort between the person with epilepsy, their family and friends, and doctors.

- managingepilepsywell.org/patients-families-nav

Ketogenic Diet Explained

The Charlie Foundation promotes ketogenic diets to treat epilepsy and other conditions. This webpage explains how and why a ketogenic diet helps control seizures for some people.

- charliefoundation.org/learn-about-ketosis

Peer support groups by and for people with lived experience

A WHO booklet to guide you in setting up and running a peer support group.

- bit.ly/WHOresource-list

Pregnancy and birth

Epilepsy and Pregnancy Medical Consortium

This organization's website provides helpful, regularly updated information and links useful for people with epilepsy and for their doctors and midwives.

- epilepsypregnancy.com

Pregnancy and Epilepsy (video)

A video produced by Epilepsy Action in the UK to answer common questions about epilepsy and pregnancy.

- epilepsy.org.uk/living/starting-a-family/pregnancy-birth-and-epilepsy

Women and Epilepsy

Hosted on the IBE website, these resources address multiple issues faced by women with epilepsy, including information about pregnancy.

- womenandepilepsy.org

Children and young people

Anti-Bullying Poster

Children for Health's free, downloadable anti-bullying poster.

- childrenforhealth.org/sdm_downloads/anti-bullying-poster

Teacher Tool Kit to Promote Well-being in Students with Epilepsy

This Canadian resource for teachers includes 2 videos (English) and 2 booklets (in 6 languages) that explain what epilepsy is, how it affects school achievement, and use of emergency medicines.

- epilepsyswo.ca/teacher-toolkit

Improving the management of prolonged convulsive seizures for children in schools: An advocacy toolkit

An IBE guide, including videos and checklists, to support schools to develop policies that promote inclusion for children with epilepsy.

- ibe-epilepsy.org/advocating-better-epilepsy-management-schools

La Historia de Juanito/ Juanito's Story (video)

This Chilean video (Spanish, with subtitles in many languages) of a puppet show educates about epilepsy, how to help during a seizure, and dispels fears and myths to promote understanding and support.

- bit.ly/la-historia-de-juanito-video

My Thinking Cap: A Coloring Book about Epilepsy

Massachusetts General Hospital produced this free, downloadable coloring book to help children understand how the brain works and what an EEG is.

- bit.ly/epilepsy-coloring-book

Seizures and Epilepsy in Children: A Comprehensive Guide, 4th edition

This comprehensive, parent-focused book covers the practical, emotional, physical, and psychological aspects of epilepsy, including medicines, side effects, testing, diets, and digital resources. Your local library may have a copy.

- bit.ly/seizures-and-epilepsy-in-children-4th-edition

Warriors of Light: Kids Yoga in Color (videos)

These 20 short videos show age-appropriate yoga techniques for self-calming through fun exercise, meditation, and relaxation.

- bit.ly/kids-yoga-in-color

Violence

Violence in a Structural and Cultural Context (video)

Emory University produced this 7 ½ minute talk to discuss structural and cultural violence.

- bit.ly/violence-in-context-video

Violence and injury (VIP) short courses

WHO offers these free, short (2 to 5 day) trainings-in-a-box that facilitators and trainers can deliver on violence and injury topics, such as child injury prevention, intimate partner and sexual violence prevention, and trauma care.

- bit.ly/WHO-VIP-courses

Glossary: Words related to epilepsy

To make this book easier to read, we used simple and clear words as often as we could. Still, the words used to talk about epilepsy can be difficult to understand. This glossary contains definitions of medical words related to epilepsy that are used in this book and in other resources on epilepsy.

Absence seizure. A seizure that causes a brief loss of awareness or alertness. The person's body does not move, but they may look like they are zoned out or staring into space. Afterwards, they usually do not remember what happened and will resume doing whatever they were doing before the seizure.

Antiseizure medicine. Medicines prescribed to people with epilepsy to prevent seizures or reduce their frequency. Taken daily, they may stop seizures from happening but do not cure epilepsy.

Atonic seizure. A type of generalized seizure that causes a person to briefly lose muscle tone. Part or all of a person's body goes limp, and the person may slump or fall. Also called a "drop attack."

Aura. Sensation or feeling in the body or mind before or at the beginning of a seizure, such as a strange smell, taste, feeling, or change in vision or hearing. Aura is a warning sign that a seizure is starting.

Automatisms. Repetitive, involuntary movements during a seizure, such as picking at clothing, lip-smacking, or eye blinking.

Complex partial seizure. A seizure that starts in a single area of the brain and causes temporary loss of consciousness, confusion, and altered awareness. Person may stare or make repetitive movements. Also called "focal impaired awareness" seizure.

Consciousness. The state of being awake, alert, and aware of oneself and the environment, involving the ability to perceive, respond, and remember what happened. When a seizure affects consciousness, a person may seem confused, unresponsive, or "not there." Afterward, they may have little or no memory of the seizure.

Convulsions. Uncontrolled, repeated, and often jerking body movements that are common to many seizures.

Cysts. Fluid-filled bumps that form in or on the body. In neurocysticercosis, cysts containing tapeworm larvae can form in the brain and trigger seizures.

Drug-resistant epilepsy. When epilepsy's seizures are not controlled after trying at least two different antiseizure medicines. Also called "intractable" or "refractory" epilepsy.

EEG (electroencephalogram). A medical test that records the brain's electrical activity to a computer using electrodes (small discs) placed on a person's scalp. Often used to diagnose epilepsy and other brain conditions.

Emergency medicine (or rescue medicine). Used to stop a seizure that lasts longer than 5 minutes (status epilepticus), which is a medical emergency. Some emergency medicines are also used as daily antiseizure medicines.

Encephalitis. Inflammation of the brain, usually caused by an infection.

Epilepsy. A brain condition that causes a person to have seizures repeatedly. Not all seizures are epilepsy, but a main feature of the condition is that seizures happen again and again.

Epileptologist. A health worker, usually a doctor, with extensive training to diagnose and treat epilepsy and seizures.

Etiology. The cause of a disease or health problem—what started it or led to it happening.

Fever (or febrile) seizure. A seizure in a child between 3 months and 6 years of age triggered by a fever above 38.3°C (101°F) from sore throat, ear infection, bad cold, or other cause. Treated with medicines to lower fever as well as to treat the cause of the fever.

Focal seizure. A seizure in one part of the brain that causes movements or sensations on only one side of the body. Sometimes it spreads to the whole brain and becomes a generalized seizure.

Generalized seizure. A seizure on both sides of the brain that affects both sides of the body. Can begin as generalized or develop when a focal seizure spreads to involve the entire brain.

Generalized tonic-clonic seizure. A seizure on both sides of the brain and body that causes sudden loss of consciousness, falls, stiffening (tonic phase), and jerking movements (clonic phase). Also called "grand mal" seizure or tonic-clonic seizure.

Genetic. Genes are the instructions inside our cells that guide how our bodies grow and work. Genetic characteristics and changes can be inherited, caused by the environment, or happen randomly.

Hereditary. Passing of genetic information (genes) from a parent to their child.

Idiopathic. When a disease or disorder has no known cause.

Infantile spasms. Seizures in babies and very young children that occur in short spasms (1 to 2 seconds), causing sudden stiffening or bending of a baby's arms, legs, or head.

Ketogenic (or "keto") diet. A high fat, low carbohydrate diet in which the body gets energy from burning fat instead of glucose (sugar). Carefully planned to meet a person's nutritional needs, a keto diet can sometimes treat seizures not well-controlled by medicine.

Lobes (frontal, temporal, occipital, parietal). These four lobes in the brain are associated with different functions: frontal (decision-making, problem-solving, speech, personality, behavior, emotion, movement), temporal (memory, hearing, language, learning), occipital (vision, face and object recognition, depth and distance perception), and parietal (sensations).

Myoclonic seizure. A generalized seizure that causes brief, shock-like jerks of a group of muscles.

Nervous system. The body's communication network, made up of the brain, spinal cord, and nerves, that sends and receives messages that control movement, thinking, feeling, and body functions.

Neurologist. A doctor who specializes in the diagnosis and treatment of brain and nervous system disorders, including epilepsy.

Neurons. Cells in the nervous system that send and receive messages between the brain and the rest of the body, allowing a person to move, feel, think, and breathe.

Paroxysmal. The sudden, uncontrolled, and intense onset of symptoms rather than a gradual worsening. Describes seizures that start and stop suddenly rather than gradually building or fading.

Psychogenic non-epileptic seizure. A seizure from psychological causes, such as stress, anxiety, or trauma. These seizures look like but are not epilepsy. Also called PNES, non-epileptic seizures, functional dissociative seizures, or conversion disorder.

Seizure. A sudden, uncontrolled, temporary disturbance to the brain's electrical activity.

Simple partial seizure. A brief seizure that occurs in a single part of the brain without causing a loss of consciousness or awareness. It can involve symptoms such as involuntary jerking, sensory changes (tingling, flashing lights), or emotional changes (déjà vu, fear). Also called "focal aware" seizure.

Status epilepticus. Multiple seizures with little or no recovery time between them. If a seizure lasts longer than 5 minutes, a person is in status epilepticus, a medical emergency.

Sudden unexpected death in epilepsy (SUDEP). When a person with epilepsy dies suddenly without a known or identifiable cause. SUDEP can affect people with all seizure types but occurs more commonly with tonic-clonic seizures.

Syndromes, Epilepsy syndromes. A grouping of signs, symptoms, and seizure types that usually begin around a certain age or set of conditions. More than 30 different syndromes affect children and adolescents, including Dravet syndrome, Lennox-Gastaut syndrome, and West syndrome.

Trauma. An emotional or physical injury. Physical trauma to the brain can cause epilepsy. Emotional trauma, caused by a terrible event experienced currently or in the past, can cause psychogenic non-epileptic seizures.

Trigger, Seizure trigger. An event or situation that causes or increases the likelihood of a seizure for a person. Triggers may include heat, flashing lights, sleep deprivation, stress, hunger, thirst, etc.

Index of seizure types, causes, and treatments

A

Absence seizure, 15, 47, **56**, 57, 60, 99, 101, 104, 108, 111, 142, 152, 185, 204, 219, 220, 245-6, 268
Add-on therapy, 96, 100, 102, 104, 107
Alcohol, 44, 47, 48, 50, 52, 53, **68**, 99, 100, 105, 111, 181, 192, 215, 253
Antihistamine, 29
Antiseizure medicines, 50, 52-56, 58, **83-123**, 153-6, 180, 184, 242
Aspirin, 28
Atonic movements, 46, 47, 48, 55
Atonic seizure, 55, 60
Aura, 51, 70, 159, 170, 186, 238, 240, 250, 260

B

Barbiturate, 105
Benzodiazepine, 100, 109, 111, 112
Birth control and antiseizure medicines, 226-7, 256
Brain diseases, 47, 50, 52, 53, 61, **63-5**, 83, 92, 114, 264, 270
Brain injury, 47, 48, 50, 52, 53, 54, 55, 57, 58, **61-2**, 63, 67, 167-8, 263, 268, 269-70, 272-4

C

Calcium, 185
Carbamazepine, 50, 56, 58, 93, 94, 95, **99**, 102, 116, 117, 118, 119, 120, 185, 208-9, 222, 226-7
Cerebral palsy, 7, **67**

Childhood epilepsy syndromes, 7, 54, 55, **60**, 147, 159, 237
Childhood seizures, 59, 168
Clobazam, 100, 226
Clonazepam, 226
Clonic convulsions, 46, 47, 48, 59
Clonic seizure, 53, 60
Clove oil, 118
Convulsions, 46, 49, 57, 70, 236, 238

D

Diabetes, 189
Diazepam, 68, **109-110**, 114, 116, 117, 120, 218, 220
Diet, see Nutrition
Diphenhydramine, 29
Dravet syndrome, 60, 237
Drug-resistant epilepsy, 76, 77, 83, **98**, 187
Drug use, see Alcohol

E

Eclampsia, 67, 204, 207, 215, **216-218**
Electrolyte imbalances, 52, 53, 65
Emergency medicine, see Rescue medicine
Encephalitis, 47, 50, 52, 61, **63**
Eslicarbazepine acetate, 226
Ethosuximide, 56, **101**, 116, 117, 222, 226
Exercise, 7, 83, **161-180**, 241, 253

F

Felbamate, 226
Fever, high, 47, 48, 50, 52, **59**, 60, 64, 65, 83, 92, 99, 147, 159, 190, 237, 270
Fever, high, medicines for, 114-15

First aid for seizures, see Seizure first aid
Focal seizure, 43, 47, **48**, 53, 54, 55, 56, 57, 58, 59, 99, 102, 104, 105, 106, 107, 108, 109, 111, 113, 177, 182, 185, 203, 219
Folic acid (vitamin B9), 207
Food, see Nutrition

G

Gabapentin, 98
Generalized seizure, 44, **47**, 52, 53, 54, 55, 56, 58, 59, 99, 104, 105, 106, 107, 108
Generalized tonic-clonic seizure, 42, **49-51**, 57, 66, 68, 93, 99, 102, 104, 105, 106, 107, 108, 174, 185, 189, 220

H

Head injury, see Brain injury
Honey, 29

I

Ibuprofen, 28, 114, **115**
Infantile spasms, see West syndrome

K

Ketogenic diet, see Nutrition

L

Lacosamide, 50, 98
Lamotrigine, 50, 52, 53, 55, 93, 96, **102-3**, 117, 119, 208-9, 223, 227
Lennox-Gastaut syndrome (LGS), 60, 100, 102, 107, 122, 237
Levetiracetam, 50, 52, 53, 54, 56, 58, 96, **104**, **111**, 116, 119, 120, 196, 208-9, 222-3, 226
Lorazepam, **111**, 114, 117, 120, 220

M

Magnesium sulfate, 218
Malaria, 47, 50, 52, 53, 59, **64**, 83, 92, 113, 264
Meningitis, 59, **65**, 83, 92, 114, 264
Metabolic disorders, 48, 53, 65, 189
Midazolam, **112**, 114, 117, 120, 220
Myoclonic movements, 46, 48
Myoclonic seizure, 15, 47, **54**, 60, 93, 104, 108, 122, 185

N

Neurocysticercosis, see Tapeworm infection
Nutrition, 83, 98, **180-191**, 207, 253
Nutrition, antiseizure medicines and, **185**
Nutrition, ketogenic diet and, 187-190, 197-200

O

Omega-3 fats, 119
Oxcarbazepine, 209, 226

P

Paracetamol (acetaminophen), 28, 114, **115**
Phenobarbital, 50, 52, 53, **105**, **113**, 114, 116, 117, 118, 119, 120, 196, 208-9, 222-3, 226-7
Phenytoin, 50, 102, **106**, **113**, 114, 116, 117, 118, 119, 120, 208-9, 226

Polysporin, 29
Pre-eclampsia, see Eclampsia
Pregnancy and breastfeeding, Antiseizure medicines during, 97, **207-212**, 222-3
Primidone, 226
Psychologically caused seizures (PNES), 52, 53, 56, **70-79**, 147, 159, 269

R

Recipes, 118, 121, 183, 197-200
Rescue medicine, 20, 57, **109-113**, 114, 120, 156, 179, 218, 220
Rest, see Sleep

S

Seizure, definition, 5
Seizure types, 34-80
Seizure, breakthrough, 89, 220, 250
Seizure first aid, 6, **15-33**, 44, 49, 130, 149, 152, 164, 167, 169, 170, 175, 176, 177, 225, 237, 238, 239, 243, 247, 251, 255, 273
Sepsis, 65
Sexual abuse, 244, 274
Side effects of medicines, 87, 92, 95, 96, 97, **116-121**, 161, 180, 181, 185, 196, 212-4, 222-3, 253
Silver sulfadiazine, 29
Sleep, 27, 62, 72-3, 83, 98, 116, 128, 181, 184-5, **192-196**, 204, 213, 215, 223, 225, 241, 254
Sleep seizures, 37, 40, 44, **58**, 194-6, 225
Status epilepticus, 19-20, 30, **57**, 60, 109-113, 123
Stroke, 47,48, 50, 52, 58, **66**, 218
Structural violence, 4, 12, 75, **263-9**, 271-5
Sudden unexpected death in epilepsy (SUDEP), 7, **57**, 123, 147, 159
Sugar, 29

T

Tapeworm infection (neurocysticercosis), 47, 50, 61, **62**, 264
Tonic convulsions, 46, 47, 48, 49, 59
Tonic seizure, 52, 60
Tonic-clonic seizure, 15, 42, 47, 57, 59, 60, 111, 113, 142, 218, 220
Topiramate, 50, 52, 53, **107**, 116, 117, 119, 208-9, 226
Treatment, access to, 4, 6-7, 9-11, 57, 97, 153-5, 156, 211, 228-231, 273, 275
Triggers, seizure, 4, 7, 20, 37, 59, 69, 71, 72, 73, 74, 77, 83, 87, 89, 98, 126, 144, 161, 163, 167, 170, 180, **181-5**, 187, 188, 192, 204, 215, 218, 223, 225, 241, 250, 251, 253, 254, 255, 269

V

Valproic acid, 50, 52, 53, 54, 55, 56, 93, 96, 102, **108**, 116, 117, 118, 119, 120, 196, 208-9, 226-7
Vigabatrin, 98
Vitamin A, 119
Vitamin B6, 104
Vitamin C, 119
Vitamin D, 108, 118, 185
Vitamin E, 119

W

West syndrome, 60, 237

Z

Zonisamide, 222-3

About Hesperian Health Guides

For more than 50 years, Hesperian has provided information and educational tools to equip individuals and community organizations to take greater control over their health and lives and mobilize to eliminate the underlying causes of poor health. Our over 300 resources present easy-to-understand, accurate, culturally respectful, and highly illustrated information on common health concerns including disease prevention and treatment, environmental health, worker health and safety, child disability, women's health, midwifery, health worker training, and community dentistry. Hesperian publications have been translated and adapted into 85 languages and are used in 221 countries and territories. According to the World Health Organization (WHO), our best-known publication, *Where There is No Doctor,* is the most widely used health manual in the world.

How this book was developed

The development of *Epilepsy and Seizures: Building Care in the Community* is the result of a collaborative editorial model that solicits extensive input and review of draft material from grassroots organizations, partners, and experts. A diverse network of partner organizations and individuals provided feedback to help us test and improve this book. Help us continue this approach—email epilepsy@hesperian.org with your ideas, feedback, and suggestions toward keeping the book relevant and up-to-date.

Support our work

Hesperian resources are published in English, Spanish, and many other languages; they are available in print and digital formats, including mobile apps, PDFs, and our free online HealthWiki.

As a not-for-profit organization, Hesperian's work is made possible through your book purchases and donations. To support further development and translations of *Epilepsy and Seizures: Building Care in the Community,* please visit hesperian.org/donate for ways to give. See some of our resources on the following pages and visit our website: www.hesperian.org

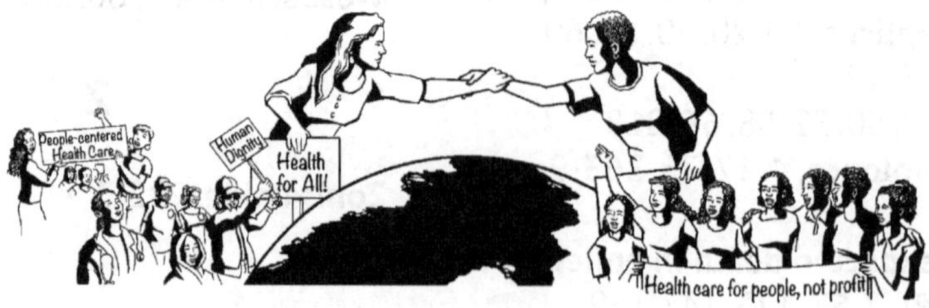
People-centered Health Care
Human Dignity
Health for All!
Health care for people, not profit

Other Books from Hesperian

Hesperian resources are available in English, Spanish, and a variety of other languages. See the Language Hub on our website (hesperian.org) to find materials in your language, or visit the Hesperian bookstore online: **store.hesperian.org**

Disabilities and Early Assistance

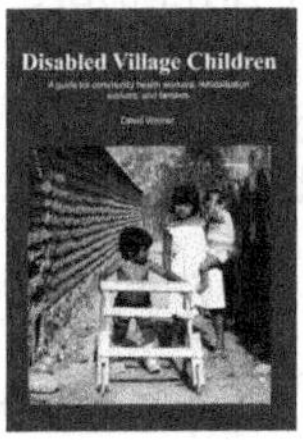

Disabled Village Children is a comprehensive resource covering common disabilities of children. It suggests community-based rehabilitation activities and explains how to make a variety of low-cost aids with local resources in mind. Emphasis is placed on how to help disabled children find a role and be accepted in the community. 654 pages, paperback.

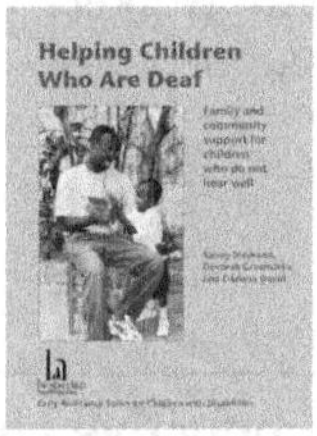

Helping Children Who Are Deaf focuses on care for young children who do not hear well and explores ways that communities can work to help children with hearing difficulties. Chapters include information to aid parents and caregivers to assess hearing loss, explore causes of deafness, and learn basic communication using both signed and spoken methods of communication. 250 pages, paperback.

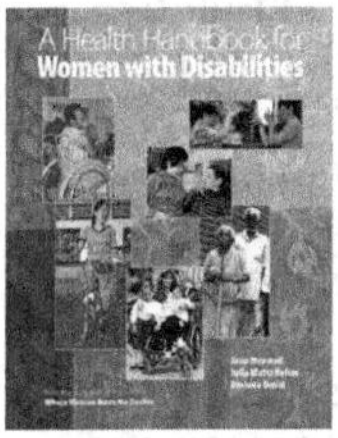

A Health Handbook for Women with Disabilities provides individuals and caregivers suggestions on caring for daily needs, healthy and safe sexual relationships, family planning, pregnancy and childbirth, and defense against violence, abuse, and stigma. This groundbreaking guide helps women with disabilities overcome barriers to poor health and advocate for better care. 384 pages, paperback.

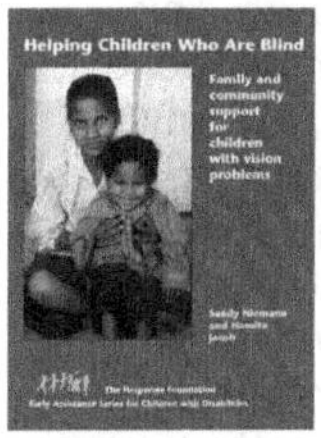

Helping Children Who Are Blind is an important aid for parents and other caregivers helping children with vision problems, starting from birth through age 5, to develop all their capabilities. Topics include assessing how well a child can see, preventing blindness, moving around safely, teaching common activities, and more. 192 pages, paperback.

Community Health Organizing and Training

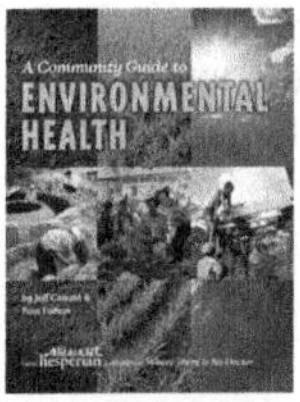

A Community Guide to Environmental Health provides tools, knowledge, and inspiration to help health promoters, activists, and community leaders take charge of their environmental health. This comprehensive guide was developed for both urban and rural communities and covers topics from toilets to toxics, watershed management to waste management, and agriculture to air pollution. Informative case studies and impactful activities address environmental health hazards where people live and work. 617 pages, paperback.

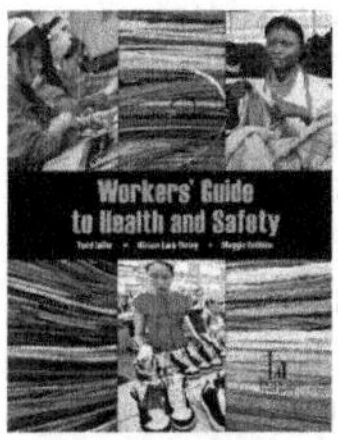

Workers' Guide to Health and Safety makes occupational safety and health accessible to those most affected by physical, social, and economic hazards—the workers themselves. Actionable tools and strategies support workers, supervisors, safety committees, and labor relations courses to improve workplace experiences and overall wellbeing for workers. The insights and techniques are useful in any factory, and especially in the garment, shoe, and electronics industries. 576 pages, paperback.

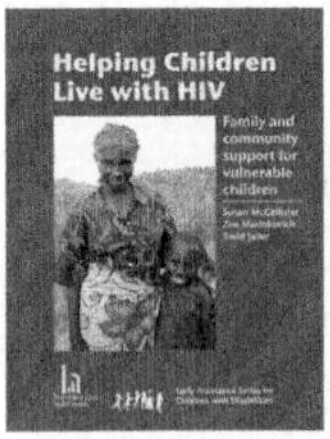

Helping Children Live with HIV is an innovative community health guide designed to ensure children with HIV can grow to adulthood and live full lives. Richly illustrated, the practical advice in this book addresses both the physical and emotional health needs of children living with HIV, and helps parents, caregivers, and health workers provide them with the love and support they deserve. 315 pages, paperback.

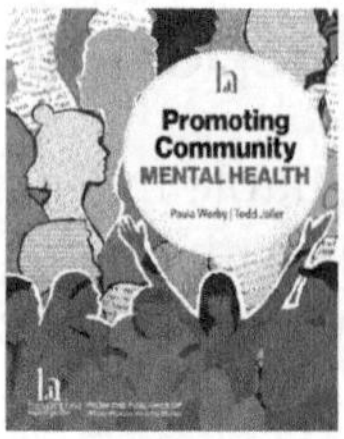

Promoting Community Mental Health offers innovative strategies and practical tools that people from all walks of life can implement in their efforts to improve the emotional and physical health of their communities. Developed with input from 26 community-led groups across the US, this concise resource helps community organizers, health workers, faith groups, and individuals integrate mental health promotion into their work and lives. 200 pages, paperback.

Reproductive and Women's Health

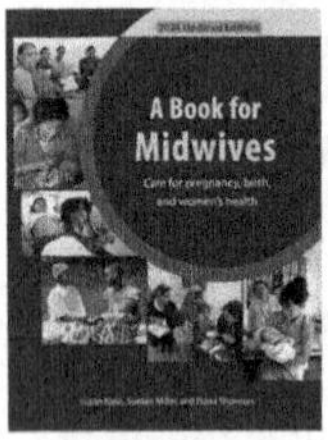

A Book for Midwives covers the essentials of care before, during, and after birth. This vital resource for practitioners, training programs, and anyone interested in safer birthing was developed with the participation of community-based birth workers. Clearly written and illustrated, this book discusses preventing, managing, and treating obstetric complications, covers HIV in pregnancy, birth, and breastfeeding, and includes reproductive health care. 527 pages, paperback.

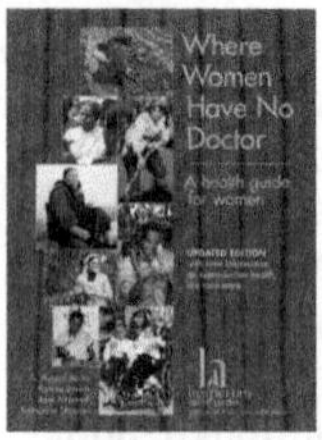

Where Women Have No Doctor combines self-help medical information with an understanding of the ways poverty, discrimination, and cultural beliefs limit women's health and access to care. Clearly written and with over 1,000 drawings, this essential resource addresses health issues across the lifespan and considers issues specific to girls, older women, women with disabilities, and refugees. 583 pages, paperback.

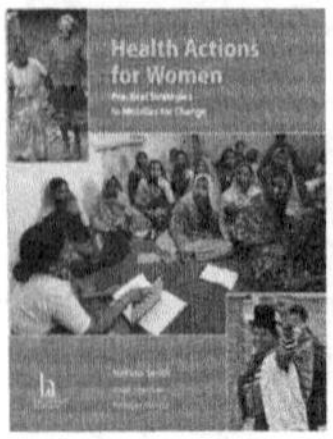

Health Actions for Women addresses social factors that prevent women and girls from enjoying healthy lives. A wealth of clearly explained and engagingly illustrated activities, stories, and strategies help women and men facilitate community discussions and action. User-tested by 41 groups in 23 countries, this resource offers proven strategies to help improve women's social status and health outcomes, even in challenging settings where organizing for women's health is difficult or dangerous. 330 pages, paperback.

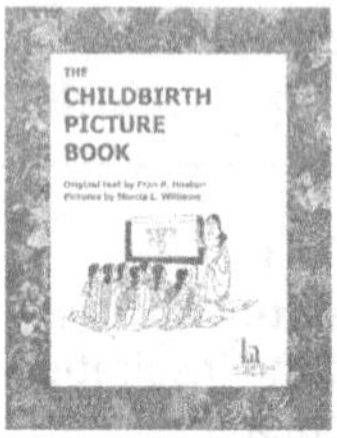

The Childbirth Picture Book provides a simple and complete guide to the basics of conception, pregnancy, childbirth, and breastfeeding. This short resource contains detailed line drawings depicting every step of the reproductive process. 68 pages, staple-bound booklet.

More Books and Booklets

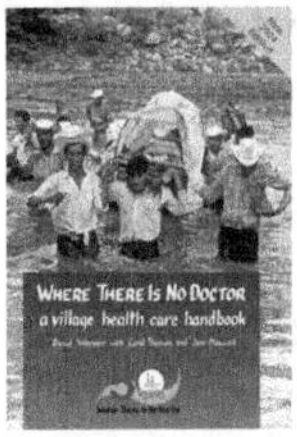

Where There Is No Doctor, perhaps the most widely used health care manual in the world, provides vital, easily understood information on how to diagnose, treat, and prevent common diseases. An emphasis is placed on prevention, including cleanliness, diet, vaccinations, and the important role of the individual and community in health care. 446 pages, paperback.

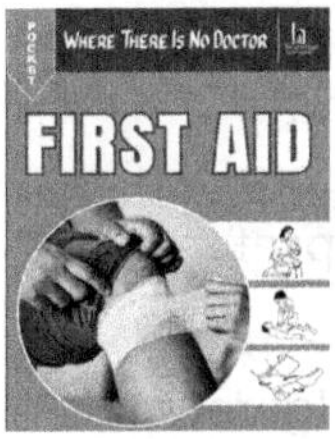

Pocket Where There Is No Doctor: First Aid supplements and expands on life-saving information from the First Aid section of Where There Is No Doctor. This convenient, portable resource is packed with easy-to-understand, actionable information and clear illustrations on emergency care for anyone who wants to feel more prepared in an emergency and better protect and care for their own health and that of their families and communities. 136 pages, trade paperback.

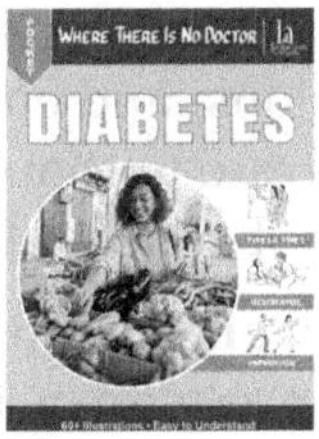

Pocket Where There Is No Doctor: Diabetes is a compact, easy-to-understand guide designed to support people living with pre-diabetes and diabetes. Addressing both the physical and social issues tied to diabetes, this book is a great tool for friends, family, health workers, support groups, teachers, and others dealing with this common health challenge to our communities. Discussion questions included. 60 pages, trade paperback.

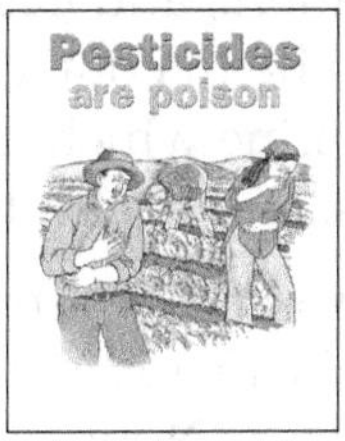

Pesticides are Poison provides detailed information about the health effects of pesticides. In addition to how to read pesticide labels, this short resource addresses how to treat people in pesticide emergencies and reduce harm caused by pesticides. It also offers alternate pest control methods that do not use harmful chemicals. Excerpted from *A Community Guide to Environmental Health.* 38 pages, staple-bound booklet.

See a complete listing with many more books and resources at store.hesperian.org

Ordering from Hesperian

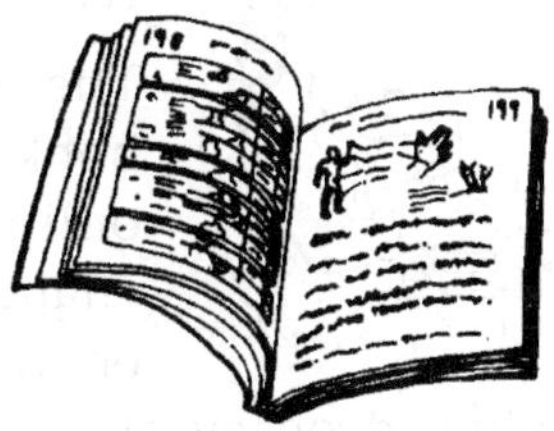

We provide bulk ordering discounts to bookstores, schools, non-profits, universities, and other organizations.

To purchase books, visit: store.hesperian.org
email: bookorders@hesperian.org
or call: 510-845-4507.

For more information about review or exam copies, or to apply for our Gratis Books Program which distributes free copies of Hesperian's community health books to health workers, teachers, and local leaders in low-income communities, please email: hesperian@hesperian.org or visit: hesperian.org.

Reproductive Health Apps

Thousands of people across the world rely on Hesperian's suite of multilingual reproductive health apps for practical, clear, and trustworthy information to make informed and confident decisions, and ensure healthier outcomes for themselves and others. The free apps operate without an internet connection or data plan once installed on a device and do not collect personal information.

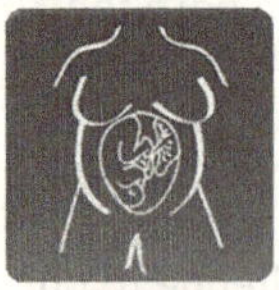

Safe Pregnancy and Birth - Find accurate, easy-to-understand information on pregnancy, birth, and care after birth. Clear illustrations and plain language make this award-winning app practical and user-friendly for community health workers, midwives, and individuals and families.

Family Planning - Designed to support frontline health workers, community leaders, and health advocates to share unbiased information on birth control options. A built-in "Method Chooser" can help determine which methods best match individual preferences, circumstances, and health history.

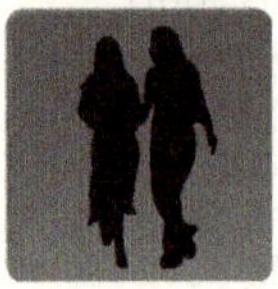

Safe Abortion - Written in easy to understand and nonjudgemental language, this is an app to help people needing or giving abortion and post-abortion care. Now in 11 languages, with a read-aloud function in select languages.

All apps can also be used online through a secure web browser at:
hesperian.org/mobile-apps

Free Health Information Online

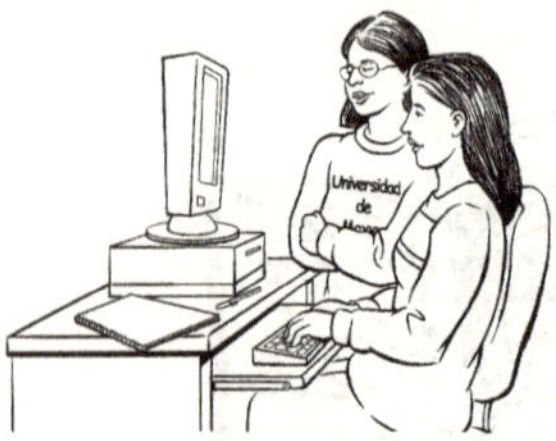

The Hesperian HealthWiki is an online library of Hesperian resources in many languages.

The HealthWiki offers free digital access to Hesperian books and fact sheets. Read essential health information online or, to easily share, print a page or download a chapter. Topics include disabilities and children's health, environmental health, reproductive health, mental health, health rights advocacy, and community organizing and training for health workers.

Share Your Story!

Please tell us how you are using Hesperian resources. We love to hear how our resources are enabling users in different settings to make positive changes. Scan the QR code or go to:
hesperian.org/share-your-story